Chronic Illness and Disabilities in Childhood and Adolescence

Chronic Illness and Disabilities in Childhood and Adolescence

Edited by
ROBERT WM. BLUM, M.D., M.P.H., PH.D.

Associate Professor
Pediatrics and Maternal & Child Health
Director, Adolescent Health Program
University of Minnesota
Minneapolis, Minnesota

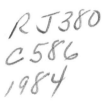

GRUNE & STRATTON, INC.

(Harcourt Brace Jovanovich, Publishers)

ORLANDO   SAN DIEGO   SAN FRANCISCO   NEW YORK   LONDON
TORONTO   MONTREAL   SYDNEY   TOKYO   SÃO PAULO

Library of Congress Cataloging in Publication Data

Main entry under title:
Chronic illness and disabilities in childhood and adolescence.
    Includes bibliographies and index.
    1. Chronic diseases in children.   2. Chronically
ill children.   3. Handicapped children.   I. Blum,
Robert W.   [DNLM: 1. Chronic Disease—in adolescence.
2. Chronic Disease—in infancy & childhood.   3. Handi-
capped.   WS 200 C5575]
RJ380.C586   1984   618.92   84-9107
ISBN 0-8089-1635-1

Grune & Stratton, Inc.
Orlando, FL 32887

Distributed in the United Kingdom by
Grune & Stratton, Ltd.
24/28 Oval Road, London NW 1

Library of Congress Catalog Number 84-9107
International Standard Book Number 0-8089-1635-1
Printed in the United States of America
84 85 86 87 10 9 8 7 6 5 4 3 2 1

To my parents,
Gladys & Moe Blum
who knew the key to
development to be in
the support of human
potential.

CONTENTS

PREFACE

The intent of the book is to assist those who work with children and youths with disabilities and chronic illnesses in understanding the core issues that these patients face in living with and adjusting to their conditions. The orientation is developmental in perspective and places youths within the multiple social contexts in which they live and receive services.

The volume provides a balance of original research reports and clinical observation with major reviews of critical issues that are confronted by youths with chronic illness and disability. The intent is not to be encyclopedic; rather, it is to focus on the generic issues that impact most disabling conditions and focus on specific illnesses that represent the majority of serious conditions affecting youths. The book can be effectively divided into four sections. The first five chapters deal with generic social and developmental considerations impacting on disabled youths: political and financial considerations, ethical issues, societal perspectives related to developing with disabilities, and issues related to the self-image of disabled youths. Chapters 6–9 explore the special needs of this population: educational, nutritional, and sexual needs, as well as compliance with therapeutic regimens. Chapters 10 and 11 review the issues faced by the dying teenager and includes a separate chapter exploring the special concerns of siblings of children who have died.

The largest section of the book (Chapters 12–23) focuses on the major chronic illnesses and disabling conditions encountered by youths: chronic pain of psychologic origin, diabetes, seizure disorders, sickle cell anemia, spinal cord injuries, cerebral palsy, developmental disabilities, genetic disorders, cancer, cystic fibrosis, chronic renal disease, and transplantation. As with all other sections, these chapters are not intended as a review of the basic pathophysiologic processes involved; nor are they intended to represent all the chronic illnesses of youth. Rather, they focus on the major physical, social, psychological, educational, and rehabilitative considerations that are critical for comprehensive and quality services for youths.

What becomes clear is that chronic conditions are complex and vary dramatically in their impact. In the chapter by Offer et al., for example, numerous myths and beliefs related to the general impact of common chronic illnesses are shattered. So, too, in the chapters by Zeltzer et al.

and Simmons et al. on youth with cancer and chronic renal disease and transplantation during childhood and adolescence, one is impressed with the resilience of the human psyche when faced with catastrophic situations. On the other hand, in Petzel et al.'s study of youth with cystic fibrosis, the devasting impact of the condition becomes clear.

Throughout the book numerous juxtapositions among and between the various conditions emerge. Conversely, in the first two sections of the book many of the common issues faced by youths with a wide variety of chronic and handicapping conditions are detailed. The book strives for a balance between highlighting the commonalities among and between conditions and those aspects that make each unique.

This work was supported in part by a grant from the Maternal & Child Health Research & Training Branch, Bureau of Health Care Delivery & Assistance, Health Resources and Services Administration, Department of Health & Human Services (MCJ000985).

With an endeavor of this size there are many people whose contributions were critical to its success and whose thanks are most well deserved. Thanks go to Elinor Beaton and Robin Meyer who typed and retyped endless chapters preparing each for final submission. And my deepest appreciation to Karen Stutelberg, the Adolescent Health Program Administrator, who followed up with contributing authors and attended to numerous production details. In addition, my thanks and appreciation go to the numerous contributing authors who attended to deadlines, complied with my editorial changes, and saw in this book a volume worthy of their efforts. Finally, to my wife Michael and my children Jamie and Alex I offer my love and gratitude for the constant support they provided me during this and every undertaking.

CONTRIBUTORS

CAROL R. ANDERSON, M.A., *Research Assistant, Department of Sociology, University of Minnesota, Minneapolis, Minnesota*

SHARI R. BALDINGER, M.S., *United Hospital Perinatal Center, St. Paul, Minnesota*

STANLEY BATTLE, PH.D., *Associate Professor, School of Social Work, University of Minnesota, Minneapolis, Minnesota*

ROBERT WM. BLUM, M.D., PH.D., *Associate Professor and Director, Adolescent Health Program, University of Minnesota Hospitals, Minneapolis, Minnesota*

JEFFREY R. BUDD, PH.D., *Instructor, Department of Health Care Psychology, University of Minnesota Hospitals, Minneapolis, Minnesota*

IRENE BUGGE, PH.D., *Instructor, Department of Health Care Psychology, University of Minnesota Hospitals, Minneapolis, Minnesota*

SARAH COLWELL, M.D., *Developmental Pediatrician, St. Louis Park Medical Center, St. Louis Park, Minnesota*

DONALD CURRIE, M.D., *Assistant Professor, Department of Physical Medicine and Rehabilitation, University of Texas School of Medicine, San Antonio, Texas*

MELISSA HAMP, M.D., M.P.H., *Assistant Professor of Pediatrics, Director of Adolescent Medicine, Children's Hospital of Pittsburgh, Pittsburgh, Pennsylvania*

KENNETH HOWARD, PH.D., *Professor of Psychology, Department of Psychology, Northwestern University, Evanston, Illinois*

SUSAN KLEIN, PH.D., *Boulder, Colorado*

SAMUEL LABARON, PH.D., *Assistant Professor, Clinical Pediatrics, University of Texas School of Medicine, San Antonio, Texas*

BARBARA LEONARD, R.N., M.S., *Instructor, Maternal and Child Health, School of Public Health, University of Minnesota, Minneapolis, Minnesota*

BONNIE S. LEROY, M.S., *Genetics Associate, Minnesota Genetic Services Program, Minneapolis, Minnesota*

MARVIN LOGEL, PH.D., *Assistant Professor of Physical Medicine and Rehabilitation, University of Minnesota, Minneapolis, Minnesota*

MARY JO MCCRACKEN, R.N., *Pediatric Pulmonary Specialist, Division of Pulmonary Medicine, University of Minnesota Hospitals, Minneapolis, Minnesota*

RICHARD NELSON, M.D., *Assistant Professor and Director, Developmental Disability Program, Gillette Children's Hospital, St. Paul, Minnesota*

DANIEL OFFER, M.D., *Chairman and Professor, Department of Psychiatry, Michael Reese Hospital, Chicago, Illinois*

ERIC OSTROV, PH.D., J.D., *Director, Forensic Psychology, Department of Psychiatry, Michael Reese Hospital, Chicago, Illinois*

SUE V. PETZEL, PH.D., *Assistant Professor, Program in Health Psychology, University of Minnesota, Minneapolis, Minnesota*

MARY ELLA PIERPONT, M.D., *Assistant Professor, Department of Pediatrics, University of Minnesota Hospitals, Minneapolis, Minnesota*

MICHAEL D. RESNICK, PH.D., *Assistant Professor, Adolescent Health Program, University of Minnesota Hospitals, Minneapolis, Minnesota*

MAYNARD REYNOLDS, PH.D., *Professor of Psychoeducational Studies, University of Minnesota, Minneapolis, Minnesota*

SUE SAUER, R.N., *Nurse Clinician, Department of Pediatrics, University of Minnesota Hospitals, Minneapolis, Minnesota*

TOMAS SILBER, M.D., *Assistant Professor and Director, Adolescent Clinic, National Children's Medical Center, Washington, DC*

ROBERTA SIMMONS, PH.D., *Professor of Sociology, Deparment of Sociology, University of Minnesota, Minneapolis, Minnesota*

MARY STORY, PH.D., R.D., *Assistant Professor, Adolescent Health Program, University of Minnesota Hospitals, Minneapolis, Minnesota*

THOMAS STRAX, M.D., *Assistant Medical Director, Moss Rehabilitation Hospital, Philadelphia, Pennsylvania*

WARREN J. WARWICK, M.D., *Professor, Department of Pediatrics, University of Minnesota, Minneapolis, Minnesota*

CAROLYN L. WILLIAMS, PH.D., *Assistant Professor, Adolescent Health Program, University of Minnesota Hospitals, Minneapolis, Minnesota*

SAUL D. WOLFSON, M.D., *Instructor in Psychiatry, Hahnemann University School of Medicine; Staff Psychiatrist, Eastern State School and Hospital, Philadelphia, Pennsylvania*

LONNIE ZELTZER, M.D., *Assistant Professor and Head, Division of Adolescent Medicine, Department of Pediatrics, University of Texas School of Medicine, San Antonio, Texas*

PAUL ZELTZER, M.D. *Associate Professor of Pediatrics, Division of Hematology/Oncology, Department of Pediatrics, University of Texas School of Medicine, San Antonio, Texas*

Chronic Illness and Disabilities in Childhood and Adolescence

Richard P. Nelson

1

Political and Financial Issues That Affect the Chronically Ill Adolescent

GENERAL PREMISES

The Phenomenon of Chronic Illness

The extent of chronic illness in American youth eludes simple description. There are no perpetual surveys or registries. The incidence of some conditions is not static. Even the definition of chronicity has no unified adherents.

Any condition, congenital or acquired, that alters expected physical growth and development and requires extended or sequential services can be legitimately defined as chronic. The pathophysiology of these conditions varies remarkably. Myelodysplasia (spina bifida), for example, results from prenatal damage to the developing central nervous system. While this process usually does not actively damage normal tissue or cause relentless disease throughout childhood, the impact of the congenital abnormality on the nervous, urogenital, and musculoskeletal systems is dynamic throughout a youth's growth to maturity. Myelodysplasia is a chronic condition.

In contrast, hemophilia, or bleeder's disease (which is also a chronic condition), may cause unpredictable and catastrophic damage from hemorrhage into vital tissues, due to the permanent intrinsic deficiency of the

CHRONIC ILLNESS AND DISABILITIES IN CHILDHOOD AND ADOLESCENCE   ISBN 0-8089-1635-1
 Copyright © 1984 by Grune & Stratton.

factor necessary for the clotting of blood that is characteristic of the disorder. Using periodic infusions of the missing clotting factor, serious disability may now be preventable despite the body's inability to manufacture the substance.

The number of chronic conditions is almost inexhaustible. Some conditions are exceedingly rare, occurring with a prevalence of approximately 1 in 100,000 youths. Others are much more common. Cystic fibrosis, a chronic disease of exocrine tissue, may occur at a rate of 1 in 400. A reasonable assumption suggests that one in four youths may have a chronic health condition. Perhaps in a majority of these youths the condition will not cause great dysfunction or require frequent or extraordinary medical care. Allergic disease may be illustrative of this type of chronic condition. Many other conditions, however, pose a measurable burden and exact a toll on the health and welfare of the youth.

Public policy has special pertinence to these youths in that it ultimately determines who receives health care, what services they obtain, and how those who provide the services are reimbursed. Health care occurs in the context of social priorities and economic realities. There must be providers and consumers. Services must be accessible, and professionals and institutions providing them must be accountable. Increasingly, the outcomes of care must be acceptable.

Adolescents are not children, nor are they adults. Just as the medical care of infants is vastly different from that of elderly persons, the care of youths is unique. Prior to discussion of policy, a brief glimpse at adolescence is essential.

The Adolescent in American Society

Growing up in America is a sociological adventure. Less than a century ago the concept of adolescence could be described from two very different perspectives. At that time, the vast majority of American youths completed their formal education at about the onset of puberty. Economic reality demanded that they find jobs to support themselves, and often their parents and siblings. For many, marriage soon followed. By the time they reached their 20th birthday, their own family was begun. The transitional period, currently known as adolescence, was completed. In remarkable contrast, a much smaller group of young people experienced the adolescent transition for well over a decade. These years were required when a young man (less frequently a young woman) left home for a boarding school, completed a prolonged course of education, entered a profession, finally married, and then became a parent in his or her own household.

Throughout the 1980s, the uneven opportunity available to young people frustrates any simplistic description of adolescence in our society.

Each year over three million teens complete high school. Only about one half will pursue a formal college or university education leading to a degree. Many other graduates will go on to other kinds of postsecondary education, including technical and vocational training. The responsibilities of adulthood descend rapidly upon many of these young people. There is the striking dilemma for over one million pregnant adolescent women each year. The vast majority of these women are unmarried and economically dependent on their own parents. They have not completed their secondary education and face difficult alternatives, none of which is necessarily satisfactory. Their transition to adulthood is abrupt.

Adolescents nevertheless possess much that is envied by older adults. Most youths are healthy and unencumbered by daily requirements for medication or any special care; they possess an enthusiasm for the future, reveling in the prospects of independence and self-sufficiency. Many of them are discovering the joy and enrichment brought by new human relationships. Opportunities for education and social mobility persist. Traditional human qualities emerge through hopeful planning and reveal themselves in adolescent growth and development.

These observations do not suggest that the milieu for all, or even most, adolescents is untroubled. The perilous status of international relations, the threat to the delicate balance in our environment, the disruption of many societal traditions, the continuing discrimination toward minorities and underprivileged groups, and the increasing demands on young people to achieve early success all cloud the adolescent mind. The burgeoning of America's elderly population has focused much public policy discussion on meeting the needs of persons who are currently retired or who will retire during the next 20–30 years. This group of Americans represents the largest single political constituency in the nation and has mobilized effectively to influence public decision makers. During a time when many parents worry about the competence of the public education system to prepare their children for a highly technical society, the traditional tax base for the support of education has eroded in communities. In many American cities the majority of households that provide the base for community property taxes are without children. It is natural that the interests and priorities of these citizens do not necessarily coincide with the needs of the young.

A clear implication then for today's youth is that his or her preparation for the future will require thoughtful individual planning and the conscious allocation of resources for education, career preparation, and the support of young families. This is a complex agenda for young people, even when they enjoy full health and physical ability, are unencumbered by any major childhood social or family trauma, and have the necessary personal resources to prepare themselves for adult life or business.

Youths with chronic illness or disability confront a much more un-certain future. Their childhood has probably created an even greater de-pendence on parents and other adults than it has for other young people. The arduous adolescent process of exploring limits, reality testing, and self-image development may be severely delayed or compromised. Future options may be perceived as dependent, not on ability or motivation, but on the status of the health condition.

In this context, public policy, which determines the extent to which necessary health care services are available, may well be a primary factor in the young person's ability to adapt to the stresses of adult life. By definition, chronic conditions are typically not curable by short-interval treatment. The continuing need to see physicians, take medication, receive treatment, and be aware of any change in symptoms forces many youths with chronic conditions into an indefinite sick role. Health care profes-sionals must therefore strive to convert their patients into persons.

The Relevance of Public Policy

All professionals or facilities with responsibilities to chronically ill or disabled youths must appreciate political and fiscal concepts that are in-herent throughout the health care and human services systems. Although there are many different perspectives on just how the political system influences the work of health care professionals, generic issues shape the posture of hospitals, government agencies, and health insurance companies and affect all children and adults with disabilities. Policies and priorities established in the political system eventually alter the care of every youth with chronic illness.

There are several hallmark principles that form the basis for assurance of services to chronically ill adolescents. They have evolved through changes in social conscience, legislation, and the courts, and they em-phasize to policy makers the need for comprehensive and appropriate ser-vices. Primary is the assertion of the right of children and youths to health care and services. In less than a generation, individual physicians have yielded their absolute authority in determining the extent and pattern of care for youths with chronic conditions. The activation of interdisciplinary teams and peer review have heightened the visibility of clinical decision making. The health care system has expanded its capabilities to provide sophisticated high-technology care. As a result of that capability, many questions are asked about consequences when a child or youth is rescued from a catastrophic illness. The special needs of that individual may be extended into decades of chronic care management.

Programs established by legislation affect young people with chronic illnesses or disabilities. The Federal Education for All Handicapped Children Act (Public Law 94-142, 1975) is civil rights legislation (see Chapter 6). This law mandates that every child in the United States be educated, regardless of disability, an opportunity that heretofore was not provided. The legislation, which grew out of a decade of sustained effort by parents, professionals, and voluntary groups assured that schools responded more appropriately to children with handicaps. The major principles of the legislation are free appropriate public education, evaluation by a multidisciplinary team, placement in the least restrictive setting, an individual educational plan, and due process provisions.

Another federal legislative act of relevance to youths with chronic conditions is Section 504 of the Rehabilitation Act, as amended. Section 504 has been described as a corollary to the Federal Education for All Handicapped Children Act, protecting the rights of adult handicapped individuals by prohibiting discrimination against handicapped persons who are attempting to gain access to programs, employment, or public buildings.

Title V of the Social Security Act has a variety of provisions that relate to children and youths, including the assurance that children have access to quality health services. The legislation provides grants to states to reduce the incidence of infant mortality and preventable diseases and handicapping conditions among children. Title V can also fund limited health care services for blind and disabled individuals under the age of 16 who receive benefits under Title XVI of the Act, the Supplemental Security Income (SSI) program. Finally, in continuing the traditional purposes of the Crippled Children's Services programs, Title V provides funds for locating and providing medical, surgical, corrective, and other services for children who have chronic conditions that potentially can result in disability.

The major federal legislation that has been critical in assuring services for the chronically ill youth is Title XIX of the Social Security Act (Medicaid or Medical Assistance). Title XIX is the largest source of public funds for health care, therapeutic services, and residential care for chronically ill youths in the United States. Due to their extraordinary health care needs, a disproportionate number of chronically ill or disabled persons are eligible for Title XIX in comparison to the entire population. Eligibility and comprehensiveness of services are at issue as budgets and priorities for public funding of health care are reviewed.

In a broad context, the federal government has been concerned with two major areas relevant to chronically ill youths: income maintenance and payment for health care for low-income persons. The federal government has guaranteed some equity for individuals caught in a system of high-cost services without adequate insurance or personal resources. States have shared the federal role in income maintenance, in health care provision, and in the guarantee of rights. States also monitor the provision of services on a programmatic or facility level and by licensure of hospitals, programs, and professionals. At the local level of government, there is responsibility for provision of some direct services, so that many individuals who require public assistance or specialized services must seek them directly from agencies that are funded and controlled by the community.

HEALTH CARE OF YOUTHS WITH CHRONIC ILLNESS OR DISABILITY

Requirements of Care

Young people with chronic illnesses or disabilities have special requirements for health care services. To be managed successfully, their conditions demand excellence in technical diagnosis and clinical monitoring. Since current principles of care cannot negate the condition (hence the chronicity), there is typically a steady progression of evaluation and management regimens. Physicians must follow the implications of recent research carefully to assure maximal outcomes for their patients. Frequently, multiple professional disciplines are necessary to facilitate comprehensive care. Commonly, these specialists may work in different clinics or hospitals, creating the need for coordination and careful communication of priorities and details to the youth and family. The specialists must recognize that the chronic condition not only alters organs or tissues, but also may interfere with normal physiological growth and development. In some situations the actual delivery of services must be adapted to accommodate emerging adolescent needs for independence and privacy.

Concepts of Health and Medical Care

Any discussion regarding the health care of the adolescent with chronic illness must first acknowledge the existence of a dynamic between the provider of care and the recipient. The nature of the dynamic is the underpinning of public policy, which is nothing more than a collective standard for the delivery of services to this select group.

There are several concepts that have implications for public policy options and comprehensive health services to youths with chronic illness or disability. The first is that health care does not occur as an isolated event in the life of a chronically ill youth. Health care is not independent of countless other events and factors that impinge on that adolescent and family but must be provided in the context of daily living.

A second concept is that disabled or chronically ill adolescents want to be as healthy as their peers and are typically reluctant consumers of care. Health care professionals may approach their work assuming that they are providing to an eager patient or client something that that person really wants, when in reality that person does not want anything that professionals have to provide. Adolescents prefer to use their time, energy, and resources for other pursuits.

Another concept links the practitioner to the delivery system in the view of the consumer. Professionals are seen, not as individual practitioners, but as part of a system of hospitals, facilities, clinics, schools, and rehabilitation centers. This system creates anxiety and often hardship. The professional or other care provider represents therapeutic regimens that are not necessarily pleasant or well received by the consumer.

A final concept centers on the complexity of a system of services interrelated by various mandates, types of funding, patterns of referral, and actions of individual practitioners. This system, which is a macrosystem of care for chronically ill or disabled youth, impinges extensively on the activities of individual providers of service and their patients.

Adolescents with chronic illness are not a homogeneous group. This large and varied population is a paradox in the health care system. Many of these youths are the beneficiaries of the remarkable advances in medical technology since the Second World War. An illustration is childhood cancer; cure is now possible for many malignant disorders, although a generation ago a rapid and fulminant terminal illness was typical. Yet success stories have limitation. Many other youths have chronic disorders that are only amenable to amelioration using current medical knowledge and skill. For these young people, life becomes an ongoing battle with their basic disease, marked by frequent encounters with the health care system, all of which is clouded by an uncertain future. Secondary to chronic illness, the adolescents and their families must endure stress that may result in greater disability than the actual physiological problem.

Interwoven genetic, biological, and environmental issues are characteristic of chronic illness in children and adolescents. Furthermore, illness, growth, and development are inextricably linked. A youth with juvenile-onset diabetes is reminded daily of his or her special need when insulin is administered. When following current principles of medical management of diabetes, a basic daily activity—namely, eating—also becomes a regimen. Since the prevalence of juvenile-onset diabetes is approximately 1 in 500 in the school-age population, it is unlikely that during everyday activity the diabetic youth encounters another youth with diabetes. Therefore, all of the aspects of the diabetic youth's medical management are unique in his or her experience: no other youth is required to use insulin, follow a diet, or do periodic urine or blood testing. If the youth does well in management and there are few complications, the regimen may be accepted through ongoing use and adaptation. If, however, that youth's condition does :.ot respond routinely and consistently to the regimen, the stress of illness intervenes. Regardless of illness, however, parents and youth must live with the constant fear that the diabetes will not remain well controlled and that there will be secondary illness, loss of school or work days, and other difficulties. Parents may also be concerned about long-term complications due to microvascular disease. There may be no evidence of these complications occurring in their child, but they are statistically predictable. These concerns lead to a permanent anxiety about the youth's future and well-being that can interfere with current family function. Parent–peer relationships, sibling interaction, and the entire family's life in the neighborhood and community can be compromised.

An Incomplete Knowledge Base

Despite the exponential accumulation of knowledge about childhood chronic illness and a rich experience throughout the nation in caring for these young people, many questions remain unanswered:

1. The true prevalence rates for many of these conditions are unknown, especially when one considers the usual spectrum of severity. Most youths with chronic illness who require frequent medical management do obtain access to a system of care. Other children with less severe, dysfunctional disease may enter the system only periodically and are even less visible. With the exception of a few rare conditions, there are no national registries or recurring surveys for most chronic diseases.
2. The outcome of many chronic illnesses is unknown. This is partly due to uneven utilization of services and limited data collection. Moreover, this lack of information on outcome for children with chronic illness is common since formal studies rarely achieve the necessary length of longitudinal follow-through. Children experience dynamic development throughout the first decades of life; the impact of any illness may not be recognized until early adulthood or even later.
3. Financial barriers and differences in quality and comprehensiveness of service are important aspects of delivery of care that are inadequately described and understood.
4. The full impact of chronic adolescent illness on families is only now coming to the attention of the research community.

These developments create a scenario of two primary issues affecting health care of chronically ill or disabled children. They can be divided broadly into these issues: gaps in service and outcome research.

Structural Gaps in Service

Historically, most public-program approaches to serving children with chronic illness have been defined based on medical eligibility determined by diagnosis and financial need. Beginning in 1935 with the passage of Title V of the Social Security Act, the federal government had the capability, acting through the states, to provide more comprehensive and accessible services to youths with chronic illnesses. Much of this effort initially centered on corrective or therapeutic treatment of youths who had the *fixed deformity* characteristic of musculoskeletal disorders and birth defects. State Crippled Children's Services programs were organized to identify such children and to assure access to service. However, due to limitations of direct service efforts in public health, an orientation to poor families, and persistently small appropriations, these programs in most states focused on only a small segment of potentially eligible children. With time, the scope of the programs included further medical diagnoses as efficacious treatments became available. An excellent illustration of the expansion of Crippled Children's Services programs was the inclusion of congenital heart disease in most of the programs in the 1950s following the introduction of successful open heart procedures with the advent of the heart–lung bypass. Chronic illnesses such as cystic fibrosis and hemophilia were also included as therapeutic approaches to these disorders evolved. Despite such changes, the programs in most cases have only 30–40 percent penetration into target populations. Thus the majority of youths with chronic illness do not benefit from these efforts.

It has been argued that not all youths with chronic illness require public health services since many families have the resources to obtain these services independently. In fact, the denominator of need for specialized health care is rarely understood. This is due in part to our lack of knowledge of the true financial burden imposed by the costs of chronic illness on many families. It is further hampered by our primary lack of epidemiological information on the prevalence and severity of many of these illnesses.

Throughout recent years there has been little public policy focused on the delivery of health care service to chronically ill adolescents. Relatively greater attention has been given to children with musculoskeletal disorders, primarily through the Crippled Children's Services programs, and to children with developmental disorders, generally through the development of university-affiliated facilities for mental retardation and through the passage of the Federal Developmental Disabilities Act. Changes in the technology of medical management, greater knowledge of outcome, and the impact of chronic illness on families increasingly suggest the need for a national policy.

Regardless of the specific pathology of the condition, most chronic illnesses share a basis of similarity for determination of public policy.

Almost by definition, chronic illness requires costly extended care that is provided by specialists in medical centers. There is a daily burden of care imposed upon families, which is accompanied by some discomfort or even pain for the youth. Frequently, these illnesses are progressive, or at least not curable, which creates a sense of uncertainty as families plan their future. Because of the low incidence of most of the conditions, both the public and the families themselves have a poor understanding of the nature of the illness.

Of most recent interest is the recognition of the effect of chronic illness on families. A number of issues have emerged from studies in the past decades, including the stress on marital relationships that results from the burden of caring for a youth who is chronically ill. Many families have limitations placed upon their mobility in seeking alternative employment, since a change might jeopardize health insurance coverage. The daily routine of care may deprive some families of leisure time and create a sense of permanent fatigue, which isolates parents and siblings from the community. The maladjustment of the chronically ill youth as well as siblings is a further cause of concern.

The health care of chronically ill youths therefore necessitates a careful review of the characteristics of current care and services. Whenever that care lacks coordination, comprehensiveness, or continuity, there is a significant risk not only that the care will be less than maximally effective but that secondary complications of the chronic illness will jeopardize the entire family. In view of the current public temperament regarding the consumption of resources in the health care system in general and the ineffectiveness of many public agencies to solve problems, it is somewhat dubious that a major new effort to reorganize the service system will be launched in the foreseeable future.

The options currently available stress the transfer of resources within the system to provide better care. In order to assure greater access and comprehensiveness, such a transfer inevitably means the shift of dollars from high-cost services (hospitalization or residential care) to lower-cost services (ambulatory or home-based care); such a transfer is not readily accomplished. The introduction of new technologies has created tremendous motivation among institutions caring for youths to maintain their operational functions and to maximize their investment in facilities and staff. Furthermore, the reimbursement system generally discourages the use of ambulatory or noninstitutional services even if it can be demonstrated that adoption of such services as an alternative to residential care is much less expensive in the long run. Redirection of providers, especially physicians and other decision makers, to alternative models is critical in the shaping of a new system. Similarly, detailed studies showing alternative financing of outpatient service are critical. Third-party payors, both public agencies and private health insurers, must be convinced that not only are such models desirable and necessary but that they might also lessen the spiral of escalating health care costs for this population of youths. Even substantially innovative financing models, such as prepaid health insurance plans targeted to chronically ill youths, may become feasible in this context.

Outcome Research

It would be misleading to imply that gaps in health care services for chronically ill youths represent the only barrier to maximal outcomes. Despite problems in financing care and organizing services, the country has invested a great many more resources in care of the chronically ill youth during recent years. There is increasing concern that some of these resources are not directed by a common strategy and that many interventions have unknown outcomes. Intervention in the course of chronic illness is designed to alter the natural history of that illness. Whether intervention is specifically medical or is oriented to family function, the entire purpose of the effort is to improve the status of the youth and the function of the youth and family. The presumption underlying this intervention is that the outcome will be superior to nonintervention. The knowledge that the use of modern medication and treatment protocols does favorably affect many chronically ill youths creates a very difficult ethical context for evaluation of the efficacy of intervention. Especially as the intervention becomes less technical and subject to scientific study, the evaluation is commensurately more difficult.

In this discussion, it is helpful to understand that as most scientists speak of the concept of efficacy, they are referring to the effectiveness of an intervention on the outcome of illness based on an expected or predicted outcome without intervention. In the real world of services, however, the measurement of efficacy becomes notoriously difficult.

Two examples may suffice for illustration. It is possible, for example, to identify youths with juvenile rheumatoid arthritis who have a similar pattern of disease. If alternative therapeutic regimens of medication and physical therapy were employed, controlling multiple variables for the purposes of analysis, one could eventually determine which specific regimen was most efficacious in favorably changing the outcome of the disease. Such a study would require careful clinical monitoring and, of greatest importance, the honest selection of patient groups of comparable clinical status prior to the onset of intervention. In arthritis, the growth and development of the youth, mobility of joints, freedom from pain, and other factors can be used to assess outcome. This example does illustrate the ability to understand outcome through careful scientific study.

An alternative example, however, demonstrates the perils of outcome research. Assume that families of diagnosed pre-adolescents with cystic fibrosis enter a patient-education program, which is provided to all families, regardless of the specific status or age of their children. (There is no discrimination according to the socioeconomic status of the family.) If, after some time, assuming that all families complete the course of education, one were to evaluate family function based upon the retention of information from the educational course, clearly there would be difficulties in establishing a cause-and-effect relationship between outcome and retention of information. This would be highly related to variability in the youth's disease status as well as to preexisting family factors that could impinge on outcome. The health educator of such a class might feel that the effort expended was justified, regardless of the effect on a specific youth or family, a conclusion difficult to objectively confirm.

While there are burgeoning additions to the literature of carefully controlled outcome studies, many more are required for the host of diseases and conditions that represent chronic childhood illness. Classic studies must be continually repeated since the outcome of disease is likely to change with the introduction of new treatment modalities. Ongoing research in this field generally will be beneficial on a continuing basis.

AN AGENDA FOR PUBLIC POLICY

Principles of Social Responsibility

The disparate nature of chronic illnesses in youths should not frustrate a basic intent to guarantee optimal health for these young people. Their intellectual and physical abilities deserve the opportunity of expression, an impossibility if they are denied care and services. Several current developments threaten accessibility to services. Each must be addressed through the articulation of policy.

Financial Difficulties

Reimbursement for comprehensive health care services is seriously incomplete. A growing number of low- and middle-income families have inadequate resources for payment of health care or specialized services and products needed by their chronically ill children. Even when reimbursement for the direct costs of service is adequate, other related expenses may create financial stress for the family. Such expenses include travel necessary to obtain specialized care, incidental expenses at health care facilities, costs of child care for siblings remaining at home, and loss of income from missed work time. Even more substantial losses may result from diminished career development or the sacrifice of a second family income due to the daily requirements of caring for the chronically ill youth.

Inaccessibility of Services

Continued geographical and cultural isolation of some youths and their families lessens the availability of services. Most specialized health care programs for chronically ill children are located at academic or major urban medical centers. Members of the professional staff at these centers rarely reflect the ethnic and socioeconomic diversity of their patient–consumers. Diseases or conditions that require highly technical care may call for extraordinarily precise interpretation by the physician or other professional to the patient and family. If contact is limited by time or language barriers, the patient motivation to follow recommendations and his or her understanding of the disease process may be limited.

Inconsistency of Resources

Resources for necessary services are fragmented among a potpourri of professionals, institutions, and agencies. The current system of care has little organizational logic. The patient can access the system at almost any level, which may not be consistent with care requirements. Formal linkages among sites of service are rare, so youths and their families must negotiate a maze of resources. The authority and ultimate responsibility for the quality of care are poorly defined. The extent of service may be arbitrary and vary considerably from facility to facility in the same community.

Financing of Care

Without correction of the inequities in reimbursement for health care, many youths with chronic illness will continue to receive incomplete care and suffer preventable complications of their diseases. A system of complementary reimbursement resources could be justified if, in fact, the vast majority of youths with chronic illness received insurance coverage or were eligible for public financing. This is clearly not the current situation. Due to mobility, underemployment, and benefit exclusions in many insurance policies or programs, the cost of necessary health care remains unaffordable for a significant number of such youths.

A clear option to provide comprehensive reimbursement would be universal entitlement. Federal and state legislators have been reluctant to embrace this principle, however, because of potential escalation of costs as well as lack of a public consensus regarding government's role in assuring health care. Most innovations in recent years have centered on cost-control programs as illustrated by prepaid plans and health maintenance organizations. Such programs attempt to ration service on a prospective basis. Assuming that a full range of necessary specialized services is available, there is no conceptual reason why youths with chronic illness or disability cannot receive appropriate health care in these programs. If, however, for reasons of economy a prepaid plan restricts referrals to a specialist or center external to its system, the outcome of care may be compromised. Public programs must redefine eligibility not strictly according to income or resource criteria but also on the basis of the needs of the client. There are encouraging models in human services that recognize the obvious status of many middle-income families whose children have extraordinary care requirements. These families do not have the additional resources necessary to purchase special care if insurance or public-funded programs are not available to them.

Recognition of the essential components of service and the commitment to finance those services are essential to the future of quality care for children and youths with chronic illness or disability. A prototype model for guaranteeing access and funding may well have similarities to the Education for All Handicapped Children Act. Clearly, the mechanism for the delivery of service and funding would be different, but such legislation might assure that youths are not denied necessary health care.

Organization of Services

Health care services have been described as a cottage industry in the United States. Despite some national and regional efforts to plan the development of new services, avoid duplication, and assure quality, most innovations in the system derive from the initiative of individual institutions, professional groups, and practitioners. Increasingly, the organization of services will reflect reimbursement availability.

There is an opportunity in this situation to rationalize care so that youths with chronic illness receive necessary services that are negotiable and practical. An emphasis on regionalization to conserve resources and stimulate the development of expertise is one potential organizational method. Regionalization has been at least partially successful in the case of several chronic conditions, notably hemophilia and cleft lip and palate. Resistance to regionalization generally originates in hospitals and professionals who lose prerogatives in their own provision of services. It is unlikely that a rigid geographical structure for regionalization can be superimposed on the current system, due to the historical placement of medical schools and other major centers and the disparate geography of many states. Incentives may have to be provided that will reward centers and groups that can meet standards of service. Other providers may then find that it is not fiscally possible to remain competitive.

Critical to the location of services will be continuation of models of care that emphasize interdisciplinary services. Physicians can provide only a segment of the care necessary for most adolescents with chronic conditions. In order that the recommendations and care provided in the health care setting be adequately translated to other service systems used by youths, including schools and community agencies, there must be a means for full communication.

Orientation to Families

Finally, it must be emphasized that youths must be cared for within the context of their family life. Immediate family members, parents and siblings, must have adequate information in order to reasonably respond to the changing needs of their chronically ill or disabled family member. Information also provides support to adolescents as they adjust to the restrictions imposed by the condition.

Community agencies that provide other human services to the youth must recognize the ambivalence of that person who is no longer a child and yet not quite an adult.

BIBLIOGRAPHY

Brandt, E.N. Block grants and the resurgence of federalism. *Public Health Report*, 1981, *96*, 495–497.

Kovar, M.G. Health status of U.S. children and use of medical care. *Public Health Report*, 1982, *97*, 3–15.

Lawton, S.E. Budget reconciliation: The new legislative process. *New England Journal of Medicine*, 1981, *305*, 1297–1300.

Nelson, R.P., & Stein, R.K. Children with special needs. In L.V. Klerman (Ed.), *Research priorities in maternal and child health*, Waltham: Brandeis University, 1981, 37–45.

Omenn, G.S., & Nathan, R.P. What's behind those block grants in health? *New England Journal of Medicine*, 1982, *306*, 1057–1060.

Select Panel for the Promotion of Child Health. *Better health for our children: A national strategy*. (DHHS [PHS] Publication No. 79-55071). Washington, D.C.: U.S. Government Printing Office, 1982.

The Surgeon General's Workshop on Children with Handicaps and Their Families (Report). (DHHS [PHS] Publication No. 83-50194). Washington, D.C.: U.S. Government Printing Office, 1983.

Zwick, D.I. Federal health services grants, 1980. *Public Health Report*, 1981, *96*, 498–502.

Tomas J. Silber

2

Ethical Considerations in the Care of the Chronically Ill Adolescent

Health professionals caring for chronically ill adolescents often are concerned with the ethical dimensions of the physician–patient relationship, particularly the moral aspects of treatment decisions. This chapter will explore these issues based on an understanding of both ethical theory and adolescent moral reasoning. The subjects addressed include the doctor's obligation to patients and their parents, consent, confidentiality, truth-telling, refusal of treatment, termination of care, and research with minors. Case reports are used to illustrate dilemmas and the principles involved in solving them.

PHYSICIAN–ADOLESCENT PATIENT RELATIONSHIP

Regardless of specialty or subspecialty, all physicians have in common an obligation to their patients. The nature of this obligation is open to controversy, ranging from technical descriptions to comprehensive medical care. All health providers, however, should be conscious of an additional subtle dimension to their relationships with their adolescent patients; it is a dimension in which they transcend the professional model and employ a model of human interaction (Silber, 1979). This occurs inevitably when one is working with the chronically ill, and it can best be understood by analyzing the physician–patient relationship.

Szasz and Hollender (1956) described three basic models of doctor–patient relationships:

CHRONIC ILLNESS AND DISABILITIES IN CHILDHOOD AND ADOLESCENCE   ISBN 0-8089-1635-1

1. *Active–passive:* The physician does something to the patient and the patient is unable to respond. The clinical application of this model can be seen in life-threatening situations, such as in the administration of anesthesia, acute trauma, coma, or delirium. The prototype of this model is the parent–neonate relationship.

2. *Guidance–cooperation:* The physician tells the patient what to do, and the patient obeys. Clinical application of this model is well exemplified in the treatment of patients with acute infectious illness. The prototype of this model is the parent–older-child relationship. It differs from the active–passive relationship in that both participants are actively contributing to the relationship and its outcomes. Although the patient is assuming some responsibility, the doctor clearly remains dominant. "The main difference between the two participants pertains to power and to its actual or potential use." (Szasz & Hollender, 1956).

3. *Mutual participation:* The physician's role is to help patients to help themselves. The patient's role is that of a participant in a partnership. The clinical application of this model can be seen in some types of psychotherapy. Its prototype is the adult–adult relationship. The participants are of approximately equal power and need each other. In different ways, the relationship will be satisfactory to both. The contracting model of patient–provider interaction in managing chronic illness approaches this model of mutual participation.

Each of the three types of doctor–patient relationship is appropriate for certain circumstances. To utilize each model appropriately for chronically ill teenagers, one must assess how the developmental tasks of adolescence are being fulfilled by the individual. Depending on where the patient is developmentally, the relationship may correspond to one or another model. To achieve a mutually constructive experience, physicians dealing with chronically ill adolescents have to undergo a process of change in the relationship, similar to another quite familiar process: ". . . the need for the parent to behave ever differently toward his growing child." (Szasz & Hollender, 1956)

Ethical Dilemmas

Chronically ill adolescents must face decisions every day. Should they share the truth about their condition with dating partners or prospective spouses? Should they be seeking a job with good health insurance instead of pursuing a vocation? How about sexual intimacy? Situations thus arise in which the doctor is asked for advice and learns about the adolescent patient's struggles and difficulties. The clinician then has to leave the role of scientific advisor and become involved in counseling. When this happens, care must be taken to avoid imposing values.

The reason for this position is both ethical and practical. Imposing values would violate the patient's autonomy, lead to a power struggle, and deprive the adolescent of an opportunity to work and exercise his or her own moral code. Adolescents should be encouraged to weigh decisions, investigate alternatives, and choose their own way. Through questioning and listening to how the individual responds, a clinician may identify each patient's stage of moral development. The questions asked may induce reflection, which may in turn promote higher levels of reasoning. This does not mean that the higher level of functioning will produce a so-called right answer or even one that is better than that produced by a lower level. It is always possible to do the right thing for the wrong reason. The point is that one role of the health care provider is to promote growth, and growth is promoted when one can articulate, examine, and challenge one's own beliefs and assumptions.

For the chronically ill adolescent, issues are frequently complex, and the patient is often called upon to make decisions governing his or her health care. The complexity of the ethical issues that may arise is illustrated by the following cases:

Joan, age 16, suffers from sickle cell disease. She discovers that she is pregnant from her only episode of sexual intercourse. She has been told that pregnancy is dangerous for women with sickle cell disease. She is anxious, desperate. She is considering the possibility of an abortion but is troubled by her religious conviction and by fear of pain. She is extremely worried about how her mother is going to feel about her. She asks for help.

John, age 14, has recurrent episodes of abdominal pain. He is hospitalized for evaluation. In the course of this hospitalization, he suffers two episodes of pain. After being examined, John is told that a medicine has been found that is going to help. A placebo is given, and the pain is alleviated immediately.

In solving moral dilemmas, familiarity with ethical theory may prove useful. This theory is an attempt to offer a rational account of a morality— a set of principles and values that guide our actions. While it does not give a concrete answer to specific problems, it does serve as a guide on how to look for an answer and how to see what factors are relevant (Melden, 1967). Often, ethical problem solving requires that one apply a logical sequence of reasoning to a situation with little immediate reliable information.

Frequently, one's moral principles are enmeshed in complicated ways. Although we may not be fully aware of them, they often point toward a preliminary decision, which then requires fine tuning. Ethical reflection helps the clinician in aiding adolescent patients concerned with moral problems. Most often, this merely involves helping the adolescents to articulate their questions. At other times, ethical theory may help by looking to see if the right question has been asked. A doctor can thus assist a patient in discerning the conflict among competing, alternative frameworks.

Bearing these issues in mind, ethical theory can be applied to the two cases summarized earlier. In the first case, Joan is faced with a choice. The unwanted pregnancy highlights a problem that is often present in the doctor–patient relationship: the need to address emotionally charged material. Some questions arise immediately: What does it mean to be nonjudgmental? What is an adolescent's responsibility? What are the provider's obligations?

It is important to stress that to be nonjudgmental does not mean to relinquish one's own values or to be blind or indifferent to personal principles. Rather, it means to do one's utmost to be objective. An essential part of objectivity is avoiding the imposition of personal judgments on the patient. In response to Joan's plea for advice, her physician helped her to continue her inquiries. Her questions included, "Is there something I ought to do? How do I feel about it? Which decisions will make me less miserable? What kind of person will this make me? Should I risk my health, my life?" There was no easy solution. Health professionals could provide some data she needed. More important, through structured questioning, they were able to help Joan to make the best choice herself. They could then be supportive of her thoughtful, autonomous decision.

In the second case, it was the doctor who had a choice. The question that came up related to his obligation toward the patient, the consequence of the action, and the best interest of the patient. In John's case, the physician had two intentions in prescribing the placebo: diagnostic, to differentiate between real and functional pain, and therapeutic, to eliminate pain. He did not contemplate the implicit deception and lack of respect toward John as a person inherent in such a procedure. He also overlooked the loss of trust resulting from the revelation of this deception (Silber, 1979).

What constituted the ethical dimension? In these, as in so many situations, a choice had to be made under circumstances where optimal solutions were not available. Decisions were made (or should have been made) after exploration of key principles of values and loyalties and after questioning the likely consequence of alternative decisions.

Adolescents suffering from chronic illness—and their parents—often have a high level of personal interaction with the doctor and other health professionals because of frequent office visits, exchange of information about the patient's progress, and the inevitable discussion of matters that go beyond the physical illness to family concerns, financial problems, and social consequences of the illness. Under these circumstances, many ethical problems arise from disagreement about recommended interventions and the role of the child or adolescent in the decision-making process.

Nondisclosure of Illness

Occasionally, parents may request that a diagnosis not be revealed to their adolescent child. This is the case, not infrequently, with an illness that is likely to be fatal. Leikin (1981) addresses this issue from an ethical perspective with clarity by stating that although the distraught parents claim a right to protect their child from this knowledge, "health care providers also have expertise in the care of sick children. Under these circumstances, the parents are not the only ones who are morally responsible." Since those who work with terminally ill adolescents know that adolescents realize its seriousness and probable fatality, it is the provider's moral obligation to establish a meaningful communication with the patient as well as with the parents to discuss the illness and its prognosis and, thus, attempt to relieve the fear, anxiety, helplessness, and loneliness that derive from partial information or conflicting nonverbal messages.

On the other hand, some children, explicitly or implicitly, do not want to be informed of the prognosis. Bluebond-Langner (1978) has described the coping mechanisms of *mutual pretense* that some adolescents with leukemia practice along with parents and staff in an attempt to maintain equilibrium. In many of these cases, to force information because of the belief that the patient needs to know the truth is to impose one's value system and risk losing the patient's trust; instead, a prudent intermediate course of waiting for the appropriate moment is indicated. In this difficult situation, all parties involved have their own attitudes and needs, which may interfere with the decision. Under such circumstances, if ethical theory is to be applied, personal beliefs must first be separated from fact. There is never assurance that one is doing the right thing (Langham, 1979). All that can be suggested is that through open discussion and interdisciplinary teamwork the system of checks and balances may be kept in existence (see Chapter 10).

Problem Patients: Noncompliance

Another moral dilemma may be presented by the adolescent problem patient:

Robert, age 16, has leukemia. He was admitted for the fourth time in one year to rule out septicemia. He misbehaved on the unit and left the ward without permission, thus missing several doses of antibiotics. He was also found smoking marijuana twice. On two occasions, while agitated, he threatened other patients. Finally, one day he hit a doctor.

Is it ever justifiable to discharge a seriously ill patient who requires inpatient treatment? To make an ethical decision, one has to analyze the medical implications, the patient's wishes, the interests of other patients, and the institutional needs (Jonsen, Siegler, & Winslade, 1982).

This patient's behavior undoubtedly has an underlying psychological reason (anxiety, denial, rage) and every effort should be made to give him counseling and guidance. An alternative might be found by admitting him to an isolated area or transferring him to a psychiatric facility. However, if this fails and he persistently interferes with his treatment, or if his actions continue to run directly counter to the goals of treatment and he interferes with the health care services being provided to others, there is no obligation to treat him.

Robert wished to continue treatment but expressed no intention of changing his abusive behavior. Medically, only one thing needs to be done: there is a medical duty to differentiate between a sociopathic origin for this behavior and a manifestation of organic illness, such as encephalopathy. Once the latter has been ruled out, there is no reason why a physician should be obliged to accept the patient's sociopathic behavior. In addition, the physician has an obligation not only to this patient but also to the other patients in the hospital. When a patient like Robert threatens other inpatients, their care is undoubtedly compromised. Finally, the hospital as an institution must provide appropriate care for all its patients. By the action of striking a doctor and threatening other patients, a patient may undermine the ability of the hospital to carry out its responsibilities.

Robert's case demonstrates ethical reasoning leading to a justification of a doctor's refusal to treat a problem patient; however, it does not apply to patients who pose problems because of simple lack of compliance. Neither does it apply to those adolescent patients who become ill as a consequence of their own behavior, as is the case with drug abuse. Such patients should receive medical care with the same attention as those who become ill through fate.

Refusal of Treatment

An even more complex problem is presented by the adolescent who refuses treatment (Schowalter, Ferhold, & Mann, 1973). It is not unusual for teenagers who are apparently well informed and who are not incapacitated to refuse recommended treatment. When the treatment is elective, there is no ethical problem; the principle of adolescent autonomy ought to be respected, even though the parents may insist otherwise. However, the situation is different when medical care is judged necessary to manage a serious illness.

Martha, age 17, suffers from anorexia nervosa. She has become severely malnourished, lethargic, hypotensive, and hypotonic. Her parents feel that if they
force her into the hospital she will never forgive them. The patient has been informed that she may die from her malnutrition, and she is afraid of dying, yet she
refuses the recommended hospitalization.

It may be argued that the doctor should permit this patient to refuse
treatment since she shows no objective sign of incompetence. This may
be disputed by considering that severe malnutrition per se may be the
cause of her irrational behavior, or even further that anorexia nervosa is
a mental disorder that renders the patient incapable of understanding the
needs of her body. A simpler moral argument, however, may be offered:
when the risk of treatment is low (feeding via behavior modification), the
benefit is high (avoiding death from starvation or electrolyte imbalance),
and the "benefits" of nontreatment are low or nonexistent, it is ethical
for the physician to probe and insist further. This case poses a genuine
moral conflict between a patient's personal autonomy and the paternalistic
value that favors medical intervention. A higher value is placed on the
principle of beneficence than on the principle of autonomy; the patient's
refusal cannot be respected, and treatment should proceed even against
her will.

Passive Euthanasia

The most traumatic ethical issue involved in the care of chronically
ill adolescents is passive euthanasia, which may include clinical decisions
such as controlling pain in a moribund cancer patient with increasing dosages of morphine or giving 100 percent oxygen to a patient with cystic
fibrosis and terminal pulmonary failure.

Jane, age 17, had suffered from multiple sclerosis since age 12. She was about
to graduate from high school when a new bout of the disease brought her to complete quadriplegia and beginning respiratory failure. Her intellect was not affected.
She was told that in order to aid her breathing she had to have a tracheostomy
and eventually be connected to a respirator. She refused and her family supported
her in this position. She also expressed her desire for an *order not to resuscitate*.
She was a Catholic and cited the Doctrine of Extraordinary Means in her support.
Her wishes were granted. She died the next day.

What are the prerequisites for ethical justification of a decision to
terminate or withhold treatment from an adolescent with a terminal illness?
If a treatment is judged inefficacious or to have a low probability for success, there is no moral obligation to perform a futile action. Thus, if no
treatment goal is attainable, treatment does not need to be initiated, or it
may be discontinued. In theory, this seems very clear. In practice, its
application is difficult. Many interventions are useful in the short run, for
example, Jane could perhaps have been successfully connected to a re-

spirator. Some medical goals, such as prolongation of life, can frequently be attained. In other cases there may be uncertainty about the efficacy of treatment. Jonsen, et al. (1982) give prudent guidelines on this difficult situation; they advise that a distinction be made between doubt over efficacy and personal trepidation or hesitation in the face of a crucial decision. There is also a need to distinguish doubt about efficacy from doubt about the ethical propriety of an act. Doubt about the rightness of a medical decision may be dispelled by a reasonable judgment that further intervention will not be useful in attaining important goals of treatment for the individual. If a patient is dying in the terminal stage of an illness, resuscitation is futile.

RESEARCH

The ethical and legal issues involved in research with children and adolescents have been described in detail (Jonsen, 1981). Adolescents may join research programs, provided the parents have given informed consent and the project has been found appropriate by an internal review board (IRB). It is every researcher's obligation to minimize risk and to notify the subject about potential risks. Clinicians should counsel their patients in this respect. Whenever a research project involves conditions for which a patient can be treated without parental consent, the adolescent may be allowed to consent (Holder, 1981).

ETHICAL OBLIGATIONS TO THE PARENTS

Ethical issues involve not only adolescents but also their parents. The clinician who is treating chronically ill adolescents knows that the parents are often themselves in need of help and support. It is not unusual for the adolescent's illness to coexist with other important and sometimes threatening events in the parents' lives, such as marital trouble, career difficulties, financial problems, or poor health. Every effort should be made to aid parents, through periodic personal contact, answers to their questions, and support for their endeavors.

However, one needs to remember that when an adolescent seeks health services, that adolescent becomes the patient. In accepting reponsibility for care of an individual, the clinician accepts an obligation (Silber, 1981). Can the obligation to the adolescent patient be reconciled with the obligation to the parents? What happens when a chronically ill adolescent wants to seek care and requests that the parents not be notified? May an otherwise dependent adolescent be considered independent when it comes to health care? These dilemmas are often expressed in terms of conflict about the issues of consent and confidentiality.

Consent is a contract between patient and physician. The physician must explain the nature of the treatment proposed as well as the existing alternatives, in return for which the patient will give permission to the physician for treatment. But in the case of the adolescent—who is neither child nor adult—who should give consent?

Confidentiality deals with the privileged nature of information provided to the physician by the adolescent. According to this, the medical history and physical findings cannot be shared with others, including parents, without the adolescent's permission. Yet when a hemophiliac becomes involved in contact sports, the adolescent with cystic fibrosis starts to smoke, or a diabetic adolescent abuses alcohol—in short, whenever chronically ill adolescents engage in activities that put their health in danger, do the parents have a right to know?

Two principles may be used in resolving such ethical questions: the principle of autonomy, which states that a person should have a say in any action that is going to affect him, and the principle of benevolence, which states that whenever something good can be done for a person it should be done, or at least no barriers should be placed to interfere with the attainment of that good.

The principle of autonomy, applied to a chronically ill adolescent, rejects the formulation that the adolescent is being protected when parental consent is requested as a prerequisite for medical care. It views insistence on parental consent as a denial of the adolescent's right as a separate person. The principle of beneficence also clearly lends support to the mature minor doctrine; many adolescents who come for medical care would never consult a doctor if they knew parental consent would be required prior to treatment. Under this principle, it is also easy to see how confidentiality can be ethically justified: lack of confidentiality would constitute a barrier to health care.

This seems to be in contradiction with the tenet that parental involvement in the care of the chronically ill adolescent is an extremely important and recognized part of the optimal health care for the adolescent (AAP, 1980). The truth is that the contradiction can be resolved by the fact that concerned clinicians do not place themselves in an adversarial position in relation to the parents when obtaining their adolescent offspring's consent or when maintaining the confidentiality of what the adolescent has revealed; the doctors share the same goal as the parents: to protect and restore the adolescent's health.

All physicians should encourage their adolescent patients to seek support from their families, sometimes to the extent of acting as intermediary in crisis situations and thus helping to restore the organization of the family. There is no question that doctors value life above confidentiality, in that they will take action and violate autonomy in cases of dangerous behavior such as hemophiliac risk-takers, adolescent epileptic automobile drivers, and depressed patients who are becoming suicidal. When such an unusual step does have to be taken, however, the physician is obliged to inform the patient about the breach of confidentiality and the rationale for it (Silber, 1981).

To conclude, the cases presented and issues discussed have illustrated how the clinician is deeply immersed in the ethical dimensions of the care of those with chronic illness. Moral education is not primarily the doctor's responsibility, but it certainly is not peripheral to his or her practice. In our society the role of moral educator of youth is not clearly assigned. Family, schools, churches, and media all have a role to play, and frequently the health care provider will become involved. When the question of what ought to be done arises, the physician transcends the profession and, as a person, becomes a role model and a model educator, for better or for worse, whether the role is desired or not. The clinician does not need to be a moralist, but ought to be comfortable in encounters with moral philosophy. From the time of Hippocrates this has been part of the clinical tradition.

REFERENCES

American Academy of Pediatrics, Committee on Adolescence. *Health assessment and health maintenance of the adolescent.* Evanston, Il: American Academy of Pediatrics, 1980.

Bluebond-Langner, M. *The private worlds of dying children.* Princeton, NJ: Princeton University Press, 1978.

Holder, A. Can teenagers participate in research without parental consent? *IRB,* 1981, *3,* 51.

Jonsen, A.R., Siegler, M., & Winslade, W.J. *Clinical ethics.* New York: MacMillan Company, 1982.

Jonsen, A.R. Research involving children: Recommendations of the National Commission for the Protection of Human Subjects of Biomedical and Behavioral Research. *Pediatrics,* 1981, *62,* 131.

Langham, P. Parental consent: Its justification and limitations. *Clinical Research,* 1979, *27,* 249.

Leikin, S.L. An ethical issue in pediatric cancer care: Nondisclosure of a fatal prognosis. *Pediatric Annals,* 1981, *10,* 401.

Melden, A.I. *Ethical theories: A book of reading with revisions.* Englewood Cliff, NJ: Prentice Hall, 1967.

Schowalter, J.E. Ferhold, J.B., & Mann, N.M. The adolescent patient's decision to die. *Pediatrics,* 1973, *51,* 97.

Silber, T.J. Ethical considerations in the medical care of adolescents and their parents. *Pediatric Annals,* 1981, *10,* 408.

Silber, T.J. Placebo therapy: The ethical dimension. *Journal of the American Medical Association*, 1979, *242*, 245.

Silber, T.J. Physician–adolescent patient relationship, the ethical dimension. *Clinical Pediatrics*, 1980, *19*, 50.

Szasz, T., & Hollender, M. A contribution to the philosophy of medicine. *Archives of Internal Medicine*, 1956, *97*, 585.

Michael D. Resnick

3
The Social Construction of Disability

The notion of a social construction of disability is based on an understanding that the lives of those with disability are intimately bound to the societal response to that disability. Why should a chapter on this topic appear in a book intended primarily for practitioners interested in diagnosis and management of chronic conditions and diseases?

The delivery of medical care services is slowly undergoing transformation from a focus on the arresting and reversing of biophysical pathology to the treatment and guidance of the whole person. This shift is seen in the expansion of the term "medical care" to "health care," or what elsewhere has been called "the coming of postclinical medicine" (Miller & Miller, 1981). This changing clinical perspective incorporates an understanding of everyday life and its relationship to health, illness, and wellbeing. The importance of this conceptual reorientation is well described by Gliedman and Roth (1980) who delineate the sociological destiny of the disabled: a greater likelihood of nonemployment or lower wages than able-bodied peers, limited upward mobility, poverty, separation and divorce, frequent hospitalization, low educational attainment, and social isolation. These outcomes are not due to physical limitations alone, but more important, to individual and societal response to disability itself. This chapter explores the origins and nature of that societal response so that health professionals working with the disabled will better understand their own attitudes and responses to disability in their clients and will be sensitive to their sociological destiny, which is an integral aspect of the everyday life experiences of those with physical disability.

29

PREVALENCE CONSEQUENCES

To understand the notion of disability as a social construction, it is best to begin with a look at its prevalence in the United States and what can be expected from its high frequency of occurrence. According to the Social Security Administration's National Survey on Disability (U.S. Department of Health and Human Services, 1978) there were 127.1 million noninstitutionalized Americans between the ages of 18 and 64. Of this group, over 21 million adults were limited in their ability to work due to a chronic health condition or impairment. In other words, 165 of every 1000 adults were disabled. Half of these disabled adults, or 10.7 million, were severely limited and could work only on a very limited basis if at all. Prevalence estimates for children and youths are somewhat more difficult since multiple data sources are typically used. From Kakalik, et al. (1973), the Rochester Survey of Pless and Roghmann (1971), and the United Kingdom National Survey of Children and the Isle of Wight Study (Charles, 1981), it can be estimated that of the approximately 84 million children and youths in the United States, at least 9.5 million, or approximately 11 percent, may be considered handicapped.

With a prevalence rate of one in ten the question must be asked: What has permitted able-bodied adults with disabled spouses, children, or classmates not merely to acquiesce in their political and social oppression, but simply not to perceive this oppression as oppression? What does the able-bodied individual see when looking at a handicapped person? Why is society so mystified by handicap (Gliedman & Roth, 1980).

Attitudes Toward the Disabled

For more than 30 years, an extensive body of literature has been developing that examines individual and societal responses and attitudes toward the disabled. Generically, this vast literature can be summarized with the observation that social expectations of the physically impaired go far beyond biomedical limitations imposed by the disability alone. To understand the sociological destiny of those with disabilities, it is necessary first to understand what those attitudes and expectations are and to understand their genesis.

Children's attitudes toward the disabled have been studied by a number of researchers. Sadly, their findings indicate that negative attitudes held by children are not restricted to childhood but rather are a prelude to the negativism, misconceptions, and fears that persist throughout adulthood. In sociometric and picture–response tests, children have indicated their preference for interacting with able-bodied children rather than with disabled children (Centers & Centers, 1963; Richardson, Goodman, Hastorf, & Dornbush, 1961; Voeltz, 1980; Weinberg, 1976). It has also been shown that negative attitudes toward the disabled tend to increase with age among children. As knowledge of disability increases, in contrast to their younger counterparts who are less knowledgeable about various types of impairment, older children show greater rather than less bias toward their peers who are disabled (Weinberg, 1978). Investigators have begun to call for a more refined examination of attitudes toward disability, with emphasis on cognitive development during childhood, not merely changes in the age. Ryan (1981), for example, has sought to understand age-related changes in attitudes as a function of evolving developmental capabilities in role-taking ability and cognition. While her study demonstrated that there tend to be inconsistencies in the age-graded relationship between attitudes toward the disabled and an individual's perception, underlying negative attitudes toward those with disability still persisted.

Attitudes of employers have been studied with the idea that such individuals are significant gatekeepers of employment opportunities as well as perceptions of employee status once a disabled worker is hired. These studies have indicated the predominance of negative attitudes (Conley, 1973; Jordan & Friesan, 1968; Phelps, 1965; Cohn, 1963). In his 1980 presidential address to the American Academy for Cerebral Palsy and Developmental Medicine, Bender (1981) noted that despite numerous federal attempts to increase the employment opportunities of the disabled, little change has transpired in either the rate of employment or the acceptance of disabled workers by the employer.

With the assumption that professionals, such as physicians, rehabilitation workers, and teachers, might hold more positive attitudes toward the disabled in light of their more frequent contact with them, a variety of attitudinal studies have been undertaken. Just as employers are gatekeepers of job opportunities, professionals are also significant gatekeepers of both services and information. As Altman (1981) notes, if professionals' attitudes toward the disabled include labeling and stereotypical thinking as reflected in other groups, the results will be the narrowing of alternatives and options considered appropriate for disabled individuals. While this literature is not extensive, the majority of studies indicate parallels between general societal attitudes and those held by social workers (Begab, 1970; Belinkoff, 1960); counselors (Dufree, 1971; Wicas & Carluccio, 1971); and physicians (Wolraich, 1982). Studies of teachers and rehabilitation workers have been noted to be of particular importance, since the expectations of these two groups toward the disabled can play a key role in the learning and rehabilitation of the disabled, with strong implications for future life chances. Bender describes the way in which rehabilitation professionals are of central importance to the disabled because of the crucial role they play in the development of new roles and self-concept for those with disability (1981). McDaniel (1976) asserts that patients' physical and emotional responses to rehabilitation are most strongly influenced by the expectations and attitudes of the rehabilitation workers themselves.

Several studies indicate that rehabilitation workers hold negative views about those with disabilities. Singleton, Cole, and Long (1979) found that the attitudes of rehabilitation professionals were more negative toward those with disability than were the attitudes of a control sample selected from the general population. Preference among rehabilitation workers for non-disabled co-workers and friends was demonstrated by DeLevi* (1966); while reviews by Yuker, Block, and Young (1966) indicate that rehabilitation staff workers exhibit increasingly negative attitudes toward the disabled as contact with them increases. More recently, Finkelstein (1980) had demonstrated that medical and rehabilitation professionals play a significant role in perpetuating negative attitudes toward the physically disabled.

Analogously, Good and Brophy (1978) attribute much of the difficulty of handicapped students within educational settings to negative attitudes and expectations of teachers. Teachers' expectations as a self-fulfilling prophecy have long been a hallmark in educational theory; this *Rosenthal effect* has recently come under scrutiny regarding the relationship between teachers and handicapped individuals. Martinek and Karper (1981) found that the teachers' expectations of handicapped students with regard to social relationships with peers were significantly lower than those for nonhandicapped students. The authors noted that this may in fact reflect realistic assessment of the interpersonal competence of those with the disability. While such assessments may be realistic, the issue of teacher expectations being a self-fulfilling prophecy cannot be dismissed. Negative attitudes of teachers toward the disabled have been documented too frequently to be dismissed as realistic assessments of disabled youths' potential (Lapp, 1957; Combs & Harper, 1967; Semmel & Dickson, 1966; Greene & Retish, 1973).

While it is distressing to note that those with important decision-making power and influence over the lives of the disabled person hold stereotypical and negative attitudes toward them, it should not be surprising. Every culture provides not only a generalized notion of the social stigmata of disabilities but also rank-ordering of various impairments (Birenbaum, 1979). The hierarchy of preferences toward various disability groups is consistent cross-age (Harasymiw, Horne, & Lewis, 1976) and cross-culturally (Safilios-Rothschild, 1970). Mental retardation and cerebral palsy are seen as least acceptable, blindness and deafness are ranked in the

---

*DeLevi, A. Attitudes of Laymen and Professionals Towards Physical and Social Disability. Unpublished Ph.D. dissertation, Columbia University, 1966.

middle together with speech defects and epilepsy, while amputation, arthritis, and wheelchair conditions are viewed as the most acceptable forms of disability (Altman, 1981). While a rank-ordering of acceptability of disabling conditions can be identified, research also indicates a generic stereotype applied to all disabled (Weinberg, 1976). This relative uniformity of response to disability is reflected in the attitudes of children born with disabilities, who tend to share negative societal values about disabilities in general (Richardson et al., 1961). Similarly, disabled adults also have been found to hold negative attitudes toward the disabled as a group (Dixon, 1977).

Goldberg (1977) has stressed that the societal reaction or social stigma association with physical disability has a more profound impact upon the happiness, adjustment, and well-being of the individual than the actual, objective physical severity of the condition itself. In his discussion of independent living arrangements for adolescents and adults with cerebral palsy, Dickman (1975) notes that other than a small group of the most severely handicapped, the way in which most people with cerebral palsy live in this country stems "not from their [physical] handicap, but from a social handicap—from society's view of them and society's attitudes." Because of the pervasive view that such individuals cannot take responsibility for their own lives, such disabled persons are relegated to the status of permanent children. Morgan of the British Spastic Society states the problem succinctly:

> . . . there is also a tendency on the part of the "normal" people to treat the basic human rights of handicapped people as privileges to be meted out to them, almost as though they were rewards to children by parents. The corollary of this is the tendency to be shocked when handicapped individuals act like adults rather than as children. . . . (Morgan, 1972).

From the repeated observation that the societal constraints imposed on the disabled go beyond the biological parameters of the disability itself, the term "handicap" has evolved as a metaphor for the additional layers of limitations heaped upon the person with physical disability (Bogdan & Biklen, 1977; Braginsky & Braginsky, 1971; Scott, 1969; Scheff, 1966; Goffman, 1963, Szasz, 1961).

Bogdan and Biklen (1977) go beyond this conceptualization to introduce a new paradigm, *handicapism*, which they propose as a framework for understanding the social experiences of those who carry with them a stigma associated with their handicap, mental illness, retardation, or other forms of deviance. Handicapism is supported by a triad of concepts: prejudice, which is an oversimplified and overgeneralized belief about the characteristics or traits of a group of persons; stereotype, which is the specific content of the prejudice that is directed toward groups or individuals; and discrimination, which is the behavioral and structural element of both prejudice and stereotype. The statement made by the Union of Physically Impaired Against Segregation clearly draws the same distinction:

> In our view, it is society which disables physically impaired people. Disability is something imposed on top of our impairment by the way we are unnecessarily isolated and excluded from full-time participation in society (thus we find) disability as disadvantage or restriction of activity caused by contemporary social organization (Bender, 1981).

Social Interaction

Before considering the roots of handicapism it is important to understand how negative social attitudes are manifest in the everyday lives of those with disabilities. Since most disabled adolescents typically have not experienced occupational discrimination, it is more age appropriate to turn to the strains and discontinuities of social interaction that occur between the disabled and nondisabled. Hastorf, Wildfogel, and Cassman (1979) note that interactions between the disabled and nondisabled are frequently accompanied by uncertainty, anxiety, and discomfort (Kleck, Ono, & Hastorf, 1966; Davis, 1961). In these interactions, able-bodied individuals tend to show less variability in their behavior, express opinions that are less representative of their actual beliefs, gesture less, and terminate the interaction sooner than they would when interacting with non-handicapped individuals (Kleck, 1968; Kleck et al., 1966). Comer and Piliavin (1972) have demonstrated that similar anxiety, discomfort, and tension are also experienced by the disabled individual. Others believe that the relative social separation of the disabled and nondisabled may account for some of the discomfort. For example, in the case of interaction with those with visual impairments, the discomfort and tension felt by the sighted persons will often carry over into linguistic fears, where the sighted individuals are "afraid that they will do or say the wrong thing . . . [such as] using the words 'look' and 'see' the same way everyone else does . . ." (Yeadon & Grayson, 1979).

The dynamic underpinning these constraints have on interaction has been articulated by Wright (1960) and Davis (1961) in their discussions of *spread effect* and *dynamic spread*. Both of these terms refer to the process by which persons focus on the individual's disability as his or her predominant characteristic. All interactions are then colored by that perception unless or until the relationship is normalized. In other words, there is the attribution of negative characteristics on the basis of the overriding label of disability itself. With spread effect, the disability becomes the focal point for interactions with others. Usually, the more obvious, unusual, or severe the disability, the more difficult it is for others to get beyond the disability so as to normalize interpersonal relationships. Simultaneously, a goal of rehabilitation is normalization, in which the disabled individual committed to culturally embedded notions of normalcy works to minimize the stigma associated with his or her disability (Anspach, 1979). For many, complete normalization is an impossible goal and, as a result, they experience frustration and a sense of failure. Part of the tension stems from handicapped peoples' perception of the discrepancy between the superficial acceptance extended to them (what Davis calls the democratic fiction that pervades society) and their awareness of the discomfort of the able-bodied individual in the interaction. What frequently results is a wide gap between expressions and responses intended and those felt—"a gap filled with profound distrust and suspicion of a rejection that may lurk beneath the facade of civility" (Anspach, 1979).

Davis describes democratic fiction as the belief that we should behave as though there were a fundamental equality of all human beings while we may believe the contrary. At the root of the awkwardness experienced in interactions between able-bodied individuals and those with disability is the conflict between mainstream definitions of normal and deviant. Given the predominant sociocultural beliefs in the United States, such awkwardness can be seen in interactions between individuals of different racial backgrounds, different religions, or even between obese and nonobese individuals. Complicating social relations between the "normal" and the "deviant" is fictional acceptance (Davis, 1961) or what social psychologists call "as if" behavior: acting or behaving as if the relationship is on a personal level when the disability is still seen as the predominant characteristic of one of the individuals. The strain in fictional acceptance is that it is built upon a facade of socially defined norms of appropriate interaction, which, all too often, is fragile; a slip of the tongue can scuttle the whole relationship.

In an interview with a wheelchair-bound 19-year-old adolescent (see Chapter 18 in this edition), the interviewer was well into the second hour of the interview, discussing dating, sex education, and sexual feelings. The question began, "Has it ever happened to you that you were just walking down a street and all of a sudden . . ." and right there the 19-year-old stopped the interview. "Can I just tell you something?" he asked. "This is the first time, and I mean the *first* time that someone outside of my immediate family has asked me a question about 'just walking down the street' without stopping in midsentence, getting flustered, back-tracking on what they meant, apologizing, or just blowing what otherwise might have been a damn good conversation." The central point is that while in the physiological sense they might not hear, see, or walk, in the social sense of everyday discourse the deaf "hear," the blind "see," and the wheelchair-bound "walk" in their own way.

One way of reducing tension between the able-bodied and the disabled is the acknowledgment of the disability. The work of Hastorf et al. (1979) indicates that acknowledging one's disability is a significant component in reducing stress in interaction. In experimental studies, the confederate who acknowledged having a handicap was preferred by experimental subjects over other handicapped confederates. The importance of the acknowledgment of handicap even applied when the acknowledging confederate acted nervous. Hastorf et al. (1979) suggest that disabled individuals may use this disclosure/acknowledgment tactic effectively even before they themselves are comfortable with such disclosure or have adjusted to their disability. Potentially, this strategy of acknowledging the handicap may reduce the discomfort, anxiety, and uncertainty that surround the nondisabled individual's interaction with the disabled person, and may allow less encumbered social relationships to evolve.

Understanding the dynamics and tensions that influence interpersonal relationships makes it easier to understand the everyday experience of disability as reported by those with physical impairments. The consequences of this strain between the disabled and nondisabled can now also be examined.

Since physical appearance is a fundamental source of information about other people, disabled persons need a repertoire of social skills to facilitate face to face interactions. In many instances, however, this will not be sufficient to offset the tendency of able-bodied persons to avoid such interactions altogether (Birenbaum, 1979). Physical appearance is particularly important during adolescence as a way of classifying and rating oneself and others. It is likely, therefore, that tolerance for differences will be lowest in this age group, resulting in a reduction in self-esteem for the physically disabled adolescent (Birenbaum, 1979). The circuitous nature of this process and outcome is insidious.

The handicap that compounds disability does not stop with strained social interactions. As previously discussed, it is understood from sociometric and experimental research that nondisabled people terminate their interactions with the disabled earlier than they would with nondisabled persons; they show less variability in their verbal behavior and tend to distort their opinions so as to make them more consistent with those presumed to be held by the disabled individual (Kleck et al., 1966; Kleck, 1968). As a result, the disabled individual receives distorted feedback in the course of interaction with others, a crucial issue in the development of interpersonal competence in adolescents. Underpinned by the generalized American norm to be kind to the disadvantaged, disabled persons frequently do not receive accurate feedback from their environment (Altman, 1981). This continuous experience of spread effect, fictional acceptance, and lack of accurate feedback means that the disabled have a restricted opportunity to develop social competence. Self-respect and self-confidence are diminished, increasing the risk that the disabled individual will come to feel deviant, different, less, and ultimately unworthy (Pless & Roghmann, 1971; Birenbaum, 1979; Anderson & Klarke, 1982). Compounding the problem is the observation that all too often those who seek out contact with the handicapped are social isolates themselves and hardly make good models for disabled children or adolescents (Birenbaum, 1979). In sum, the lack of social skills in a disabled person more reflects experience with negative social encounters and weak role models than unwillingness, lack of interest, or incapacity.

Origins of Societal Response to Disability

Despite extensive documentation of the devalued status and stigmatization of the disabled (Shattuck, 1976; Winthrop & Taylor, 1957; Greenbaum & Wang, 1965; Hollinger & Jones, 1970; Harasymiw et al., 1976) it is difficult to identify the source of these negative attitudes. The prejudice is historical and cross-cultural in nature (Wright, 1960; Barker, Wright, Meyerson, & Gonick, 1946; Thoreson & Kerr, 1978). As such, these beliefs are ubiquitous and difficult to trace. An example is the attitudes toward blindness. Yeadon and Grayson (1979) state that the underpinnings of negative societal responses to the blind are deep, variegated, and complex. Such attitudes, they contend, may be understood in light of:

1. Biblical beliefs that blindness was a punishment for sin
2. The association between loss of vision and castration fears
3. The ambiguity of expectations of the sighted person toward the visually impaired, accentuated by the impaired individual's particular way of moving and mannerisms
4. The association of blindness with venereal disease
5. The fear that blindness is possibly contagious

Hastorf et al. (1979) address the issue of interpersonal discomfort as stemming in part from the nondisabled person's realization of vulnerability to disability. There is a further fear described by Goffman (1963) as the fear of stigma—being discredited by others for associating with the disabled.

Gellman (1959) has described the underlying sources of negative attitudes toward the disabled as including the belief, rooted in Judeo–Christian thinking, that handicaps represent punishment for evil behavior, thereby making the disabled individual evil and dangerous, and the corollary assumption that the disabled person has been punished unjustly with his disability and is therefore likely to seek redress for the injustice through retribution, making that individual dangerous.

In a related light, Livneh (1980) contends that the core of peoples' rejection of the disabled lies in the basic existential fear of death. Others, however, have focused on more tangible sources of handicapism in society, such as the media (Reichel, 1975; Safilios-Rothschild, 1977; Thurer, 1980). Thurer notes that the portrayal of the disabled in the media is typically negative, including Cain, Oedipus, Richard III, Captain Ahab, and a wide range of children's characters such as Pinocchio. Thurer also notes that on the other hand, the disabled are romanticized in the media by conveying the impression that they are more in touch with their inherent humanness, more insightful and self-reflective, and more sensitized to themselves and all humanity than are others. Taylor (1981) cites such recent films as *The Elephant Man, Whose Life is This Anyway?, Ice Castles, Voices,* and *The Other Side of the Mountain* as examples of this romanticized portrayal of the handicapped. Weinberg and Santanna (1978) found that in the depiction of comic-book characters, the physically disabled are never ordinary individuals but rather are either very good or very evil. Such a portrayal leads to the implicit conclusion that there is a close correspondence between physiological characteristics and personal traits. They note, ". . . a physically distorted person in a neutral role perhaps distracts from the major theme since people would assume that if an individual's appearance were extreme, his behavior could not be neutral." In a content analysis of 45 books from middle-school libraries, Baskin (1974) found that persons with physical disabilities were portrayed as either incompetent and helpless or possessing extraordinary capabilities and skills. Taylor's (1981) conclusion is that if such portrayals persist, the stereotypes will continue to endure and the more accurate association of ordinariness with disability will be more difficult to establish.

Others agree. Bogdan and Biklen (1977) make reference to the selective reporting of news stories by reporters; the tendency is to ignore those events including the disabled that counteract or contradict our stereotypical expectations. By failing to jar our mind-set, preferential attention is given to stereotype-enforcing events such as telethons.[a] In an examination of the relationship between physical attractiveness and crime as reported in several forms of media, Needleman and Weiner (1974) found that physical difference is frequently associated with the reporting of violence and other forms of criminal activity. Walt Disney constantly rein-

---

[a]See, for example, Anspach, 1979 for a perceptive discussion of political activism on the part of the disabled, a mobilization that she calls "identity politics".

forced this stereotypical association between deformity or difference and violence (Bogden & Biklen, 1979).

Finally, researchers have analyzed the content of jokes and humorous exchanges as a reflection and perpetuator of underlying negative attitudes toward the disabled. Barker and associates (1946) found that in humor directed at persons with physical handicaps, 80 percent of the jokes deprecated disabled persons. This contrasted with humor directed toward farmers, dentists, judges, and physicians, in which slightly over 40 percent of those subjects were derogated. The everyday language of children, less constrained by the norms for politeness, clearly reflect the devalued status of the disabled—gimp, crip, spaz, mental retard.

While it may never be possible to isolate or causally identity the genesis of handicapism in American society, an understanding of how such negative definitions and perceptions are constructed, adding handicap to disability, is essential not only for gaining greater insight and understanding among practitioners but also as a prelude to working with disabled individuals in order to expand their repertoire of coping skills.

THE SOCIAL CONSTRUCTION OF REALITY

As an approach to understanding the origins and perpetuation of negative attitudes toward the disabled, the perspective that reality exists only to the extent that there is a consensus that it is true has been adopted (Berger & Luckmann, 1966). What this conception assumes is social reality and not scientific reality. The social construction of reality is really a definition of a social activity involving consensus. That is, through a common medium of communication, people systematically arrange and build ideas about events that happen. These events can include whether or not someone is considered good or bad, whether a nation has won or lost a war, or whether in fact a room is a horrible mess. What this concept assumes is that the subject of discussion is social reality and not scientific fact. The difference is analogous to that between a camera and a canvas—the former records without interpretation, the latter records and interprets simultaneously. The construction of subjective reality occurs when people observing physical events evaluate these actions and behaviors by assigning meanings to them as they happen. Consider the following example: Objective reality might be the eruption of Mt. St. Helens volcano. The social construction around this event might be that the event is "fantastic, beautiful, marvelous" or that it is "catastrophic, a tragedy, a disaster." From one objective reality come multiple interpretations.

Normally socialized human beings learn to evaluate objective reality as a nonconscious activity in terms of its impact on themselves and perhaps on others as well. While it is possible to describe events objectively, it is the nature of human socialization that people evaluate as they describe. Evaluation is a function of language acquisition (Mead, 1934). As we learn the language of description, we are taught and we learn the language of evaluation: "that is nice," "that is good," "that is bad." Indeed, when the dispassionate viewing of events by human beings is desired in a given situation, it requires a deliberate effort to remove the evaluative component from the language that is used to describe it.

Switching to the issue of disability, it is important to understand that the evaluations made of physical impairment or difference need to be understood in light of mainstream cultural values as well as individual interpretations of those values. A quick glance at the advertisements in any popular magazine would emphasize the tremendous value placed on the body whole, the body young, and the body beautiful (Litman, 1964). Through the socialization process in this culture, Americans have come to acquire very strong values in terms of beauty, youth, work, and productivity. It is against these values that people and events are seen and instantaneously assessed in their compatibility or discordance with the mainstream values. Given the societal focus on being well, vital, mobile, and young, it is no accident that those who cannot keep pace are devalued. From these negative assessments cascade the flood of restrictive experiences that appears to be the sociological destiny of the disabled (Gliedman & Roth, 1980)—social, vocational, and educational limitations resulting in low self-esteem, depression, and unfulfilled potential. With such culturally embedded negative expectations, the disabled are presumed to be capable of assuming but a limited repertoire of social roles (Safilios-Rothschild, 1970). One such role is that of the patient. Implicit expectations of the patient role are compliance and passivity. Birenbaum (1979) notes that children who are constantly treated as sick or who, because of social attitudes, are placed in a permanent sick role may never be given the opportunity to prove themselves. The consequence of playing out this role, Birenbaum notes, is that their physical impairment becomes their life's central focus. Embracing the sick role as one's social identity typifies the disabled patient role; in such a role one no longer strives for normalization.

In a similarly constraining role—that of the helped person—disabled people find themselves the constant recipient of help, more often than they actually need it based solely on physical limitations. Well-intentioned but often misguided assistance comes from concerned parents, health professionals, teachers, strangers, and in fact from anyone with whom the helped person comes in contact. To be a helped person in this culture, which values self-reliance and independence, includes subtle yet pervasive expectations in terms of dependency and gratitude; the ramifications of such a social identity are enormous.

The public relations representative is a role played out by disabled individuals who find that the relative uniqueness of their condition and the associated ignorance of others place a constant burden of explanation and interpretation upon them. This is what elsewhere has been referred to as being a "professional cripple,"* where one's primary role is to explain, discuss, and clarify what it means to be disabled.

Finally, closely linked with this role is the model disabled person, what Wright (1960) called the salutory aspects of disability. With the model disabled person, interaction centers around the admiration of others for how well they cope with their disability, amazement at their accomplishments despite their disability, how sensitive they are, how happy, and how much they get out of life. The consequence of this overriding expectation toward the disabled, despite its superficially flattering appearance, is a variation of spread effect. This role, like all others described, permits only a limited, circumscribed range of behaviors, repertoires, and opportunities for the disabled person in the eyes of others. Each role provides a set of expectations that limit options. These limiting kinds of expectations, along with the negative societal reactions to physical disabilities previously described, are what constitute handicapism—and the process by which handicap is layered upon the physiological limitations of the disability itself.

CHANGING ATTITUDES

Given the pervasive nature of handicapism in American society, it becomes evident that no single strategy will suffice for the overwhelming task of changing such negative reactions and stereotypes. The ubiquity of ideas that lead to the social isolation and stigmatization of the disabled suggests that a public relations campaign alone will do little to alter the overriding perception of those with physical disability in a society that places great value on beauty and physical wholeness. Bender (1981) recommends education plus structured contact between the disabled and nondisabled in order to begin combating negative stereotyping. Yuker et al. (1966) have indicated that as many as one half of the studies reporting the impact of education about the disabled on nondisabled persons' attitudes show no significant change whatsoever. Visits to institutions and agencies, and other related superficial forms of contact between the disabled and nondisabled, result in little or sometimes negative attitudinal change.

Positive attitudinal change is more likely to occur with extensive contact, on the basis of equal status, between those with and those without

---

*Owen, R. Personal communications. Sister Kenney Institute, March, 1982.

disability. According to Bender, such contact on an equal footing plus educational information is the most powerful way of bringing about desired attitudinal changes. Finkelstein's (1980) recommendations are more sweeping. He sees the key to elimination of stereotypes and destructive expectations as substantial material changes in the environment (i.e., architectural design) and fundamental questioning and transformation of social roles and role relationships between the disabled and the nondisabled, as well as extensive educational campaigns. Others however, have criticized such calls for widespread societal transformation as both radical (Siller, 1980) and unrealistic (Kerr, 1980).

Since much of the literature has drawn analogies between the minority status of the disabled and the political situation of blacks, women, and other groups in America, it is probably most useful to learn from the experiences of these other populations. The creation of attitudinal and social change in America is a slow and incremental process that must be supported by legislation in the domains of employment, training, public assistance, and education. The development of positive interactions in community and school settings is seen as critical for the development of positive or at least neutral attitudes toward the disabled by nondisabled children (Voeltz, 1980). Such a recommendation suggests the importance of the development of a new generation of citizens unencumbered by the pervasive negativism of handicapism. The media would play a primary role in this process of societal transformation, through the elimination of stereotypical portrayal of the disabled, through the normalization of roles, personality types, and characteristics of those with physical disability, and through an end to the current tendency to romanticize the personal strengths of the disabled. There is need to expand research to include macrosociological and structural determinants of the devalued status of the disabled in American society (Bynder & New, 1976). A continued focus on microsociological concepts (i.e., problems of interaction between the disabled and nondisabled) would continue to divert attention away from institutional and political changes that could give rise to a more humanistic incorporation of those with physical disability into the mainstream of everyday American life.

The practitioner then has the unique opportunity to be involved on both the societal and individual levels of effecting change. On the individual level, it is imperative that the clinician acknowledge and address the interpersonal and self-esteem issues that derive from social stigmatization and isolation. An adolescent who has lived with disability for any length of time will be an expert in recognizing the looks, stares, rejections, and the thousands of overt and covert insults that occur as a result of negative societal attitudes. What may not be as immediately evident to that young person, however, are ways in which he or she can deal with and address such manifestations of handicapism. One major clinical task is to help disabled youths reject the labels imposed by society. Young persons can be helped to understand that there are ways of talking that encourage the confusion of objective reality with evaluations of that reality. By expanding the repertoire of responses that an adolescent may make in an interaction, adolescents can quickly learn how their own emotional and verbal responses help establish others' responses to them. Role playing and the learning of social skills are especially effective tools. Perspective-taking skills training can help the adolescent develop the insight that there are choices of response to any situation. Rather than feeling locked-in to a limited set of negative responses to an unpleasant situation, the adolescent can begin to redefine his or her situation.

Humor can be an extremely potent weapon in the normalization of strained interactions. For adolescents who are cognitively still locked-in by limited conceptual capabilities, it is possible to rehearse a set pattern or repertoire of responses to certain types of situations. The role modeling and rehearsing of specific responses by the adolescent can enhance his or her ability to satisfactorily resolve uncomfortable situations. Furthermore, identification of a disabled role model—or a Big Brother or Big Sister model—would provide the adolescent new alternatives.

On a macrosociological level, the practitioner should play a major role in facilitating linkages between the disabled client and community resources, such as employment opportunities, political mobilization, and lobbying efforts. While it may be argued that the linkage of the individual with such community resources may fall outside of the practitioners' role, to effectively improve the functioning of those with disabilities such public involvement is fundamental. On both the macrosociological and microsociological levels, it is believed that the practitioner can be instrumental in the promotion of positive outcomes for the disabled individual in terms of specific physiological and psychological issues, while contributing to the mobilization of the physically disabled along with their nondisabled counterparts who seek to effect humanistic and progressive change in American society.

REFERENCES

Altman, B.M. Studies of attitudes towards the handicapped: The need for a new direction. *Social Problems,* 1981, *28* (3), 321–337.

Anderson, E.M., Klarke, L., & Spain, B. *Disability in adolescence.* London & New York: Methuen, Inc., 1982.

Anspach, R.R. From stigma to identity politics: Political activism among the physically disabled and former mental patients. *Social Science and Medicine,* 1979, *13* (8), 765–773.

Barker R., Wright, B., Meyerson, L., & Gonick, M. *Adjustment to physical handicap and illness: A survey of the social psychology of physique and disability* (Rev. ed.). New York Social Science Research Council: No. 55, 1946.

Baskin, B.H. The handicapped child in children's literature themes. In D. Bergsma & A.E. Palver (Eds.), *Developmental disabilities: Psychologic and social implications.* New York: Alan R. Liss, Inc., 1974.

Begab, M.J. Impact of education in social work students' knowledge and attitudes about mental retardation. *American Journal of Mental Deficiencies,* 1970, *74,* 801–808.

Belinkoff, C. Community attitudes toward mentally retarded. *American Journal of Mental Deficiencies,* 1960, *65,* 221–226.

Bender, L.F. 1980 Presidential address to the American Academy for Cerebral Palsy and Developmental Medicine. *Developmental Medicine and Childhood Neurology,* 1981, *23,* 103–108.

Berger, P.L., Luckmann, T. *The social construction of reality: A treatise in the sociology of knowledge.* Garden City, New York: Doubleday, 1966.

Birenbaum, A. The social construction of disability. *Journal of Sociology and Social Welfare,* 1979, *6* (1), 89–101.

Bogdan, R., & Biklen, D. Handicapism. *Social Policy,* 1977, *7* (5), 14–19.

Braginsky, D., & Braginsky, B. *Hansels and Gretels.* New York: Holt, Rinehart and Winston, 1971.

Bynder, H., & Kong-Ming New, P. Time for a change: From micro to macro sociological concepts in disability research. *Journal of Health and Social Behavior,* 1976, *17* (March), 45–52.

Centers, L., & Centers, R. Peer group attitudes toward the amputee child. *Journal of Personality and Social Psychology,* 1963, *61,* 127–132.

Charles, M. Stark reality. *Nursing Mirror,* October 14, 1981.

Cohn, J. Employer attitudes toward hiring mentally retarded individuals. *American Journal of Mental Deficiencies,* 1963, *67,* 705–712.

Combs, R.H., & Harper, J.L. Effects of labels on attitudes of educators toward handicapped children. *Exceptional Children,* 1967, *33,* 399–403.

Comer, R.J., & Piliavin, J.A. The effects of deviance upon face-to-face interaction: The other side. *Journal of Personality and Social Psychology,* 1972, *55,* 33–39.

Conley, R.W. *The economics of mental retardation.* Baltimore/London: Johns Hopkins University Press, 1973.

Davis, F. Deviance disavowal: The management of strained interaction by the visably handicapped. *Social Problems,* 1961, *9,* 120–132.

Dickman, I.R. No place like home: *Alternative living arrangement for teenagers and adults with cerebral palsy.* New York: United Cerebral Palsy Associations, Inc., 1975.

Dixon, J.K. Coping with prejudice: attitudes of handicapped persons toward the handicapped. *Journal of Chronic Disorders,* 1977, *30,* 307–322.

Dufree, R. Personality characteristics and attitudes toward the disabled of students in the health professions. *Rehabilitation Counseling Bulletin,* 1971, *15* (1), 37–44.

Finkelstein, V. *Attitudes and disabled people: Issues for discussion.* New York: World Rehabilitation Fund, Inc., 1980.

Gellman, W. Roots of prejudice against the handicapped. *Journal of Rehabilitation,* 1959, *25* (1), 4–6.

Gliedman, J., & Roth, W. *The unexpected minority: Handicapped children in America.* New York: Harcourt Brace Jovanovich, 1980.

Goffman, E. *Stigma: Notes on the management of spoiled identity.* Englewood Cliffs, N.J.: Prentice-Hall, 1963.

Goldberg, R.T. Rehabilitation research on disability. *Journal of Rehabilitation,* 1977, *42,* 14–18.

Good, T., & Brophy, J. *Looking in classrooms*. New York: Holt, Rinehart & Winston, 1978.

Greenbaum, J.J., & Wang, D.D. A semantic-differential study of the concepts of mental retardation. *Journal of Genetic Psychology*, 1965, *73*, 257–272.

Greene, M.A., & Retish, P.M. *A comparative study of attitudes among students in special education and regular education*. Training School Bulletin, 1973.

Harasymiw, S.J., Horne, M.D., & Lewis, S.C. Disability social distance hierarchy for population subgroups, *Scandinavian Journal of Rehabilitative Medicine*, 1976, *8*, 33–36.

Hastorf, A.H., Wildfogel, J., & Cassman, T. Acknowledgement of handicap as a tactic in social interaction. *Journal of Personality and Social Psychology*, 1979, *37* (10), 1790–1797.

Hollinger, C.S., & Jones, R.L. Community attitudes toward slow learners and mental retardates: What's in a name? *Mental Retardation*, 1970, *8*, 19–23.

Jordan, J., & Friesen, E. Attitudes of rehabilitation personnel toward physically disabled persons in Columbia, Peru, and the United States. *Journal of Social Psychology*, 1968, *74*, 151–161.

Kakalik, J.S., Brewer, G.D., Dougharty, L.A., Fleischauer, P.D., & Genensky, S.M. *Services for handicapped youth: A program overview*. Santa Monica: Rand Corporation, 1973, (Appendix A).

Kerr, N. *Commentary on Finkelstein's attitudes and disabled people: Issues for discussion*. New York: World Rehabilitation Fund, Inc. 1980.

Kleck, R. Physical stigma and nonverbal cues emitted in face-to-face interaction. *Human Relations*, 1968, *21*, 19–28.

Kleck, R.E., Ono, H., & Hastorf, A.H. The effects of physical deviance upon face-to-face interaction. *Human Relations*, 1966, *19*, 425–436.

Lapp, E.R. A study of the social adjustment of slow-learning children who were assigned part-time to regular classes. *American Journal of Mental Deficiencies*, 1957, *62*, 245–262.

Litman, T. An analysis of the sociologic factors affecting the rehabilitation of physically handicapped patients. *Archives of Physical Medicine and Rehabilitation*, 1964, *45*, 12.

Livneh, H. Disability and monstrosity: Further comments. *Rehabilitation Literature*, 1980 (November/December), *41* (11–12), 280–283.

Martinek, T. J., & Karper, W.B. Teachers' expectations for handicapped and non-handicapped children in mainstreamed physical education classes. *Perceptual Motor Skills*, 1981, *53*, 327–330.

McDaniel, J.W. *Physical disability and human behaviour*. New York: Pergamon, 1976.

Mead, G.H. In C.W. Morris (Ed.), *Mind, self and society: From the standpoint of a social behaviorist*. Chicago: University of Chicago Press, 1934.

Miller, A.E., & Miller, M.G. *Options for health and health care: The coming of post clinical medicine*. New York: Wiley-Interscience, 1981.

Needleman, B., & Weiner, N. *Faces of evil: The good, the bad and the ugly*. New York: Department of Sociology, Oswego State College. Presented at the Conference on Sociology and the Arts, Oswego, New York, 1974, (mimeographed).

Pless, I.B., & Roghmann, K.J. Chronic illness and its consequences: Observations based on three epidemiologic surverys, *Journal of Pediatrics*, 1971, *79*, 351–359.

Phelps, W.R. Attitudes related to the employment of mentally retarded. *American Journal of Mental Deficiencies*, 1965, *69*, 575–585.

Reichel, E.A. Changing attitudes toward the disabled. *Journal of Applied Rehabilitation Counseling*, 1975, *6*, 188–192.

Richardson, S.A., Goodman, N., Hastorf, A., Dornbush, S. Cultural uniformity in reaction to physical disabilities, *American Sociological Review*, 1961, *26* (2), 241–247.

Ryan, K.M. Developmental differences in reactions to the physically disabled. *Human Development*, 1981, *24*, 240–256.

Safilios-Rothschild, C. Prejudice against the disabled and some means to combat it. In J. Stubbins (Ed.), *Social and psychological aspects of disability*. Baltimore, Maryland: University of Park Press, 1977.

Safilios-Rothschild, C. *The sociology and social psychology of disability and rehabilitation*. New York: Random House, 1970.

Scheff, T.J. *Being mentally ill: A sociological theory*. Chicago: Aldine Publishing Co., 1966.

Scott, R. *The making of blind men*. New York: Russell Sage Foundation, 1969.

Shattuck, N. Segregation versus nonsegregation of exceptional children. *Exceptional Children*, 1976, *12*, 235–240.

Semmel, M.I., & Dickson, S. Connotative reactions of college students to disability labels. *Exceptional Children*, 1966, *32*, 443–450.

Siller, J. *Commentary on Finkelstein's attitudes and disabled people: Issues for discussion*. New York: World Rehabilitation Fund, Inc., 1980.

Singleton, G., Cole, J., & Long, M. *The attitudes of rehabilitation professionals, their colleagues and other disciplines*. Paper presented at 56th Annual Session of American Congress of Rehabilitation Medicine: Honolulu, Hawaii, 1979.

Szasz, T.S. *The myth of mental illness*. New York: Hoeber-Harper, 1961.

Taylor, J. Portrayal of persons with disabilities by the media. *Mental Retardation Bulletin*, 1981, *9* (1), 38–53.

Thoreson, R.W., & Kerr, B.A. The stigmatizing aspects of severe disability: Strategies for change. *Journal of Applied Rehabilitation Counseling*, 1978, *2*, 21–26.

Thurer, S. Disability and monstrosity: A look at literary distortions of handicapping conditions. *Rehabilitation Literature*, 1980, *41*, 12–15.

U.S. Department of Health and Human Services. *Work disability in the United States: A chartbook*. (SSA Publication No. 13-11978). Social Security Administration: December 1980.

Voeltz, L.M. Childrens' attitudes toward handicapped peers. *American Journal of Mental Deficiencies*, 1980, *84* (5), 455–464.

Weinberg, N. Social stereotyping of the physically handicapped. *Rehabilitation Psychology*, 1976, *23* (4), 115–124.

Weinberg, N., & Santana, R. Comic books: Champions of the disabled stereotype. *Rehabilitation Literature*, 1978, *39*, 327–331.

Wicas, E., & Carluccio, L.W. Attitudes of counselors toward three handicapped client groups. *Rehabilitation Counseling Bulletin*, 1971, *15* (1), 25–33.

Winthrop, H., & Taylor, H. An inquiry concerning the prevalence of popular misconceptions relating to mental deficiency. *American Journal of Mental Deficiencies*, 1957, *62*, 344–348.

Wolraich, M.L. Communication between physicians and parents of handicapped children. *Exceptional Children*, 1982, *48* (4), 324–329.

Wright, B.W. *Physical disability—A psychological approach*. New York: Harper & Row, 1960.

Yeadon, A., & Grayson, D. *Living with impaired vision: An introduction*. New York: American Foundation for the Blind, 1979.

Yuker, H., Block, J.R., & Young, J. *The measurement of attitudes toward disabled persons*. Albertson, New York: Human Resources Center, 1966.

Thomas E. Strax
Saul D. Wolfson

4

Life Cycle Crises of the Disabled Adolescent and Young Adult: Implications for Public Policy

THE TASKS OF ADOLESCENT DEVELOPMENT

The psychosexual and psychosocial development of an individual proceeds in a succession of stages, each of which incorporates the preceding stage as a foundation for new physical and psychological forces. These forces create conflicts that need to be resolved by the close of that stage if healthy development is to progress. The process can be arrested at any maturational phase due to a variety of causes. Physical disability certainly has a high potential for inducing arrest in development. This chapter will focus mainly on how disability affects the adolescent phase of development. The discussion will be limited to physically disabled children of normal intelligence with intact families.

Adolescence is a period characterized by biological, social, and emotional changes. Adolescents have four major developmental tasks:

1. Consolidation of their identity
2. Achievement of independence from their parents
3. Establishment of new love objects outside of the family
4. Finding a vocation

The actual time period of adolescence varies from culture to culture. Among the poor, it can be an extremely short period of time, with the adolescent becoming independent between ages 15 and 18. In the middle class, adolescence might extend through college or even graduate school, with the individual still being controlled and supported by the family mantle (Oettinger, 1968).

Achieving the four major developmental tasks during a period of biological stress is extremely difficult for the normal individual; these tasks are even more arduous for those with a physical disability.

The disabled individual almost always has a prolonged adolescence for several reasons:

1. The disabled adolescent has been overprotected and sheltered.
2. Most psychological growth occurs within the nuclear and extended family because experiences with peers are limited.
3. The identity crisis is even more profound than in able-bodied peers because of a dearth of appropriate role models (Martin, 1975; Friedman, 1974; Richmond, 1973; Waldhorn, 1972).

Maturation and the achievement of adolescent goals do not occur smoothly, but progress in a jerky, chaotic fashion.

The establishment of one's identity is a process that undergoes constant revision. Frequently, the lability and changes that occur at mercurial rates during adolescence appear mind boggling to adult observers, especially parents. The adolescent's struggle to achieve an individual identity and gain distance from parents generates anxiety and tension. This anxiety is manifested in behaviors that offer an outlet from the tension. Some typical adolescent behaviors, such as new hair styles, musical taste, and dress code, are easily recognized. In order to master anxiety, the adolescent assumes various identities and then discards them when they are no longer functional. If there is too much anxiety or too weak a psychic structure, the psyche's controls can be overrun and antisocial behavioral manifestations such as delinquency, truancy, sexual promiscuity, and drug abuse may result.

Disabled adolescents are at a disadvantage in attempting to deal with the developmental demands of adolescence. Their limited mobility interferes with peer relationships. Furthermore, the excessive caring they may have received often contributes to producing passive individuals who are reluctant to be on their own. In contrast, some disabled adolescents may be rebellious and may perform antisocial acts as a way of overcompensating for their psychological passivity and as a means of gaining peer and social recognition.

For the disabled adolescent, the teenage years are a particularly troublesome time. While he or she may have had concerns about identity prior to this stage, they were not as central as they are now. The disabled adolescent may feel the limitations and restrictions of the physical disability more acutely in comparison with physically normal peers who are engaged in many activities. There is substantial risk for self-destructive behavior stemming from depression or compensatory acting out.

In order to deal with the painful realities of rejection, scorn, and embarrassment, the disabled adolescent will resort to devices such as fantasy and denial. Depending upon their intensity and frequency, these defense mechanisms need not be pathological (Dorner, 1973; Freeman, 1970).

Identity and Society

In order to find one's identity, one must first have an intact image of one's own body, be able to fantasize different identities, and see how various roles fit. The first identity figures are parents. As adolescents enlarge their horizons, the choice of identities goes beyond the family to musicians, presidents, lawyers, doctors, and other visible people. The availability of heroes and role models depends upon culture, economic status, and exposure. Disabled children in wheelchairs do not often get a chance to attend baseball games or wander around downtown. They are also limited as to the number of individuals they can fantasize being and still relate to reality—somebody in a wheelchair cannot be a baseball player.

How we see ourselves in relationship to the perceived ideal of our society is extremely important. Tringo (1970) investigated the attitudes of nondisabled high school students, college undergraduate and graduate students, and rehabilitation workers toward 21 specific disabilities. He found that subjects with higher educational levels showed less rejection of disabled persons. There were nine possible ratings from which to choose ranging from "would marry" to "would put to death." Increased educational level seems to decrease reported social-distance scores. Furthermore, familiarity and experience with specific disabilities may have been responsible for the ratings assigned them. Cancer, stroke, and heart disease are common in all families, and were accorded high affiliation ratings. Alcoholism (despite its prevalence) and criminal behavior tended to have low positions in the study.

Yuker, Block, and Young (1970) found that close personal contact with a disabled person resulted in greater acceptance of that person's specific disability. On the other hand, persons having disabled family members and professionals working with the disabled showed little change in their attitudes with increased contact. It was felt that a rehabilitation setting provided information that stressed the limitations of the disabled and disallowed for personal contact with patients.

Friedman (1974) studied the effects of modeling on choosing acceptable playmates among nondisabled, disabled children in wheelchairs, and facially disfigured children. His models represented the highest, the middle, and the low preferential groups. He studied children from the 7th to the

11th grade. Nondisabled children, those who were wheelchair bound, and the facially disfigured all modeled identically—they chose as friends nondisabled first, wheelchair bound next, and facially disfigured last of the three groups.

Self-acceptance must be achieved by the disabled individual before acceptance by others can occur. These studies demonstrate two aspects of rejection; the first is the reluctance of the physically normal child to accept a physically disabled counterpart into the peer group. As a result, the disabled adolescent is deprived of a valuable tool for working out adolescent problems. The ostracizing of the disabled by the normal adolescent appears to be based, in part, on lack of experience with the disabled and fear that disabilities are contagious. The second aspect of rejection evidenced by the studies is the rejection of self. By the time physically disabled children become adolescents, they are aware of society's ideal physical image. Like their normal peers, they will reject another physically disabled adolescent, and they will also reject themselves. An individual's self-image is usually based on society's norms. (Seidel, 1975; Brutten, Richardson, & Mangel, 1973; Schooler, 1973).

People look better and more perfect in their dreams. An example of this is the dissatisfaction most people experience when first hearing their voice taped or seeing their face on film. On the other hand, it is difficult to deny one's physical disability when one walks toward a reflecting image or enters a crowd of people with similar disability. It is our personal and professional experience that paraplegics and other disabled individuals with marked gait problems see themselves in their dreams as walking normally.

The most anxiety-producing summer that I* ever had was that between my second and third years in medical school. I had been offered—and had accepted—a summer fellowship to work with disabled children. Most of the children had cerebral palsy, and I was forced to face issues about myself that I had previously rejected or denied.

The Parent–Child Relationship

Independence from parents has two elements; one is emotional and the other is financial. The disabled child is usually pitied and coddled more than the able-bodied child and, therefore, is much more dependent upon the parents. There is a greater fear of loss of parental love and of the eventual loss of the parent than is true of able bodied children. Parents

---

*Dr. Strax has athetoid cerebral palsy, and the experiences described are his (Editor's note).

who encourage progressive independence in normal adolescents often overprotect and baby their physically disabled teenager (Waldhorn, 1972; Caplan & Lebovivi, 1969).

The child who has been overprotected grows into an individual who feels in need of special protection. He or she may not have to live up to the same rules and regulations that control the lives of other family members (Grinberg, & Grinberg, 1974; Freeman, 1970). The combination of real and fantasy needs of the physically disabled may encourage an infantile and immature personality.

When they finally enter the outside world, schools segregate such youths into special classes. Peer groups will not admit them; without friends they find life extremely lonely. In an attempt to find friends and attract attention, the disabled are more prone to turn toward inappropriate behavior such as loud talking and foolish behavior. The normal adolescent who uses this type of behavior usually gets instant negative feedback from family, teachers, and peer group members. Frequently, this is not the case with the physically disabled.

Children who are considered disabled by their parents and have not been admitted to peer groups have substantial difficulty in school. They usually need some special attention because of coordination, writing, and speaking problems. They feel that they are inferior and may fail to meet their parents' expectations. This, coupled with their inability to be accepted within a peer group, leads to social withdrawal. Many of the parents we see are afraid to allow their disabled child to be integrated into society. They feel that their child can only be hurt. The parents of a normal child expect him or her to eventually leave home. This is not so with the parent of the physically disabled child. This child is expected to remain a child and is forever protected.

I was extremely lucky. My parents felt that the most important thing they could give me was the ability to exist in society on my own two feet. To do this, I had to be integrated into society. When the Cub Scouts would not take me, my mother started her own pack for the children in the neighborhood. When the schools would not accept me, my parents went to court. When the bus driver would not let me ride, they forced him to take me (through the president of an affiliated union).

Parents should, if possible, encourage their disabled child to grow and be treated as any other child. It is important, for emotional maturation, to be accepted into a neighborhood peer group.

The School Setting

The next problem is what to do with the severely physically disabled individual who cannot move around in a school situation and, therefore, needs a special class or a special school. This child must also be given an opportunity to be integrated into society if he or she is to live a life within that society.

Segregation versus integration of the disabled is a difficult problem. Neither special schools nor an isolated environment is being advocated. There have been studies to show that the disabled child can learn better in a homogeneous peer group, instead of having to meet the demands of a 40-pupil class that is moving at a rate he or she cannot handle. The problem with this type of isolation is that at some point the individual must be integrated into society. This is difficult if integration has not been an ongoing process.

Normal children are able to increase contact with the world between ages one and two when they start to walk and talk. Lessons learned during these early experiences are needed for later maturation. By age five or six, the normal child is ready for school and knows how to make friends and play with other children. The physically disabled child may not be walking until age five or six and is therefore denied outside stimuli and influence of a peer group. By the time of adolescence, such a child is far behind the emotional maturation of his or her physically normal peers and lacks the experience of handling social and sexual peer relationships. It is agonizing for a physically disabled or uncoordinated youngster who has trouble dancing, conversing, or participating in sport activities to join in with other teenagers.

At the onset of puberty, a child's life is centered in the family, but shortly thereafter it shifts to close friends. Intense friendships are made first with members of the same sex and later in adolescence with members of the opposite sex. Assimilation into a peer group provides the adolescent with a vehicle for separation from the home. The earlier the entry into a peer group, the quicker the emotional milestones needed for independence will be met (Oettinger, 1968; Caplan, & Labovivi, 1969; Brutten et al., 1973; Blaine, 1973).

Isolation and Depression

Williams[16] discussed the alienation syndrome in adolescence. He pointed out that the American society reinforces narcissistic, competitive individualism with emphasis on performance, achievement, and productivity at the expense of relationships between young people. Yet, unless there are successful relationships both in the family and with peers, successful relationships cannot be established later in adolescent and adult life.

A fast-moving, high-achievement, need-oriented society does not have a place for a slow individual. It is not fashionable to have disabled friends or to slow down for someone who needs some help. Dorner (1975) found that the nonhandicapped friends of preadolescent spina bifida youngsters were lost during adolescence. About half of the adolescents with spina bifida in his sample were judged to be severely socially isolated. In his group, the more mobile the spina bifida adolescent was, the less social isolation he or she experienced. Depression was extremely common in his study. Thirty-one percent of the girls and 15 percent of the boys had persistent periods of depression and suicidal ideas. Anxiety about the future was extremely common, primarily over employment, independence from the family, and the possibility of marriage.

Late Adolescence

The functions of late adolescence and adulthood are to establish new love objects outside of the nuclear family and to establish a vocational goal. These functions cannot really be undertaken until the adolescent has been able to

1. Consolidate an identity
2. Achievement of independence from the family
3. Gain acceptance into a peer group (Waldhorn, 1972; Brutten et al., 1973; Centers & Centers, 1963; Tringo, 1970).

Disabled individuals enter adulthood socially deprived and immature. They do not know how to approach or relate to others of the same sex, let alone someone of the opposite sex. The social aspects of school and peer-group activities have usually been absent.

To the above problems add the additional concerns of an individual who is

1. An outcast, not acceptable to society
2. Frequently egocentric and filled with self pity
3. Most likely to have rejected him or herself

The physically disabled are less mobile and, therefore, have less chance of meeting and courting appropriate mates in the usual fashion available to the able-bodied members of their peer group. If the disabled person has developed the emotional maturity, self esteem, and confidence needed to find a mate, he or she must now deal with the problem of not being acceptable to people of the opposite sex. Often the disabled person is uncertain of whether his or her defective body will function.

Employment

Besides the social stigmata of having a physical disability, there are practical problems. A study done in 1977 by the Social Security Administration found almost 18 million disabled adults between the ages of 18 and 64. Forty percent of them needed some help in their activities of daily living, which was usually provided by an immediate member of the household. In half of the cases, the help was provided by a spouse or child. Only ten percent had paid help, and this was only for one day or less weekly. Of those who needed help, 27 percent received none. It is very difficult for someone to be a lover, a provider, and a patient at the same time (Hershkowitz, 1977).

For the disabled, finding a vocation—and through it, economic independence—is extremely difficult, if not impossible. Many potential employees with disabilities are turned down simply because they are physically disabled. In mid-1974, Sylvania refused to hire 53-year-old Lawrence Katz for a technical writing job because the company doctors noted that his treatment for Hodgkin's disease one year earlier made him a poor insurance risk. Mr. Katz filed a complaint with the United States Department of Labor, charging discrimination. Six months later, with the help of the Department of Labor, Mr. Katz was hired.

According to the 1970 census, 1.5 out of 7.0 handicapped individuals of employment age were unemployed. At that time, there were 121 million adults living in the United States who were between the ages of 16 and 64. This number excluded those in institutions or in military service. Women constituted 51 percent of this group. 11.2 million people were found to have disabilities lasting longer than six months; one in every 11 Americans was disabled. Arkansas led the list with one in seven, and Hawaii had the fewest, with one in seventeen. Six percent more handicapped than nonhandicapped persons had earnings below $2000/year. Seven percent fewer handicapped than nonhandicapped persons had earnings over $7000/year. The $7000/year barrier was difficult for the handicapped to cross. Only 58 percent of handicapped males are employed, compared with 76 percent of all males (Hershkowitz, 1977).

The Rehabilitation Act of 1973 (Sections 501 and 504) requires affirmative action for the employment and advancement of qualified handicapped people in a contract in excess of $2500 entered into by any federal department or agency for the procurement of property and services. This provision also applies to subcontractors. Every government contractor or subcontractor holding a contract of $50,000 or having 50 or more employees, must prepare and maintain an affirmative action program, which is to be set forth in an affirmative action plan.

Employers give many reasons for not considering handicapped people. These are usually based upon myths such as "Our insurance rates will skyrocket," or "We would have to treat them differently, give them special privileges," or "Our present employees would not accept them." One of the best ways to evaluate all of these statements is to review a study done by the DuPont Corporation (Wolfe, 1974) which has had extensive programs for hiring handicapped employees. They found no increase in workmen's compensation costs as a result of hiring the handicapped. Another study, by the United States Chamber of Commerce and the National Association of Manufacturers, found that 90 percent of 279 companies experienced no increase in their insurance costs as a result of hiring handicapped individuals. Adjustments in the work place have been minimal in most companies that hire the handicapped. These usually consist of simple changes, such as lowered work space, special desks, entrance ramps, or minimal doorway modifications. DuPont found that the disabled worker was a safe worker; 96 percent of the 1,400 handicapped employees had better safety records than their able-bodied counterparts. They also did not find that their disabled employees wanted to be treated differently from their able-bodied employees.

Fellow employees did not consider special parking spots for paraplegics to indicate executive privilege. The DuPont study, covering a 30-year period, showed that the disabled employee was competitive with the unimpaired worker in productivity, attendance, job stability, safety, and cost of employment. Seventy-nine percent of the employees had better attendance records, and 93 percent had average or better turnover rates (Wolfe, 1974).

PUBLIC POLICY CONSIDERATIONS

Before long range planning can be discussed or considered, there must be complete and accurate data on who the handicapped are and their needs. This is not currently available; too frequently, it has become necessary to look at data that has been gathered for other purposes and extrapolate from these data the limitations of function and personal experiences of handicapped people. The Office of Handicapped Individuals (OHI) must begin to fill the data gap on handicapped persons. This can be done in conjunction with the National Center on Health Statistics.

Federal, state, and local governments must have a long-range plan for dealing with the problems of the disabled. The task is too great for local governments alone. Money must be set aside for the following:

1. Programs for the training and establishment of regional mini-team centers should be created. These teams should consist of health, social, and professional personnel who will go into communities and evaluate disabled individuals. This will establish what their medical and social needs are and what programs might benefit them.
2. Attitude reassessment programs should be designed, developed, and packaged to tackle attitudinal problems in a particular group. For

example, there should be a program to help parents understand their attitudes toward their disabled children, a program for teachers to help facilitate integration of disabled youngsters into the regular school system, a program to help employers and employment agencies reevaluate their attitudes toward disabled employees, and a program for the disabled themselves, so that they can reevaluate themselves. These programs should be factual and informative and should provide a basis for people taking these courses to examine their own attitudes and beliefs.

3. Resource teams should be trained to help employers facilitate affirmative action programs and evaluate the skills of disabled employees.

4. There should be regional evaluation centers, probably in rehabilitation facilities or departments of vocational rehabilitation, to evaluate job qualifications of handicapped workers.

5. A civil rights bill is also needed for the physically limited. This should include the right to use public transportation, and it should require that public transportation contain facilities for physically disabled individuals.

6. A welfare system that encourages a person to seek and obtain as much self-sufficiency and independence as possible is vital. This system should provide for a transition period that will be flexible enough to allow an individual to work part-time if he or she is not capable of working full-time.

7. Barrier-free public housing is a necessity.

8. Halfway houses are needed for those disabled who are not completely independent in activities in daily living but could be with the aid of a paid, able-bodied helper. This would keep these people out of institutions, thereby reducing costs.

9. A national advocate for the disabled is needed.

10. The services provided by the Committee on Prosthetics Development must be expanded to evaluate and develop many self-help aids to enable the more severely disabled to become independent in activities of daily living, and to develop new industrial equipment to allow neurologically impaired individuals to operate precise equipment.

CONCLUSION

If disabled individuals are treated specially they will continue to remain dependent and retain the image of second-class citizens.

For the disabled, the time from adolescence through young adulthood is a period of self-examination and rejection. Hopefully, it will be followed by a healthier, more realistic acceptance of themselves, their handicaps, their limitations, and their strengths. This usually happens when there is a supportive family unit and later, understanding peers and adequate medical, social, and vocational services.

REFERENCES

Blaine, G.B., Jr. Meeting the challenge of today's adolescent. *Delaware Medical Journal,* 1973, *45,* 193–195.

Brutten, M., Richardson, S., & Mangel, C. *Something's wrong with my child.* New York: Harcourt Brace Jovanovich, Inc., 1973.

Caplan, C., & Lebovivi, S. *Adolescence: Psychosocial perspective.* New York: Basic Books, Inc., 1969.

Centers, L., & Centers, R. Peer group attitudes toward the amputee child. *Journal of Social Psychology,* 1963, (Suppl. 29), 24–26.

Dorner, S. Psychological and social problems of families of adolescent spina bifida patients: A preliminary report. *Developmental Medicine and Child Neurology.* 1973, (Suppl. 29), 24–26.

Dorner, S. The relationship of physical handicap to stress in families with an adolescent with spina bifida. *Developmental Medicine and Child Neurology,* 1975, *17,* 765–776.

Freeman, R.D. Psychiatric problems in adolescents with cerebral palsy. *Developmental Medicine and Child Neurology,* 1970, *12,* 64.

Friedman, R.S. Modeling behavior of nondisabled and disabled adolescents based upon social preference for and similarity to nondisabled and disabled models (Ph.D. dissertation, Hofstra University, 1974). Hempstead, Long Island, New York.

Grinberg, L., & Grinberg, R. Pathological aspects of identity in adolescence. *Contemporary Psychoanalysis,* 1974, *10,* 27–40.

Hershkowitz, M. *One in eleven handicapped adults: A survey based on 1970 census data,* Washington, D.C.: U.S. Government Printing Office, 1977.

Martin, H.P. Parental response to handicapped children. *Developmental Medicine and Child Neurology,* 1975, *17,* 251–252.

Oettinger, K. *Normal adolescence,* New York: Scribner Library, 1968.

Richmond, J.B. *The family and the handicapped child.* (Clinical Proceedings: Children's Hospital National Medical Center), 1973, *25* (July–August), 156–164.

Schooler, J.C. (Ed.) *Current issues in adolescent psychiatry.* New York: Brunner-Mazel, 1973.

Seidel, U.P., Chadwick, O.F.D., & Rutter, M. Psychological disorders in crippled children. A comparative study of children with and without brain damage. *Developmental Medicine and Child Neurology,* 1975, *17,* 563–573.

Tringo, J. The hierarchy of preference toward disability groups. *Journal of Special Education,* 1970, *4,* 295–306.

Waldhorn, H.K. *Rehabilitation of the physically handicapped adolescent.* New York: John Day, 1972.

Williams, S.S. Alienation of youth as reflected on the hippie movement. *Journal of the American Academy of Child Psychiatry,* 1970, *9,* 251.

Wolfe, J. *Disability is no handicap for Dupont.* President's Committee on Employment of the Handicapped, Washington, DC, 1974.

Yuker, H.E., Block, J.R., & Young, J.H. *The measurement of attitudes toward disabled persons,* New York: Albertson, 1970.

Daniel Offer
Eric Ostrov
Kenneth I. Howard

5

Body Image, Self-Perception, and Chronic Illness in Adolescence

The purpose of this chapter is to explore the self-images of groups of physically ill adolescents and to compare these self-images with those of groups of normal (i.e., nonpatient) teenagers.

Self-image is an important aspect of the psychological functioning of adolescents. It has been found to correlate significantly with other important aspects of their functioning, such as personality development, interpersonal relationships, family relations, coping abilities, mood, and physical health (Offer, Ostrov & Howard, 1981a). Self-image can be measured reliably and validly (Offer, Ostrov & Howard, 1982); it represents a psychological dimension along which psychiatrically disturbed, delinquent, and normal adolescents are clearly separated. Gender differences in self-image also can easily be explored; these differences have been used to elucidate differences between male and female adolescent development in American culture (Offer, et al., 1981a).

Studies of the self-image of adolescents with physical illness are sparse. Notable among them are the studies of Campbell, Hayden, and Davenport (1977) on patients with myelodysplasia, and Landon, Rosenfeld, Northcraft, and Lewiston (1980) on patients with cystic fibrosis. The first large-scale study on the relationships between psychological states and various physical illnesses among adolescents was done by Kellerman, Zelter, Ellenberg, Dash, and Rigler (1980). Comparisons were made between 349 physically healthy adolescents and 168 randomly selected patients receiving treatment for six various chronic and serious illnesses.

Kellerman's study found no support for the notion of psychological deviance concomitant with serious and chronic disease. Specifically, in self-esteem measures, no differences were found between the physically ill and the healthy adolescents. Their finding that anxiety was correlated negatively with time elapsed since diagnosis indicates the existence of increased development of coping skills. Where adolescents with certain types of diseases expressed feeling significantly lower levels of control over their health than did their healthy peers or their cohorts with different diseases, there was a realistic basis for their feelings. Those patients who were able to exert some degree of control over their illness and symptoms, through self-administered medication, manipulation of diet, or other methods of dealing directly with their illness rather than passively receiving medical services exhibited perception of greater levels of control over their health, regardless of actual medical prognosis.

Zeltzer, Kellerman, Ellenberg, Dash, and Rigler (1980), in an extension of the preceding study and using the same population, attempted to clarify adolescents' perceptions of the impact of illness on their life. These authors report that total impact of illness (leukemia or colds) did not differ between ill and healthy respondents, and the nature of adolescent concerns was similar in both groups. Restriction of freedom was reported as the major disruption brought about by illness; other areas of impact included relations with peers, siblings, and parents. Kellerman et al. concluded that it is not accurate or useful to consider the seriously ill adolescent as inevitably exhibiting psychopathology (see Zeltzer et al., Chapter 20 in this edition).

METHOD

The Offer Self-Image Questionnaire (OSIQ)*

The OSIQ was constructed to measure the self-concept of adolescent boys and girls between the ages of 13 and 18. Self-concept is a particularly crucial personality dimension for adolescents and, empirically, has been directly correlated with their mental health and adjustment. In addition, self-concept has been shown to be a relatively stable personality trait from adolescence onward. Because it has been clinically observed that adolescents who can master one aspect of their environment often fail to adjust in other areas, the OSIQ was constructed with 130 items to evaluate adolescents' functioning in 11 content areas and five different aspects of

---

*The OSIQ, its manual, and the scoring system are available from the senior author.

self, important in the psychological world of the teenager. These categories are as follows:

1. Psychological self
   Impulse control
   Mood
   Body image
2. Social self
   Social relations
   Morals
   Vocational and educational goals
3. Sexual self
   Sexual attitudes and behavior
4. Familial self
   Family relations
5. Coping self
   Mastery of the external world
   Psychopathology
   Superior adjustment (coping)

Reliability and validity have been discussed elsewhere (Offer et al., 1981a). The OSIQ has been administered to over 20,000 teenagers in the United States, Australia, Holland, Indonesia, Taiwan, Ireland, and Israel. The populations sampled include males and females, younger and older, normal, psychiatrically disturbed, delinquent, rural, urban, and suburban adolescents.

Standard Scoring

OSIQ scores are presented in the form of standard scores, which show the amount by which individuals differ from a reference group average. The reference groups (total N = 1385) are composed of normal youths tested in 1979 and 1980 in schools across the United States. A standard score of 50 corresponds to a subject's having a raw scale score equal to the mean of the appropriate control group's mean. A standard score higher than 50 reflects better adjustment with scores lower than 50 reflecting poorer adjustment.

Since these standard scores are derived by comparing raw scores to like-age, same-sex control groups, average standard scores do not reflect age or sex-linked differences in OSIQ scores in the general population, though age or sex effects specific to the particular group being studied still could be present.

In the present study, to increase the number in each group, younger adolescents (from 13 to 15 years of age) and older adolescents (from 16 to 19 years of age) in the various groups of physically ill adolescents were combined. Other research (Offer et al., 1981a) has shown that age generally has little effect on self-image scores. Because physical illness might have very different effects upon boys than it does upon girls, and because these effects might exist over and above the differences in self-image by sex usually found in normal groups, girls' and boys' group means were calculated separately. To graphically show the differences between physically ill adolescents' group means and those of normal adolescents, profiles were drawn presenting means on each OSIQ scale in relation to the control group mean of 50. To explicate scale score differences, percent affirmations were compared at the item level. A percent affirmation for a group, with respect to an item, is the percent of subjects in that group responding positively to that item. As a result, percent affirmations can range from zero to 100 percent (see Table 5-1).

Comparisons between physically ill adolescents' group means and those of normal adolescents were made by use of two-tailed t tests. Differences at the .05 level or less were considered significant. A difference in percent affirmation with respect to any given item between a group of physically ill youths and a control group was considered notable only if it exceeded ten percentage points.

Description of Samples Studied

Asthma

These data were collected by M. Ostrov in Connecticut in 1982. Subjects were part of routine, out-patient clinical practice and suffered from mild to severe asthma. Only two subjects needed to be hospitalized at any time for this condition. Approximately half of the patients were mild asthmatics who used medication on an as-needed basis. They needed medication when under physical or emotional stress, but this occurred rarely. The disease did not affect their life appreciably. The other half of the patients in the study group were on cortisone. However, they were also free to engage in all activities, with the exception of strenuous activities such as basketball. The physician would lower the dosage when side effects were noted. There were no self-image differences between the two groups; therefore, results from the two groups were pooled and analyzed together. The subjects came from lower-middle-class backgrounds. Their disability was from none to mild and moderate; there were no severely disabled adolescents in this group. The physician noted that in his opinion, the females were generally more mature (see Results).

Cancer

These data were collected by R. Freeman (1983).* Most of the patients in this group were diagnosed as having leukemia. There were a few who had Hodgkin's disease. These subjects all were outpatients who had had recent episodes, and they were undergoing active chemotherapy or radiotherapy. None had the illness for longer than one year. Their disability was moderate and only occasionally severe. Socioeconomically, they were middle class.

Children of Parents with Multiple Sclerosis

Data were collected by S. Solomon (1981).† In this case, subjects comprised children with one parent who suffered from multiple sclerosis. All of the children were normal. The parents were mildly to moderately impaired and had had the condition for a minimum of five years. None of the parents had been hospitalized within the past year. They all came from middle- to lower-middle-class family backgrounds.

Cystic Fibrosis

Regarding these subjects, data were collected by Landon et al. (1980). This condition is a congenital disease that had affected these children for years (see McCracken, Chapter 21 of this edition). There had been multiple hospitalizations and serious medical problems throughout the years. These were middle-class children with severe disability.

RESULTS

Standard Score Profile

Asthma

Results showed a normal profile for the males and an above normal profile for the females (see Figs. 5-1 and 5-2). The female asthmatic group scored significantly higher than the normal control group on all but two scales: sexual attitudes and family relationships. These asthmatic adolescent girls had superior self-images as compared with the normal adolescent

---

*Freeman, R. The self-image of adolescents with cancer. Unpublished Ph.D. Thesis, Northwestern University, Chicago, 1983.

†Solomon, S. The self-image of adolescents with one parent suffering from multiple sclerosis. Unpublished Master's thesis. Department of Psychology, University of Saskatchewan, Saskatchewan, Canada, 1981.

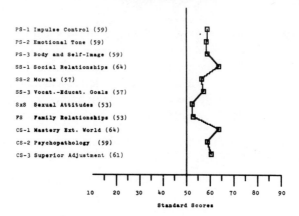

Figure 5-1. Asthma (females). Offer self-image questionnaire. Numbers in parentheses are standard score values for each scale. (Data collected by Dr. M. Ostrov, Middlebury, CT., 1982.)

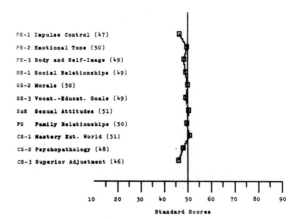

Figure 5-2. Asthma (males). Offer self-image questionnaire. Numbers in parentheses are standard score values for each scale. (Data collected by Dr. M. Ostrov, Middlebury, CT., 1982.)

girls. They saw themselves as excellent copers with no significant emotional or other problems. An interesting question arises as to whether their high self-image was at all related to the asthma or whether it was an independent finding. The superiority of their self-image could be a fact that was independent of their asthma.

Cancer

The profiles of this group of subjects, suffering from acute leukemia and Hodgkin's disease, were also essentially normal (see Figs. 5-3 and 5-4). Again, the girls fared better than the boys. The adolescent girls were superior on two scales: social relationships and psychopathology (high on this scale means a lack of psychopathology). The males similarly showed significantly less psychopathology than the normal controls and were significantly low on only one scale: body image. This interesting finding will be further examined in the item analysis.

Children of Parents With Multiple Sclerosis

This group is of special interest because, although they were not physically ill themselves, they had lived with physical illness for at least five years (see Figs. 5-5 and 5-6). The males had extremely low sexual self-image. In one area, morals, they were significantly higher than the normal. The females, in contrast, had two areas in which they were significantly lower than normals: morals and vocational and educational goals.

Cystic Fibrosis

The self-image of this group of severely ill and impaired adolescents was significantly lower than that of normals in a multitude of different areas (see Figs. 5-7 and 5-8). The males were high in morals and significantly lower than normals in emotional tone, body image, social relationships, sexual attitudes, and psychopathology. The females were significantly lower than normal in 7 of the 11 scales. Even seriously ill psychiatric patients do not present as low a self-image as do adolescents with cystic fibrosis.

Item Level Analysis

It is a fact that a scale score can be misleading. If a subject chooses extreme positive and negative responses, the result can be an artificially "normal" score. The item level analysis can, therefore, throw light on the findings for asthmatic and cancer patients. In addition, how subjects answered a few selected items that were directly relative to their illness is of interest. How extreme item responses led to average scale scores would, of course, be less relevant to the cystic fibrosis sample, who will be left out of this analysis. Since the children of the multiple sclerosis

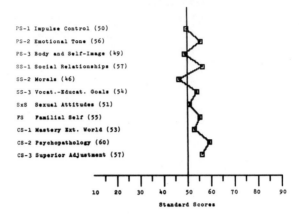

Figure 5-3. Cancer (females). Offer self-image questionnaire. Numbers in parentheses are standard score values for each scale. (Data collected by Dr. Freeman, Chicago, IL., 1981.)

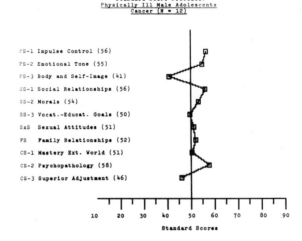

Figure 5-4. Cancer (males). Offer self-image questionnaire. Numbers in parentheses are standard score values for each scale. (Data collected by Dr. Freeman, Chicago, IL., 1981.)

66

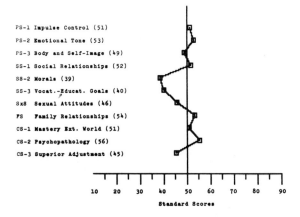

Figure 5-5. Youth with a parent with multiple sclerosis (females). Offer self-image questionnaire. Numbers in parentheses are standard score values for each scale. (Data collected by Dr. Solomon, Saskatchewan, Canada, 1981.)

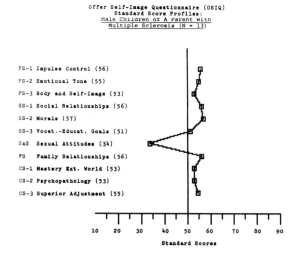

Figure 5-6. Youth with a parent with multiple sclerosis (males). Offer self-image questionnaire. Numbers in parentheses are standard score values for each scale. (Data collected by Dr. Solomon, Saskatchewan, Canada, 1981.)

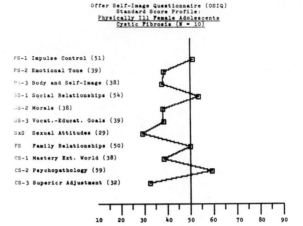

Figure 5-7. Cystic Fibrosis (females). Offer self-image questionnaire. Numbers in parentheses are standard score values for each scale. (Data collected by Dr. Landon, Palo Alto, CA., 1980.)

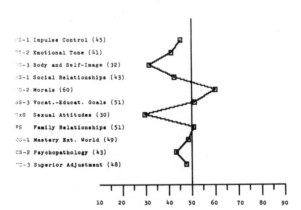

Figure 5-8. Cystic Fibrosis (males). Offer self-image questionnaire. Numbers in parentheses are standard score values for each scale. (Data collected by Dr. Landon, Palo Alto, CA., 1980.)

68

group were used as a special control group in this study, they also will not be investigated in the item analysis.

It was found that in most of the 130 items, the research subjects with asthma and cancer had similar responses to the normal control group. For the percent affirmation, or endorsement, the first three responses of each item were collapsed to mean affirmation, or endorsement. Responses of the last three choices were collapsed to mean no affirmation, or no endorsement.

Two phenomena were sought in this analysis: first, how do physically ill compare to normal adolescents on items where they should objectively (because of their illness) not feel as well; and second, how do physically ill patients compare to normals on items that normals have characteristically stated caused them emotional problems?

Item 27 in Table 5-1 clearly shows that adolescents with asthma and cancer are aware of their physical condition; as a matter of fact, cancer patients are considerably more worried about their health than are asthmatic adolescents. The answers to items 16, 54, 68, and 117 demonstrate the concern physically ill adolescents have about how to handle their sexuality and maturation. Item 54 has been used in the past to ascertain how open adolescents were in the questionnaire study. This question is endorsed by over 50 percent of normal teenagers. Adolescents who deny

Table 5-1
Percent Endorsement of Individual Items

Item	Normal		Asthma		Cancer	
	Male	Female	Male	Female	Male	Female
16. It is hard for a teenager to know how to handle sex in a right way.	23	31	33	21	33	40
27. In the past year I have been very worried about my health.	22	27	48	37	50	60
42. The picture I have of myself in the future satisfies me.	81	80	90	95	100	73
54. I am so very anxious.	54	54	57	47	67	53
68. I enjoy life.	90	89	90	89	100	100
117. Sexual experiences give me pleasure.	85	68	90	53	92	50
128. I am fearful of growing up.	20	20	33	0	33	40

Number of the item refers to its number in the original questionnaire. Items are shown only if asthma or cancer group showed meaningful differences from normals with respect to above items.

their feelings would not endorse this item. Physically ill adolescents were found to be identical to the normals in this respect. In one subgroup (males with cancer), they were actually higher.

Some of the adolescents seemed to exaggerate their positive feelings—their optimism—which seems to be out of proportion to the normal (see items 1 and 4). When that occurs, it is only on a few items; it does not emerge as a specific pattern.

DISCUSSION

The Self-Image in Three Groups of Physically Ill Adolescents

In recent years, the primary aim of medical care has shifted from the treatment of acute (mostly infectious) diseases to the continuous care of chronic ailments. Obviously, some diseases are more serious than others; some are more debilitating, and still others cause severe problems in the patient's social field. The four groups of physically ill adolescents studied by different investigators using the Offer Self-Image Questionnaire (OSIQ) can be compared with the original large normative sample. Findings in this study are similar in principle to those of Kellerman et al. (1980). Those in the asthmatic group look essentially like normal teenagers. Based on these data, the psychosomatic theory, which speculates that patients with asthma are suffering from specific psychological conflicts, is not tenable. (See, for example, French & Alexander, 1941.) If these patients have psychiatric difficulties, they exist in addition to the asthma. In other words, asthma is not caused by underlying psychological conflicts, nor are there significant secondary psychological problems caused by the physical illness.

Similarly, the cancer group has a normal self-image. Only the males had a low body image. As can be seen throughout this study, males are more sensitive to impairment of their bodies. The acuteness and severity of the illness does not seem to have affected males with cancer seriously. This is not to say that these adolescents have no problems with their body image, their affect, or their peers. Neither is it saying that adolescents have no anxiety associated with their illness. What is clear is that more often than not the adolescents studied have coped successfully with their fears and worries. There is no doubt that one often finds adolescents who cannot cope with having cancer. The point of this study simply is that one way to find out how adolescents with severe illnesses feel is to ask them to assess their own self-image. Since it has been found earlier that 20 percent of normal adolescents state that they do not feel positive about themselves (Offer et al., 1981a), it would follow that in this same 20 percent minority preexisting psychological problems may reemerge and be exacerbated by the cancer and its treatment.

To answer an obvious question, the authors do not believe that such adolescents are simply denying their overwhelming anxiety, fear, and loss of a sense of self. As has been shown in the sample item analysis (see Table 5-1), cancer patients do not differ from controls in significant emotional items. They also do not have the restricted response spread one might expect among persons using denial. In other words, the data make statistical, as well as psychological, sense.

The group of adolescents who grew up in a home in which one of the parents had multiple sclerosis for a period of at least five years showed definite problems in their sexual self-image. In addition, the girls had low vocational and educational goals and some problems with coping. It is interesting that a chronic crisis, such as a sick parent, appears to have relatively more impact on adolescent self-image than mild chronic illness or acute, very serious illness. Lingering pressure, particularly when it is physically visible, is most stressful on the self-image system.

Cystic fibrosis is a lethal genetic disease in which chronic respiratory and digestive problems delay growth and sexual development. Adolescents who suffer from cystic fibrosis have major difficulties with their self-image. Indeed, for both males and females, the only part of the self-image system that remains intact is the familial self. All other aspects of the self are disturbed: the psychological, the social, the sexual, and the coping aspects. The findings are similar to those of Boyle, di Sant'Angnese, Sack, Millican, and Kulczycki (1976) who showed that patients with cystic fibrosis have a higher frequency of emotional disturbances than does the general population (See Chapter 22 in this edition).

Medical Care and the Adolescent: A Comment

These data clearly demonstrate that in two important physical illnesses—chronic mild to moderate asthma and acute severe cancer—adolescents have a normal self-image. Adolescents with cystic fibrosis have a decidedly disturbed self-image. The physician treating adolescents from the first two groups has to communicate clearly why treatment is instituted and do whatever he or she can to develop a good personal relationship with the teenager. The reason compliance is so often an issue in the treatment of adolescents is that the adolescent sees himself or herself as normal and, therefore, not in need of treatment. If treated as if he or she is disturbed, the teenager will be alienated and consequently lost.

Adolescents, like adults, have to be individually evaluated. If an adolescent is disturbed, it most probably is not caused by the physical illness itself but is in addition to the physical illness. The majority of adolescents, again like adults, can cope relatively well with chronic mild or acute crisis. There is no reason to believe—and more important, there are no data that lend support to the idea—that they cannot cope with their illness.

One speculation is that in illnesses in which the social stigma is easily noticed by others (i.e., cystic fibrosis), the self-image system is impaired. The greater the stigma, one might assume, the greater the impairment. However, even if parts of the self-image system are damaged, other parts remain intact. The physician needs to know which is which in order to determine when the impairment is severe enough to require professional mental health care; when self-image is only mildly impaired, how to help the teenager with support, encouragement, and empathic understanding; and which parts of the self-image remain intact. These are the areas that should be strengthened. They will help the physician in working with the adolescent. For example, the male with cystic fibrosis has normal mastery, family relationships, morals, and vocational and educational goals. Support of the teenager's aspirations in these areas can be particularly helpful.

In all of this the authors would like to underscore the importance of gender differences. Social class should also be kept in mind as an important independent variable.

It should be remembered that studying the relationships between physical illness and psychological problems on a truly random basis is just beginning. Statements like the one by Schenker (1976) that "any real or imagined threat to body-image during adolescence can be more traumatic and difficult to cope with than at any other time of life" are just not supported by data.

Last, normal development is more complex than psychopathological development (Offer & Sabshin, 1984). It has a variety of differential patterns that are not mutually exclusive. These patterns present adolescents with a multiplicity of coping styles and psychological profiles. In the next decade it will be the task of the behavioral scientist to elucidate these patterns, to describe them, and to relate them to the adolescent population. Most adolescents pass through the teen years without ever being seen or studied by either a physician or a behavioral scientist. It is important to study as many of the variations they present as is possible in order to gain a better understanding of adolescents in health as well as in illness.

ACKNOWLEDGMENTS

The authors are grateful to Mrs. Shiaomay Young and Mr. David Parrella for their assistance in preparing this manuscript, and to Dr. S. Gottoff for his helpful comments. The authors are particularly grateful to the following investigators who graciously shared their data with us: Drs. M. Ostrov, R. Freeman, S. Solomon, and C. Landon.

REFERENCES

Boyle, I.R., di Sant'Agnese, P.A., Sack, S., Millican, F., & Kulczycki, L.L. Emotional adjustment of adolescents and young adults with cystic fibrosis. *The Journal of Pediatrics*, 1976, *88*, 318–326.

Campbell, M.M., Hayden, P.W., & Davenport, S.L. Psychological adjustment of adolescents with myelodysplasia. *Journal of Youth and Adolescence*, 1977, *6*, 397–407.

French, T.M., & Alexander, F., et al. *Psychogenic factors in bronchial asthma*. Washington, D. C.: National Research Council, 1941.

Kellerman, J., Zeltzer, L., Ellenberg, L., Dash, J., & Rigler, D. Psychological effects of illness in adolescence. I. Anxiety, self-esteem and perception of control. *The Journal of Pediatrics*, 1980, *97*, 126–131.

Landon, C., Rosenfeld, R., Northcraft, G., & Lewiston, N. Self-image of adolescents with cystic fibrosis. *Journal of Youth and Adolescence*, 1980, *9*, 521–528.

Offer, D., Ostrov, E., & Howard, K.I. *The adolescent: A psychological self-portrait*. New York: Basic Books, Inc., 1981a.

Offer, D., Ostrov, E., & Howard, K.I. *The Offer self-image questionnaire for adolescents: A manual* (3rd ed.). Chicago: Michael Reese Hospital, 1982.

Offer, D. & Sabshin, M. *Normality and the Life Cycle*. New York: Basic Books, Inc. 1984.

Ostrov, M., & Ostrov, E. The self-image of adolescents with asthma. Manuscript to be published, 1983.

Schenker, I.R. Medical care of adolescents in a suburban community. In E. Fuchs (Ed.), *Youth in a changing world: Cross cultural perspectives on adolescence*. The Hague: Mouton Publishers, 1976.

Zeltzer, L., Kellerman, J., Ellenberg, L., Dash, J., & Rigler, D. Psychologic effects of illness in adolescence. II. Impact of illness in adolescents: Crucial issues and coping styles. *The Journal of Pediatrics*, 1980, *97*, 132–138.

Maynard C. Reynolds

6

The Educational Needs of Disabled Children and Youths

THE EDUCATIONAL RIGHTS OF DISABLED YOUNG PEOPLE

Educators have been exceedingly busy recently implementing new policies for the education of students who are temporarily or permanently disabled. These policies have been expressed variously through court decisions, state and federal legislation, and statements of professional organizations and advocacy groups. The most important and comprehensive document for the purposes of schooling is Public Law 94-142, the Education for All Handicapped Children Act. This law was passed by Congress and signed by President Gerald R. Ford in 1975, and it became fully effective in the fall of 1978. The major assumptions underlying this legislation are that all children have the right to education, and all children, no matter how profoundly handicapped they may be, can learn.

The law, in sum, mandates the states to provide free, appropriate education for all handicapped children in minimally restrictive environments and with the concurrence of the parents. Specifically, the provisions of the law make the following requirements of public schools:

1. Search out all handicapped children, even those with the most profound handicaps
2. Make a multidisciplinary assessment of each such child on the basis of which an individualized educational plan (IEP) must be formulated

CHRONIC ILLNESS AND DISABILITIES IN CHILDHOOD AND ADOLESCENCE   ISBN 0-8089-1635-1

3. Place the student according to the IEP in an instructional setting
    (preferably a regular classroom) that will enhance the student's de-
    velopment
4. Monitor the student's educational progress according to the IEP, and
    make annual reassessments of the student's development
5. Facilitate the participation of the student (when appropriate) and par-
    ents or guardians in the educational planning
6. Observe the principles of due process in all major decisions, including
    the right of parents to appeal placement and other decisions for their
    disabled children

Most public school personnel have made massive efforts to comply
with the new mandates, yet in 1982 no state was judged to be in full compliance (U.S. Department of Education, 1982). All states have conducted
child-find searches for handicapped and chronically ill students who may
not be in school at all or for whom only minimal education has been provided. These searches have been successful on the whole and few, if any,
known handicapped children are out of school. Most residential institutions
for children have had to upgrade their educational programs and initiate
conferences with parents and local school authorities to make educational
plans for the children in their care. The least restrictive environment principle requires that special education and related services be delivered to
handicapped children in regular-education classrooms whenever possible.
Thus, handicapped students may be placed in special classes or schools
only when the placement can be justified and, even then, only for a limited
time; the programs provided in such settings must have specific goals and
objectives. This principle, popularly known as mainstreaming, has required
major changes in the roles of regular school teachers and principals and
new adaptations in the services provided by special education teachers,
school psychologists, school social workers, and other specialists. In response to these changes in functions and roles, colleges, schools, and
departments of education have had to begin revising their preparation
programs for all school personnel (Reynolds, Birch, Grohs, Howsam, &
Morsink, 1980).

It is notable that the schools of the nation have been given the responsibility of locating every handicapped child or youth and arranging
a multidisciplinary diagnostic study for each. In many countries the responsibility for children with disabilities is carried mainly by health or
social agencies. It is interesting to speculate on why the primary responsibility in the United States was assigned to the public schools. At least
since the Brown decision in 1954, schools have been recognized as one
of the principal instruments for achieving equality of opportunity for all
persons. For this reason, perhaps, political interventions in schooling seem

to be more numerous and penetrating than ever before. In no aspect of schooling are such interventions more evident than in the provision of education for students with disabilities; it is here that Public Law 94-142 is having important and pervasive effects.

Obviously, full understanding of a handicapped child and of the child's family depends upon the additional participation of health professionals, social service personnel, and other specialists, many of them not employed in the schools. Achieving the necessary coordination of services among the various professions and the agencies in which they are employed is a major problem. Special projects undertaken by the American Academy of Pediatrics and the American Society of Allied Health Professions illustrate some of the efforts being made by professional groups to achieve such mutual understanding and coordination.

Related Services Interpreted

Under Public Law 94-142 the schools are responsible for making special education and related services available to handicapped children. Special education needs no definition, but related services do. The law defines related services as "transportation . . . developmental, corrective, and other support services." The phrase other support services holds much difficulty for the schools. There is no doubt that it covers the services of audiologists and psychologists, for example, but what about specialists who provide recreation? Psychotherapy? Parent counseling? Medical services? In one midwestern community, equestrian therapy (horseback riding lessons) became an issue. During the years the law has been in effect, physical therapy, occupational therapy, and corrective physical education programs have increased rapidly in many communities, not only in special schools but also in mainstream settings. Inasmuch as physicians do not usually participate in the supervision of such programs, it is clear that some allied health professions are forging new degrees of independence in their practices within the school setting.

Judicial interpretations of related services have tended to broaden rather than limit the definition (FOCUS, 1981). Some observers feel that this broadening stems not directly from Public Law 94-142 but indirectly from the expanded concept of the purposes of education—to enhance one's life—which follows from the enrollment of all children, including those with severe and profound handicaps, in school. Obviously, in some cases the provision of appropriate education requires schools to teach severely handicapped students to walk, to feed themselves, to use the toilet on their own, and other such basic skills, in addition to the cognitive skills of reading, writing, and arithmetic.

It was not too long ago that one of the de facto tests to determine a child's admissibility to public schools was whether he or she was toilet trained. Sometimes a child was admitted on condition that the parents provided the help for toilet training. Should the term *other support services*, therefore, be interpreted to include taking a student to the toilet? Changing soiled clothes? Catheterizing a child with kidney problems? What about making sure that a child's hearing aid is functioning properly?

Obviously, the interpretation of related services is a potential source of problems for school curricula and budgets. It raises many detailed questions on the responsibilities and relations of schools, health and social service agencies, and families; it is certain to continue receiving the attention of the courts as well as school administrators.

PREVALENCE RATES OF HANDICAPS*

Public Law 94-142 was based on estimates that the percentage of children with handicapping conditions in the United States is about 10–12 percent of the total school-age population. The federal government pays each state slightly more than $200.[†] for each student who is identified as handicapped and in need of special education, up to 12 percent of the state's population of children. In fact, the percentage of handicapped students reported by states has been increasing but is still below 12 percent; during the early 1980s the figures were nearer nine–ten percent. About 4.2 million IEPs were prepared during the 1981–1982 school year (U.S. Department of Education, 1982).

At most, only about three percent of children can be judged to have distinct and chronic handicaps; the remainder, up to a total of about 12 percent at any one time, comprises mainly those children who display relatively mild or moderate—and often transient—conditions, such as learning, speech, or behavior problems, or mild mental retardation. The United States Department of Education estimated in its report to the Congress that currently only 13 percent of the children considered handicapped

---

*The term prevalence indicates the number or percentage of students needing services at any one time; incidence indicates the number of those who may need services at some time in their lives. Incidence rates, thus, are higher than prevalence rates.

†The authorizations under Public Law 94-142 are much higher but full funding has never occurred. Under the law, federal supports for handicapped children were to rise gradually to a level representing 40 percent of the average per-child cost of education nationally. By the 1981–1982 school year, the level of federal supports was approximately 12 percent of such cost. Many legislators and President Ford, at the time he signed the bill, commented on the extreme unlikelihood that Public Law 94-142 would ever be fully funded. More than 90 percent of the cost of educating handicapped students is covered by state and local school district funds.

for the purposes of schooling are severely handicapped (U.S. Department of Education, 1982). Yet, from kindergarten through sixth grade, as many as 40 percent of children may manifest some learning or behavioral problems at one time or another, and this cumulative figure goes higher if the adolescent group is included (Rubin & Balow, 1971). It should be noted, consequently, that the incidence rates for handicapping conditions go up markedly when children with temporary handicaps are included, and especially when the time intervals[‡] used for counting incidence are expanded.

For the 1980–1981 school year, the national incidence rates for the largest categories of handicap were as follows[5]:

	Percentages of total	Cumulative percentages
Learning disabled (LD)	36	36
Speech impaired (SI)	30	66
Mentally retarded (MR)	19	85
Emotionally disturbed (ED)	8	93

These data are based on unduplicated counts; that is, each child was counted only once according to what was considered to be the primary handicap. As can easily be seen, 93 percent of the total population of handicapped children and youth as reported to the United States Department of Education by the states were in four categories. The large majority (but not all) of the children were only mildly handicapped. Only seven percent of the cases were students with physical and sensory impairments.

Some noteworthy data on prevalence of handicapping conditions by categories and sex follow:

1. In six states more than half the total number of reported handicapped students were classified as learning disabled (LD).
2. The number of cases of learning disability increased for the nation as a whole by 48 percent between the 1977–1978 and 1980–1981 school years. In the same three-year period, the rates for mental retardation decreased by ten percent.
3. Males exceeded females by almost two and a half to one in the learning disability category.
4. Males exceeded females by three to one in the seriously emotionally disturbed category.
5. Overall, 64 percent of students reported as handicapped were male and 36 percent were female.

[‡]The national figures (now showing that about nine–ten percent of school-age children are handicapped) are the count on a single day (December 1) of each year and, thus, do not show the larger incidence figure that would result from a count made over a longer time span.

SPECIAL EDUCATION IN SECONDARY SCHOOLS

The clearest mandate of the new educational policies is that the schools be opened to all young persons, no matter how exceptional their educational needs may be. This has proved to be a larger challenge to secondary schools than to those serving younger students. At this time, only about 75 percent of all high school age adolescents receive diplomas. There are about one million fewer students enrolled in the 12th grade than attended the 5th grade eight years earlier. Although there is no unequivocal evidence that a disproportionately large number of students who dropped out of school before graduation were exceptional, it is reasonable to assume that many were having learning problems, were unable to adjust adequately to school, or were finding school to be unfriendly and uninteresting. It should be noted that the period for compulsory school attendance in most states now ends at age 16, about grade ten; nevertheless, students have a right to education beyond age 16 although they are not compelled to seek it.

An adolescent with special needs is much less likely to be provided with adaptive education and related services than is a younger student whose needs are comparable. Data for the 1978–1979 school year show that only 29 percent of the students receiving services under Public Law 94-142 were in grades 7–12; 67 percent of students for whom IEPs were written were age 12 or lower. The overwhelming reason for referring the majority of secondary students for special education is learning disability or emotional disorder (U.S. Department of Education, 1982, p. 21). Although services to youths ages 18–21 may be increasing at a higher average rate than those for younger students, the total rate for services in secondary schools and beyond is still relatively low (U.S. Department of Education, 1982).

The relative lack of services in secondary schools and for adolescents probably results from a number of factors, including (1) the greater self-dependence of eligible students and, thus, lesser need for special services, (2) the difficulties of accommodating special services in the complex structure of the secondary schools, (3) the lack of knowledge to serve the special needs of teenagers, and (4) the relative recency of the attention that is given to secondary school programs for students with special needs.

Many current problems in secondary education affect all students, but it is likely that those with handicaps are especially affected. Such problems are reflected by many teenagers in their lack of feelings of accomplishment, frequent absences from school (as high as 25 percent each day in some schools), and behavioral problems. A recent study based on interviews with students in seven different secondary schools showed that 21 percent could not think of anything that happened in school that generated a feeling of accomplishment; an additional 31 percent could not think of anything related to the curriculum that gave them a sense of accomplishment; and 20 percent cited sports or extracurricular activities, and 11 percent cited socializing with friends as their main sources of school-related satisfaction. Only one student in five reported "a sense of accomplishment from the essential business of schooling" (Shaw, 1982, p. 704).

It is necessary to remember that each day many secondary school teachers see 150 or more students in about five instructional periods. Those five periods are separated by approximately five-minute intervals that usually are spent in quick conferences with individual students. Class loads have been going up rapidly in recent years as education appropriations have been diminished and enriching curricular offerings reduced. Such conditions do not facilitate careful individual instruction for anyone, much less for those with special needs.

It should be added that the preparation of most secondary school teachers tends to be oriented to particular subject matter. Generally, such teachers are still prepared in a four-year baccalaureate program that includes at least two years of general education and a one-year-plus major in a subject such as chemistry, history, English, or mathematics. The amount of professional preparation is limited and, at least in some places, less than what was required 30 years ago. In an interesting analysis, in which teacher education was reduced to a typical 40-hour work week equivalency, Yarger et al. estimated that the professional training of the average secondary school teacher occupied slightly more than six weeks (Howey, Yarger & Joyce, 1978). Secondary teachers rarely have special training in normal human development, and they have even less training in handling students with disabilities.

Classification

For students to be eligible for special education and related services and for school districts to qualify for compensating funds, children must be classified as handicapped according to the limited set of categories specified by state and federal governments. The problem is that these specified categories often lead to the attachment of stigmatizing labels to students and even to gross misclassifications (Hobbs, 1975). It is hard, for example, to imagine a more diverse group than students with cerebral palsy (CP), insofar as educational needs are concerned. Yet the label CP is often applied in a largely undifferentiated or stereotypical manner. Teachers are not unusual in this tendency to stereotype; it is a major problem in our society and is a primary complaint of disabled adolescents. They want and deserve to be thought of as individuals (see Resnick, Chapter 3 in this edition).

The classification system used by schools has been described as scandalously unreliable, especially for students with only mild handicaps (Scriven, 1983). Glass (1983) likened the system to that of the psychiatric diagnosis of schizophrenia several decades ago. In an illustrative anecdote, he told of two seemingly competent psychiatrists who diagnosed new admissions to the same hospital as schizophrenic at 90 and 10 percent rates, respectively (Glass, 1983). Given so little reliability in classification, how can specific diagnoses or treatments be created or discovered? The question must also be asked of some parts of the special education enterprise.

Nevertheless, educators persist in using simplistic schemes of classification, perhaps because that is how they must proceed to receive funds. Most states and the federal government categorically issue funds to school districts only after students have been assigned to a handicap category. Funding also may be the reason for the threefold increase in the number of school-related disorders listed in the third revised *Diagnostic and statistical manual* (DSMIII; American Psychiatric Association, 1979) as compared with the second edition. The new listing includes *shyness disorder, overanxious disorder, academic achievement disorder, specific academic or work inhibition, and specific arithmetical disorder* among others. The third edition thus transforms common adolescent problems and school-related difficulties into mental disorders with labels and code numbers. Next, one fears, comes "treatment" at high expense. Can labeling what may be developmental problems as mental disorders help young people to solve them, or will the practice cause additional problems?

Clearly, the classification systems that are appropriate in the schools may be quite different from those that are relevant in other settings. Indeed, procedures for human classification always have varied greatly from agency to agency, time to time, and culture to culture. The approach used in a particular setting must be understood in its historical, political, moral, and economic context, as well as in terms of the technical requirements for professional services; often the classification systems in use serve the people who are categorized poorly, if at all.

Classification systems ought to be designed for specific purposes, and in the schools that means instructional purposes. For example, a student should be considered blind only if the methods and materials he or she needs for reading do not require the use of sight (Braille or optacon would be the method of choice.) It is noteworthy that such an approach to classification differs from that used for other purposes, such as specifying etiology or making a general prognosis; it is certainly unlike the method used to qualify the blind for income tax exemptions. Similarly, a deaf child for educational purposes is one for whom the usual audito–oral processes are functionally absent and cannot be used for instruction.

The instructional approach to classification in the schools has led to some categories, such as *learning disabled* or *educable mentally retarded*, which are only rarely used in other settings. It also means that some disabilities with major medical significance may receive only slight attention in the schools because they require few special adaptations in educational programs. For example, the programs necessary for many children with orthopedic problems, cancer, diabetes, or other chronic health problems may differ little from those common to the general run of students. Of course, teachers may need to understand the health problems to facilitate necessary health-related treatments during school hours or to provide records for physicians, parents, and health managers, but often it is a serious mistake to try to classify such children in any special way for instructional purposes. It is even more of a mistake, and illegal in many cases, to place such students in special classes or schools simply because they have medical problems. Students themselves tend to deeply resent being labeled or assigned to special schools unless such placement is absolutely essential.

For purposes of instructional classification, teachers are mainly concerned with their students' current levels of academic performance and psychosocial development and with the conditions needed to facilitate further growth. When teachers seek help, the intent is usually to redesign classroom environments and activities to make them more helpful for an individual student's learning. However, when health professionals and psychologists classify children according to specific categories (e.g., orthopedically handicapped, dyslexic, hyperactive, disturbed, attention deficient), the labels have little intrinsic value for teachers. The valuable assessments are those related to the student's instructional needs.

The literature of education often uses terms in a special way to refer to students' problems. Stevens (1962), for example, urged certain distinctions in the use of the terms "impairment," "disability," and "handicap." In his definitions, *impairment* refers to an actual defect in tissue, as in the absence of fingers or a severed nerve; *disability* refers to a loss of function, as when a person does not have the finger dexterity necessary for typing; and *handicap* refers to the extent to which an impairment or disability interferes with the person's normal living. Many students have impairments or disabilities that are not handicaps. A student who uses a wheelchair but is able to attend a regular school and follow an ordinary curriculum is not classified as handicapped for instructional purposes. Although health-related management may find it necessary to focus on an impairment or disability, in the schools limited attention is given to such a condition, and attempts are made to minimize the handicapping effects.

Interprofessional Communications

When IEPs must be designed for students with special needs, the participants other than the parents usually include several professionals from different fields who specify the kind of special education and related services that should be provided. Unfortunately, the professionals often are unable to communicate clearly with each other; sometimes their language is overly technical or even idiosyncratic; sometimes they lack experience dealing with colleagues in other professions; and sometimes their point of view is psychological, medical, or psychiatric rather than educational.

One method of analyzing the problems of communication among different professionals is to use the concept of *orders of dispositions* suggested by Sellars (1958). The concept is applicable when a syndrome has a complicated chain of cause and effect, and members of the different professions tend to focus on particular aspects (Meehl, 1972). For example, consider the case of a child with phenylketonuria (PKU). First there is the genetic factor that interacts with diet (too much phenylalanine) to produce mental retardation, which in turn limits the ability to learn to read and, consequently, narrows the individual's vocational opportunities as an adult. The several orders of disposition here are genetic, dietary, cognitive, literacy, and employability. The knowledge base for all five dispositions combined is formidable, even if all parts are not yet complete. This fact is relatively unimportant because only particular parts of the knowledge base are relevant to particular decisions. Thus, the teacher who is trying to teach the PKU child to read may need to know only that the child is on a special diet and how the child functions cognitively. Other parts of the knowledge structure are not essential to the teacher's instructional decisions.

A common pattern of multi-professional discourse on educational problems is for each professional to elaborate on the dispositions he or she knows most about; for example psychologists often describe a student in terms of cognitive predispositions (attention, memory, perception) and personality factors, on the assumption that this information is essential to instruction. The next, more remote level of dispositions is to describe the child in neuropsychological terms, as if to say that the educational problem is imbedded in neurological problems. Unfortunately, not much is known about how to relate neurologically and psychologically based dispositions to specific instructional strategies, although considerable time seems to be spent on these various orders of disposition by different professionals. Communication has hardly begun between educators and the other professionals with whom they consult, although a number of suggestions for improving communication have been offered by Braga (1972), Cromwell, Blaskfield, and Strauss (1975), Hunt and Sullivan (1974) and Reynolds (1979).

Neglect of Prevention

A greatly dispiriting and unfortunate problem in the schools is that special attention usually is given to students after their problems are full blown, although earlier attention might have prevented them in whole or part. Special education laws and regulations permit the use of categorical funds only when children are severely disturbed or display severe discrepancies between ability and achievement. For some years, however, many school programs have demonstrated that attention to problems at incipient stages reduces the rate of serious problems later (Far West Laboratory, 1980). For example, good preschool programs for high-risk children have been shown to reduce by half the number of students requiring intensive and expensive special education programs later (Lazar, 1981).

Education thus shares with many other fields of human service the responsibility of using public resources to prevent major casualties. The problem is not primarily technical—a great deal is known about how to provide early, efficient preventive school programs—but rather it is political and economic. Systems of funding, accountability, and new modes of leadership are required. Not only educators but public policy leaders as well must lead the movement toward earlier, more efficient, and more humane intervention.

Resistance by Minority Groups

Much of special education is suspect, these days, in minority communities. Even the largest of the special education programs tend to label children with negative terms, such as retarded, disturbed, and disabled and disproportionately high numbers of children so labeled are from minority families. The parents want necessary services for their children but not at the expense of demeaning and sometimes permanent labels.

Clearly, there are differences in the extent to which various ethnic or racial groups are represented in special education programs. For example, data for the 1978–1979 school year show that 41 percent of all black students in special education programs were classified as educable mentally retarded compared with 18 and 10 percent for white and Asian–American students, respectively. Data on the learning disability category show an obverse pattern: 38 percent of white and only 23 percent of black special education students were in this category (General Accounting Office, 1981, p. 62).

Numerous class action suits, such as that of Isaac Lora versus the Board of Education in New York City, have centered on the discrepancies in racial or ethnic classification rates and procedures. In the case of Isaac, a minority student, the court decided that the procedures that were used to refer, classify him as emotionally disturbed, and place him in a special school were inappropriate. To repair the situation, Isaac and all of his class were returned to mainstream schools, and all teachers in the school system (70,000 of them!) were ordered to undergo two years of part-time in-service training on proper procedures for dealing with students such as Isaac.

School personnel find class action suits of this kind extraordinarily difficult. Not only are many school operations changed and new expectations for services established, but also, the time limits on making the necessary changes tend to be very short, and there is no outside help. For example, a court decision may require changes in the placement of hundreds of students who have presented major behavior problems, but the legal mandate is directed only at the schools; existing mental health or corrections agencies are not affected, and the court makes no provisions for the costs its order entails.

Finding answers to the difficult problem of serving minority children with special needs will not be easy. A lot of people are trying to devise assessment and classification systems that are fair or nondiscriminatory, but it is hard to define these terms, let alone satisfy everyone as actual practices are changed. Probably the answers will come through procedures that address instructional issues immediately and do not include the kinds of simplistic and mostly irrelevant testing and classification procedures now required to obtain funds.

Budget Cutbacks

Particularly worrisome to the schools are the current reductions in education and other human services appropriations. Agencies that should be cooperating with schools to serve handicapped children and their families are being forced to draw apart. In one medium-sized city, for example, funds and services amounting to about $500,000./year were recently withdrawn by several health and United Fund agencies from a large public school service for handicapped students. The rationale was that because the legal mandate to assess, teach, and serve such students is addressed to public schools, they should provide the money. This kind of decision occurs more and more often as all agencies experience declines in resources and expanding demands for services. Although the coordination of health, education, and social service agencies should be strengthening, political expediencies are forcing each to return to its isolated traditional function.

Effective cross-agency planning and coordination are essential but will be achieved only if leaders at the highest levels in state and community agencies recognize the problem and strengthen the efforts for coordination. It has been suggested that governors or legislative leaders, who operate at a level above that of the separate service departments, create a *children's budget*; funding would be based on an examination of the services that are needed by children and their families and the principle of the optimal coordination of services.

Working With Parents

An area in which improved planning and service are specifically needed is in work with the parents of handicapped students. Teachers are now required by law to meet with parents to plan handicapped children's school programs. Any information on the children in the teachers' possession must be made available to the parents, if requested, for use in formulating what they see as their children's needs and plans. This new relation is an unfamiliar one for both teachers and parents, and at times it is threatening to all concerned. Neither the teachers nor the parents have been prepared for consultation and sometimes they feel they have reasons for mutual distrust. Good efforts at collaboration seem to pay off, but problems of great complexity are frequently brought to the surface. When parents themselves have serious problems and need training or counseling, whose responsibility is it to help them? Should schools provide the in-depth services? If not, who should do the job? Many agencies seem to have some of the necessary resources for this work, but often it is not available on call; thus, parent–teacher conferences frequently result in frustration and embarrassment because problems have been revealed, but there is too little follow-through by the parent and family-serving agencies.

SOME PROMISING DEVELOPMENTS

Despite the numerous problems currently plaguing the schools, there are many creative developments that hold promise for the future.

Systems Procedures

An important innovation in education is the application of broad systems procedures in the regular schools; they make it feasible to deal with the increasing diversity of students in mainstream classrooms. For example, Wang (1980) described an Adaptive Learning Environments Model (ALEM) that depends upon an intricate system of assessments and correlated instructional activities to make certain that every student in a classroom is engaged at his or her proper instructional level in basic subjects. ALEM also includes a curriculum for teaching students to take increasing amounts of responsibility for planning their own studies over increasing periods of time. Management of the system is facilitated by computers in which detailed records are kept for use by students, teachers, and parents when they review progress and make plans for the future. In effect, the system provides something like a daily updated IEP on every student. Detailed staff development and program-monitoring procedures are part of the total system, thus making certain that a high quality of operation is developed and maintained.

Several key ideas should be noted about such systems in relation to students who have special needs: First, the systems create a new kind of school environment in which all students are served optimally. Everyone's program is individualized; that is, for each student, the program is organized to fit with his or her developmental level in each subject. Such individualizing does not mean that a student works alone—in the ALEM system there is no less group instruction than with ordinary classroom procedures—but the group instruction offered by the teacher always brings together students who are at a similar achievement level and, thus, share similar needs. When ALEM is in operation, the special education teachers, school psychologists, and other staff members are drawn into the mainstream classrooms to assist handicapped students as part of a total system. Because they have less need to remove selected students to resource rooms, clinics, or special classes, they are able to avoid all discontinuities in programming for both students and teachers that call for endless communication about who is doing what, with what materials, and with what results. The special education program is simply the most intensive aspect of a broader, fully coordinated system for instruction (Reynolds & Wang, 1981). Systems procedures, such as ALEM, offer advantages to disabled students on both social and academic variables.

The End of Isolation

In the past, regular teachers and education specialists usually operated in separate ways and places. Indeed, schools of the past can be described as following a *two-box* system: on the one side were regular classes with "normal" students, regular teachers, and ordinary school supervision and funding, and on the other side were special classes for "exceptional" students, conducted by special teachers, supervised by special education administrators, and supported by special categorical funds. Between the two boxes were the school psychologists, counselors, and social workers who functioned as gatekeepers; they labeled each student and sent him or her to one box or the other, and they labeled each teacher to match. This resulted in educable mentally retarded (EMR) students, EMR classes, teachers of EMR pupils, supervisors of EMR classes, and EMR funds. That kind of arrangement still exists in many places but not for much longer.

A more complex administrative model for the organization of special education programs began to emerge in the 1960s and peaked after the enactment of Public Law 94-142. It is sometimes described as a cascade or continuum of administrative arrangements. Some of its features are shown in Figure 6-1, and can be expanded upon as follows:

1. Regular classrooms are the primary instructional setting for all children, with particular adaptations made to meet the special needs of particular students.

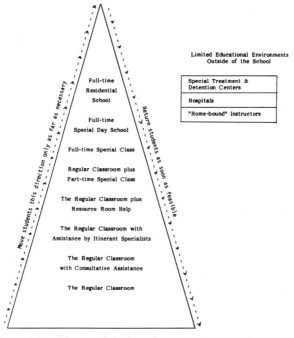

Figure 6-1. The special education cascade. (Reprinted from Reynolds, M.C., & Birch, J.W., *Teaching exceptional children in all America's schools* (rev. ed.). Reston, VA: The Council for Exceptional Children, 1982, p. 39. Permission granted by Reynolds.)

2. Children are not classified and given special placements on a per-
    manent basis but rather are moved to special stations only for as long
    as necessary and then are returned to regular classrooms as soon as
    is feasible. As a result, indelible labels are avoided. The total number
    of children served in special settings over time greatly exceeds the
    number served at any given time.
3. The boundary lines between special education and regular education
    are renegotiated and opened so that students can pass back and forth
    easily, as dictated by their educational needs.
4. Regular and special education staff members become more interactive
    or collaborative in their daily work through sharing responsibilities
    for students, rather than isolating themselves in separate centers and
    classrooms.
5. Careful justification is required to move a student out of the regular
    school environment, especially when the removal would take the stu-
    dent from both home and neighborhood school environments for
    placement in a residential center.

A visitor to public schools today is likely to encounter something like
this broad continuum or cascade of instructional arrangements. Not only
are children being moved about the cascade arrangement, but specialized
personnel are as well.

Specialized staff members, such as braille teachers, school psychologists, learning disability teachers, and many others are coming "down"
to the regular classroom base of the cascade to provide their particular
services. The recognition is growing that not all specialized instruction
need go on in special places and, in fact, that it is likely to be disadvan-
tageous to confine children to special places, which tend to be very limiting
environments, for long periods of time.

Special teachers, psychologists, and other special staff members are
drawn into the mainstream at the base of the cascade where they work
with students as the coprofessionals of the regular teachers. This new
relation creates the consultation challenge. For the first time, many school
staff members are expected to work in environments in which they must
engage in face-to-face consultation with other professionals. They share
an obligation to create a school environment that is democratic and serves
all its students well; that is, an environment in which no one is stigmatized
for being different, every member is valued equally, everyone is assisted
in learning and developmental activities, and all help to maintain the setting.

As a result of such changes, the topic of consultation is taking on
key importance in teacher preparation. All school staff members must
understand and be skilled in using specialists to solve professional prob-

lems. They must know about the special kinds of contracts that are possible when two or more professionals decide to work together on a problem, not by referral or shifting responsibility to someone else, but by addressing the problem together in a common environment. They are learning to recognize that a call for consultation with a specialist is not a sign of weakness but, rather a sign of professional commitment and concern. Programming for handicapped students is probably the most frequent topic for consultation among school personnel, as well as for consultation with parents, health professionals, and community specialists.

In Figure 6-1 a seperate box takes note of the fact that some children are placed in special settings outside of the schools. Some young people violate the law and are placed in detention or retraining centers; others are ill and in hospitals; and still others have chronic health problems or disabilites and remain at home. In all such settings it is common for the schools to provide instructors and to attempt to keep students up to date in their studies to the extent that this is possible. Special devices, such as telephones connected to regular classrooms, are often used to maintain contact with classmates and teachers; this is especially common in the case of homebound students.

All of the placements in these special cases are made by persons other than educators. Judges or physicians usually have ordered the placements, and the schools are simply accommodating these decisions and respecting the students' rights to education.

Even under the best of circumstances, instruction provided in these special environments tends to be very limited, and educators favor the return of students to regular school environments as soon as possible.

Cooperative Goal Structures

Another idea of growing importance in the schools is the establishment of social environments that are characterized by cooperation and mutual understanding among students. Traditionally, schools have been dominated by individualistic and competitive modes of management and evaluation. Students sat in rows looking at the backs of heads of students in front of them and toward the teacher, the primary authority figure. When students looked at one another they were reprimanded, and if they talked to neighbors they might be suspected of cheating. Grading usually was based on social comparisons, and it was a "zero-sum game." A few high scorers in the class lowered the chances for good grades among others.

Today, classrooms increasingly are broken into small groups in which students are expected to work together, to be mutually helpful, to understand other group members well, and to work for group as well as individual goals. In the simplest case, a teacher might say, "If everyone in the group reaches the 80 percent correct level on the test, there will be an extra 10 points for everyone; and all those over 95 will get an A." Such procedures encourage positive rather than negative interdependencies among students; they help to avoid the isolation of particular students; and they make it essential that students understand each other well within the positive frame of concern. It is truly notable that the research findings on cooperative goal structuring consistently show strong advantages on achievement as well as social variables, such as acceptance and appreciation of handicapped students (Johnson & Johnson, 1975). Indeed, the research also shows that social structures built on cooperation markedly improve the opportunities for students who are different.

No one is arguing for a total restructuring of school procedures to cooperative arrangements, because it is important that students also learn to work and achieve individually and to recognize the realities of competition in our society. Nevertheless, there is a strong trend toward emphasizing cooperation in the classroom. American industry shows a similar trend, with much attention given to Japanese models, in which workers and managers cooperate for quality improvements and efficiencies as well as humane working conditions.

Deliberate Psychological Education

Another promising trend in curriculum is toward what can be called *deliberate psychological education*. Sprinthall (1980) contrasted two methods of teaching a high school course in psychology. In the first, the subject is taught strictly as a science. Students are expected to learn facts, procedures, and theories about sensation, perception, learning, human development, social psychology, abnormal psychology, and so on. In effect, the course is a simplified version of a college or professional general introduction to psychology. In the second method, more emphasis is given to application of psychological principles to the students' life situations. For example, they are taught about human development by being made aware of their own stages or levels of development and those of their siblings, parents, or friends. They study learning not only by reading about Pavlov, Thorndike, and Skinner but also by learning how to do peer-tutoring with a classmate, in professional style. This second approach is one kind of deliberate psychological education.

Another important facet of deliberate psychological education is the work on moral development by Kohlberg (1969) and others. Their procedures include the assessment of students' current levels of moral development; then they proceed through an appropriately scaled curriculum, with discussions of moral dilemmas to encourage awareness of higher principles that might be applied.

As students are assisted in becoming more mature psychologically, they increase their knowledge of and skill in relating to classmates, especially peers who may be different and thus can be easily dismissed from awareness. Deliberate psychological education has not yet become the object of mass curriculum changes in the schools, but interest in it is rapidly growing, and it may become a significant subject in the future. It is part of a larger set of changes that promise more opportunities for handicapped students, especially during the adolescent years when peer understanding and support are so critically important.

BUT WON'T IT ALL GO AWAY?

In 1981, President Reagan proposed the repeal of Public Law 94-142 and proposed instead *block granting* of the funds provided under the law with other categorical support programs. Although his effort failed, it is quite likely that the same suggestion will be made again. Most observers consider Public Law 94-142 and its principles to be sturdy and able to withstand even strong political assaults. Even if Public Law 94-142 should be repealed, or if it is administered only weakly in the future, the many layers of legislation and judicial decisions at both state and federal levels will continue to uphold its principles.

In the meantime, events are moving quickly: deinstitutionalization has reduced the rolls of public residential institutions, and enrollments in special schools have declined substantially. Schools are changing in response to Public Law 94-142 faster than are the training programs for personnel. As a result, teacher-preparation educators are reevaluating teaching candidates, teacher-preparation curricula, and the length of training programs.

As a profession, the moral development of education has been raised a degree over the past few years as the problems of serving handicapped children have been confronted. Increasing numbers of school personnel have had to face the potentially catastrophic experience of dealing with rejection that is experienced by some handicapped students and their families. Increasing numbers of educators realize that they have a duty to model in the schools the kind of inclusiveness that must prevail in a generally deinstitutionalized society. There is no reason to expect adults to show concern with, decency toward, and genuine helpfulness for disabled people if children have no experience with those sentiments during their school years.

REFERENCES

American Psychiatric Association. *Diagnostic and statistical manual* (3rd ed.). Washington, DC, 1979.

Braga, J. Role theory, cognitive dissonance theory and the interdisciplinary team. *Interchange*, 1972, *4*, 69–78.

Cromwell, R.L., Blaskfield, R.K., & Strauss, J.E. Criteria for classification systems. In N. Hobbs (Ed.), *Issues in the classification of children: A handbook of categories, labels and their consequences*. Los Angeles: Jossey-Bass, 1975, 4–25.

Far West Laboratory for Educational Research and Development. *Educational programs that work* (7th ed.). San Francisco: Author (1855 Folsom St., 94103), 1980.

FOCUS on special education legal practices, 1981, *1* (2).

General Accounting Office. *Disparities still exist in who gets special education*. Washington, DC: Author, 1981.

Glass, G. Effectiveness of special education. In M. Reynolds & J. Brandl (Eds.), *Policy Studies Review* (special issue entitled Public Policy and the Education of Handicapped Persons), 1983, in press.

Hobbs, N. *The futures of children*. Los Angeles: Jossey-Bass, 1975.

Howey, K. R., Yarger, S.J., & Joyce, B.R. *Improving teacher education*. Washington, DC: Association of Teacher Education, 1978.

Hunt, D.E., & Sullivan, E.V. *Between psychology and education*. Hinsdale, IL: The Dryden Press, 1974.

Johnson, D.W., & Johnson, R.T. *Learning together and alone*. Englewood Cliffs, NJ: Prentice-Hall, 1975.

Kohlberg, L. Stage and sequence: The cognitive-developmental approach to socialization. In D. Goslin (Ed.), *Handbook of socialization: Theory and research*. New York: Rand McNally, 1969.

Lazar, I. Early intervention is effective. *Educational Leadership*, 1981, *38* (4), 303–305.

Meehl, P. Specific genetic etiology, psychodynamics and therapeutic nihilism. *International Journal of Mental Health*, 1972, *1*, 10–27.

Reynolds, M.C. On the implications of mainstreaming in the USA. *McGill Journal of Education*, (Fall) 1979, *XIV* (3), 317–325.

Reynolds, M.C., Birch, J.W., Grohs, D., Howsam, R., & Morsink, C. *A common body of practice for teachers: The challenge of Public Law 94-142 to teacher education*. Washington, DC: American Association of Colleges for Teacher Education, 1980.

Reynolds, M.C., & Wang, M. *Restructuring "special" school programs: A position paper*. Pittsburgh: Learning Research and Development Center, University of Pittsburgh, 1981.

Rubin, R., & Balow, B. Learning and behavior disorders: A longitudinal study. *Exceptional Children*, 1971, *38*, 293–299.

Scriven, M. Comments on Glass. In M.C. Reynolds & J. Brandl (Eds.), *Policy Studies Review* (special issue entitled Public Policy and the Education of Handicapped Persons), 1983, in press.

Sellars, W. Counterfactuals, dispositions and causal modalities. In H. Feigl, M. Scriven & G. Maxwell (Eds.), *Minnesota studies in philosophy of science* (Vol. 2). Minneapolis, MN: University of Minnesota Press, 1958.

Shaw, R.A. High school students' feelings of accomplishment. *Phi Delta Kappan*, June 1982, *63* (10), 704.

Sprinthall, N.A. Psychology for secondary schools: The sabertooth curriculum revisited? *American Psychologist*, 1980, *35* (4), 336–347.

Stevens, G.D. *Taxonomy in special education for children with body disorders*. Pittsburgh: Dept. of Special Education and Rehabilitation, University of Pittsburgh, 1962.

U.S. Department of Education. *Fourth annual report to Congress on the implementation of Public Law 94-142*. Washington, DC: Author, 1982.

Wang, M.C. Adaptive instruction: Implications for improving school practices. *Theory into Practice*, March 1980, *19* (2), 122–127.

Mary Story

7

Nutritional Needs of Adolescents with Chronic and Handicapping Conditions

Nutrition is increasingly recognized as an essential component in the total care of adolescent patients who have chronic and handicapping conditions. Nutrition-related problems occur frequently in these children and youths, and adequate nutrition is important for both prevention and treatment. Strong evidence now exists that recovery can be accelerated in many chronic disorders, resistance to infections can be strengthened, and duration of hospitalization can be decreased if close attention is paid to the nutritional status of the patient throughout the entire course of illness (Krieger, 1982). Early assessment of nutritional status, followed by counseling, intervention, and surveillance in the area of nutrition will substantially help ensure the health and well-being of youths with chronic and handicapping disorders. Regardless of the nature of the disease or disorder, the individual's growth and development to his or her full capacity must be promoted (Baer, 1982).

This chapter outlines some of the major nutrition-related problems of chronically ill and handicapped adolescents and discusses their nutritional assessment. To discuss normal nutritional needs of adolescents is beyond the scope of this paper; and the reader is referred elsewhere (Dwyer, 1981; Heald, 1979; Hegsted, 1976; Lucas, 1981; Marino and King, 1980; McGanity, 1976; Tanner, 1962).

GENERAL NUTRITION-RELATED PROBLEMS AND CONSIDERATIONS

The nutritional requirements of young people with handicaps or chronic illnesses may be significantly altered by either the medical condition or the therapy necessary to control the disorder. These youths face a greater risk than average for nutritional problems, resulting from their condition, and indeed, nutrition-related problems occur frequently among children and adolescents with chronic and handicapping conditions. Examples of frequently reported nutritional problems and factors contributing to high nutritional risk are presented in Table 7-1. This table is not meant to be inclusive; it should be kept in mind that considerable individual variation exists among the patient population.

Obesity

Obesity is common in youths who suffer from chronic and handicapping disorders. It is frequently seen in those with Prader-Willi, Carpenter, Cohen's, Laurence-Moon Biedl, and Down's syndromes, myelomeningocele, and other syndromes or conditions that limit activity. In addition to reduced activity as a major factor contributing to obesity, excessive calories may be ingested through offerings of overprotective parents or through eating out of frustration and boredom. Obesity may be psychologically induced, resulting from emotional disturbances or psychological trauma stemming from the illness. For some, food and overeating may be among the few pleasures they have in life. Food and eating may also be used to express independence, as a means of control, or an expression of conflict with parents.

Spina Bifida

Obesity is a frequent complication in adolescents with spina bifida. There is a wide variation in the degree of paralysis encountered in these individuals. Obesity can impair the ambulation potential of a spina bifida patient to such a degree that an individual who could be ambulatory may be wheelchair bound due to excessive weight (Rickard, Brady, & Gresham, 1977). An example is those individuals who, because of lower muscle weakness, are unable to straighten their legs completely during weight bearing. If the knee can only be extended to 45 degrees, a mechanical disadvantage is imposed that requires a muscular force equivalent to three and a half times the body weight for ambulation. Under these circumstances, any increase in body weight increases the muscle force requirement 350 percent above normal (Rickard, Brady, Hempel, & Gresham, 1976).

The problem is complicated by an early trend toward obesity. Nu-

Table 7-1

Frequently Reported Nutrition Problems and Factors Contributing
to High Nutritional Risk of Children with Handicapping Conditions

Diagnostic classes of conditions/diseases	Examples of frequently reported nutrition problems and factors contributing to high nutrition risk
Infective and parasitic diseases	1, 9
Neoplasm	1, 2, 7, 10, 12
Allergic, endocrine system, and nutritional diseases (e.g., asthma, PKU, rickets, diabetes, etc.)	1, 2, 3, 4, 6, 9, 11, 12
Diseases of blood and blood-forming organs (e.g., sickle cell anemia, etc.)	2, 4, 7, 10, 12
Mental, psychoneurotic and personality (e.g., sickle cell anemia, etc.)	1, 3, 5, 8, 10, 11, 12
Disorders of nervous system and sense organs (e.g., cerebral palsy, epilepsy, hearing impairment, etc.)	1, 2, 3, 4, 5, 7, 8, 10, 11, 12
Diseases of circulatory system	1, 2, 3, 7, 11, 12
Disease of respiratory system	1, 6, 7, 10, 12
Diseases of digestive system (e.g., cystic fibrosis, chronic inflammatory disease)	1, 2, 4, 5, 9, 12
Diseases of genito-urinary tract (e.g., nephritis, etc.)	2, 10, 14, 15
Diseases of bone and organs of movement (e.g., muscular dystrophy, scoliosis, etc.)	1, 5, 8, 11, 12
Congenital malformations (e.g., cleft palate and lip, spina bifida, circulatory system, etc.)	1, 3, 4, 5, 8, 11, 12
Certain diseases of early infancy (e.g., brain injury, etc.)	1, 8, 10, 11, 12
Accidents, poisoning and violence (e.g., amputations, burns, etc.)	1, 2, 8, 11

Nutritional problems and factors contributing to high nutritional risk

1. Altered energy needs/intake
2. Altered nutrient needs
3. Condition of oral cavity hampers food intake and/or indicates nutrition problems
4. Nutrient deficiencies
5. Constipation/diarrhea
6. Food allergies
7. Lack of nutritional knowledge/ vulnerability of misinformation
8. Poor appetite
9. Delayed feeding skill development/mechanical feeding problems
10. Malabsorption
11. Nutrient–drug interactions
12. Maladaptive behaviors

Modified from Nutrition Services for Children with Handicaps. *A manual for state title V programs.* M.T. Baer, project director, December, 1982, With permission.

tritionists at the James Whitcomb Riley Hospital for Children, Indianapolis, Indiana have observed a trend toward overweight in children with mye-lomeningocele that can be recognized as early as six months of age. Fur-thermore, over 90 percent of their teenage population with myelomen-ingocele are overweight (Rickard et al., 1977). Although obesity is an extremely visible disorder, the true extent of excess weight in children with myelomeningocele can be easily overlooked if conventional means of measurement are used. In spina bifida children there is a pronounced difference in distribution of body fat, which comprises a greater proportion of body mass. A greater percentage of fat is found in the lower limbs and is apparently associated with lower-limb paralysis (Hayes-Allen & Tring, 1973). Because of differences in body fat, standard weight and height cri-teria may tend to underestimate the extent of obesity. Therefore, it has been recommended that a combination of skinfold measurements—triceps, subscapular, suprailiac, biceps, and calf—is the most reliable method for assessing body fat distribution in spina bifida patients (Hayes-Allen & Tring, 1973).

The concept of obesity prevention should be introduced during the initial hospitalization for operative repair of the spinal cord defect. Obesity, once established, is notoriously difficult to treat, and since there is a marked tendency for perpetuation, the ultimate aim should be prevention. Increased parental education, awareness of inappropriate eating, elimi-nation of food rewards, limitation of high calorie–low nutrient foods, and greater school involvement may spare some children the burden of be-coming overweight with all its attendant problems.

Regardless of their disorder or condition, weight reduction for ov-erweight adolescents should be reserved for those who have finished their growth period. A goal for adolescents who are growing is the prevention of further gain in body fat (monitored through skinfold measurements). For those who have completed their growth, the treatment plan may in-clude actual weight reduction. Adolescents with serious defects and ex-tensive paralysis who have limited activity will require fewer calories for appropriate energy balance or weight loss than their active peers. With limited physical activity, an intake of only 800 to 1000 kcal/day may be needed to induce weight loss. When less than 1000 kcal/per day are pro-vided, careful attention should be paid to the nutritional adequacy of the diet. A weight-loss goal of one-fourth or one-half pound per week would be a reasonable expectation.

Prader-Willi Syndrome

The Prader-Willi syndrome is characterized by obesity, hypogon-adism, hypotonia, and mental retardation. Sequalae associated with obes-ity, such as diabetes and respiratory impairment, have high morbidity and are often responsible for the premature mortality associated with this syn-drome (Bistrian, Blackburn, Hallowell, & Heddle, 1977). Attempts to control the obesity by dietary management have frequently been unsuccessful. Hyperphagia, coupled with the mental retardation associated with the syndrome, makes intervention exceedingly difficult (Coplin, Hine, & Germican, 1976).

Conventional dietary treatments aimed at the reduction of obesity in Prader-Willi patients have generally proved to be unsuccessful. Children with Prader-Willi require fewer calories than normal children of comparable age to maintain their weight, and they require more drastic reductions to lose weight (Coplin et al., 1976). Thus, it becomes difficult to reduce calories to a level that promotes weight loss.

Bistrian et al. (1977) successfully treated obesity in four older Prader-Willi adolescents using a protein-sparing modified fast consisting of 1.5 g of meat protein/kg of ideal body weight, plus vitamin, mineral, and fluid supplements. Positive nitrogen equilibrium was sustained in spite of starvation ketosis. Clinical diabetes mellitus in two subjects was rapidly ameliorated by this regimen. Short-term weight loss greater than 18 kg occurred in three of the four subjects, and reduced weight persisted during observation periods of 26 to 55 months. The researchers suggested that the modified, protein-sparing fast may eliminate or reduce hunger, a feature of concern in the Prader-Willi syndrome, since a hypothalamic disturbance of satiety has been postulated.

Behavioral treatment approaches have also been shown to be promising in achieving weight loss in these individuals (Altman, Bondy, & Hirsch, 1978). Regardless of the treatment program used, a firm commitment from the family or care giver is needed, and family involvement is imperative. Ideally, obesity should be prevented before food habits are established or health complications become evident.

Cerebral Palsy

Nutritional problems are common in infants, children, and youths with cerebral palsy (CP) (American Dietetic Association, 1981; Eddy, Nicholson, & Wheeler, 1965; Ruby & Matheny, 1962). In spastic paralysis there is an increase in stretch reflexes and irritability of muscles. An attempt to move a leg in one direction may be prevented by contraction of antagonist muscles. This blocks an intended motion and generally limits physical movement of any kind in the spastic patient. Because of limited activity, caloric requirements will be lowered (Calvert & Davies, 1978). Obesity, which further impedes mobility, is a common problem in children and youth with spastic palsy.

On the other hand, adolescents with athetoid CP have involuntary motor activity and consequently have very high energy needs. These adolescents may have difficulty consuming adequate energy intakes and consequently, many athetotic youth are extremely thin. Futhermore, poor function of the mouth, tongue, and throat may make eating a slow, laborious process and normal mastication of food difficult. Phelps (1951) estimated that an athetotic 17-year-old male would require about 6000 cal/day to maintain ideal weight for height. Conversely, a male of the same age with spastic palsy may require only 1500 cal/day to maintain ideal weight, and a normal 17-year-old needs about 3000 cal/day.

Providing adequate nutrition for CP patients is of concern to the health care provider; for those with spastic palsy who have low energy requirements, care must be taken to ensure that the diet is nutritionally adequate, and for those with athetoid palsy, consideration must be given to increasing the food intake.

Undernutrition and Growth Failure

Recently, accumulating data have pointed to the role of chronic malnutrition in chronically ill adolescents who have growth impairment. Studies have documented that nutritional therapy promotes positive nitrogen balance, weight gain, and frequently, acceleration in growth. Most of the research on malnutrition and growth failure in children and youths with chronic illnesses have focused on cystic fibrosis and inflammatory bowel disease; consequently, it is these two disorders that will be reviewed here. However, the information presented can be applied to other chronic malabsorptive states, as well as chronic liver and renal diseases.

Cystic fibrosis. Cystic fibrosis (CF) is the most prevalent inheritable chronic disease in white children and occurs in about 1 of 2000 live births (Chase, Long & Lann, 1979). Medical advances have improved the life span of CP patients; 70 percent are expected to live to age 17 (Robinson & Norman). However, in spite of the great strides made toward improving the survival rate and arresting pulmonary deterioration, impaired growth and malnutrition affect a significant number of those with CF (Solomon, Wagonfeld, Rieger, Jacob, Bolt, Horst, Rothberg, & Sandstead, 1981).

The importance of malnutrition in the disease process remains unknown; however, studies have indicated that relative underweight (weight corrected for height) is a major factor adversely affecting survival in CF patients (Kraemer, Rudeberg, Hadorn, & Rossi, 1978). Shepherd, Cooksley, and Cook (1980) have shown that adequate nutritional support can favorably affect growth, clinical status, and the course of chronic pulmonary disease in some patients.

Pancreatic insufficiency leading to fat, protein, fat-soluble vitamin B_{12}, and malabsorption of minerals, such as iron and zinc, is nearly universal among those with CF (Chase et al., 1979). Patients are generally administered water miscible forms of fat-soluble vitamins and pancreatic enzymes, which ameliorates but does not completely resolve the problem of malabsorption; poor growth and malnutrition persist.

One recent study (Solomons et al., 1981) compared several biochemical indices of nutrition between a group of 18 juvenile CF patients and 40 normal controls. The results revealed among the CF patients an overall reduction in the mean concentration of many nutrients, many of which were at deficient levels. Water-soluable vitamins were minimally affected, whereas levels of the fat-soluble vitamins, Vitamin A and 25-OH-chole-calciferol, were significantly depressed. These effects occurred despite outpatient management that included pulmonary physiotherapy, inter-mittent antibiotics, a low-fat, high-protein diet, pancreatic enzyme re-placement, and multivitamin supplementation with water miscible fat-sol-uble vitamins.

Patients with CF have been commonly characterized as having vo-racious appetites; however, studies have repeatedly shown that these pa-tients usually have dietary intakes that are inadequate for their needs (Chase et al., 1979; Hubbard & Mangrum, 1982; Shwachman, 1981). Pa-tients with CF need an energy intake of about 150 percent of the RDAs for a healthy person of their age and sex to compensate for the increased nutrient loss and increased energy expenditure due to infections or fever as well as to the additional energy needs for respiration and performance of physical therapy (Hubbard & Mangrum 1982).

Growth failure and undernutrition are frequently reported in CF pa-tients. Sproul and Huang (1964) studied 110 CF patients between the ages of 6 and 18 and reported that the majority had significant weight and height deficits and that the more severe the pulmonary process, the greater the height and weight impairment. Lapey, Kathwinkel, DiSant'Agnese, and Laster (1974) found this to be true and concluded that the degree of growth failure and the state of nutrition were more closely correlated with the degree of severity of pulmonary disease and its relapses than they were with pancreatic insufficiencies. Shepherd et al. (1980) studied the effects of nutrition therapy on growth and in the clinical, nutritional, and respi-ratory status of 12 undernourished CF patients from six months before to six months after a period of supplemental parenteral nutrition. Nutrition therapy consisted of hypercaloric intake for 21 days. Results showed that a "catch-up" growth in weight and height occurred and that there was a significant reduction in the rate of infections as well as a sustained im-provement in respiratory function. The researchers concluded that ade-quate nutritional support can favorably affect growth, clinical status, and the course of chronic pulmonary disease in CF patients. Although this is encouraging, studies will need to further elucidate the potential impact of nutrition on growth retardation in CF.

When oral intake of nutrients is insufficient to reverse malnutrition, nasogastric and parenteral nutrition offer feasible alternatives. Poor food intake is common when there is poor pulmonary function or during active lung infection. Poor appetite may be as important a determinant of un-dernutrition and growth failure in CF as is nutrient loss from malabsorption and increased energy needs (Shepherd et al. 1980). Labored breathing, made worse by lung infections, may cause fatigue and anorexia. Conse-quently, energy and nutrient intake are reduced at a time when the need for them is the greatest (Hubbard et al., 1982). During such times, parenteral nutrition or nasogastric feeding may be warranted.

Studies that have investigated the role of nutrition in maintaining optimal growth and clinical status in CF patients have noted the importance of accurate and ongoing nutritional assessment throughout all phases of the disease process. Nutritional status should be monitored via anthropometric and biochemical measurements, clinical evaluation, and dietary assessment at regular intervals; the individual nutrition plan should be revised as necessary.

Nutritional guidelines for CF patients generally include a high-protein, high-energy, moderate- to low-fat dietary intake, supplemental vitamins, and individualized use of pancreatic enzymes. In adolescents and young adults with CF, the symptoms of malabsorption appear to be less prominent, and the need for dietary fat restrictions less marked, than in younger children (Lapey et al., 1974). Adolescents with CF should be free to adjust their diets instead of being bound to a strict regimen. They usually know how much fat and what combinations of food will cause gastrointestinal distress, and they should be encouraged to regulate their own diet on the basis of symptomatology, with help from the nutritionist when needed (Hubbard et al., 1982; Lapey et al., 1974).

Chronic inflammatory bowel disease.   Crohn's disease and ulcerative colitis are two chronic illnesses of unknown pathogenesis with periods of clinical remission and exacerbation. While both disorders affect the colon, only Crohn's disease extends into the ileum, which may in some cases be the sole site of involvement. The inflammatory process in ulcerative colitis involves the mucosa, which infiltrates and abscesses and tends to be widespread (Krieger, 1982). The two disorders share a number of clinical manifestations, including mucoid or bloody diarrhea, abdominal pain, anorexia, fever, weight loss, growth failure, and delayed puberty (Krieger, 1982). Although there are many similarities, long-term management and prognosis tend to be different.

Growth failure is a well-known complicaton of inflammatory bowel disease (IBD) and is difficult to treat. Growth failure and delayed sexual maturation have been described in 20–30 percent of IBD patients under the age of 21, particularly those with Crohn's disease (McCaffery, Nasor, Laurence, & Kirsner, 1970). Growth retardation may preceed clinical manifestation of IBD by years and may be unrelated to the severity of the disease.

The etiology of abnormal growth remains unknown: endocrine function does not appear to account for the severe growth impairment. Recent reports have emphasized that chronic malnutrition is the major factor contributing to growth retardation in adolescents with IBD (Davidson, 1982; Grand, 1981; Kelts, Grand, Shen, Watkins, Werlin, & Boehme, 1979;

Motil, Grand, Matthews, Bier, Maletskos, & Young, 1982). Inadequate intake, excessive losses, malabsorption, and increased nutrient requirements are all factors leading to the chronically malnourished state (Kelts et al. 1979).

Inadequate intake may be caused by disease-induced anorexia or by voluntary restrictions (Davidson, 1982). Patients may restrict food consumption voluntarily because of increases in diarrhea associated with the ingestion of food or due to exacerbation of abdominal pain by meals (Grand, 1981).

Decreased absorption of nutrients and increased losses also occur in patients with IBD. Steatorrhea occurs in approximately 40 percent of Crohn's disease patients and reflects mucosal injury, bacterial overgrowth, bile salt deficiency, and reduction of bile salt pool as a consequence of ileal disease (Grand, 1981). Calcium and magnesium losses are increased when steatorrhea is present. Excessive losses of blood and protein in stool as well as hypoalbuminemia are also common. In addition, decreased levels of folic acid, iron, and vitamin B_{12} are frequently observed (Davidson, 1982; Grand, 1981; Kelts et al., 1979).

Alterations in zinc metabolism in adolescents with IBD have also been reported. Zinc deficiency is known to be associated with growth failure and delayed sexual development (Sandstead, 1982a). Although only a limited number of patients with Crohn's disease or ulcerative colitis show laboratory evidence of zinc depletion, testing is complicated by the fact that currently no unequivocal diagnostic laboratory tests for zinc deficiency exist. Keeping this limitation in mind, zinc levels should be assessed in patients with IBD. Even in the face of normal laboratory values, a carefully controlled therapeutic intervention trial with zinc supplementation may be warranted if zinc deficiency is suspected due to growth failure, impaired taste, or anorexia. Zinc supplementation should be limited to two or three times the RDA unless otherwise medically indicated (Sandstead, 1982b). In summary, known nutrient deficiencies commonly encountered in adolescents with IBD include calcium, magnesium, zinc, iron, vitamin B_{12} and folate, the fat-soluble vitamins, and protein.

Several studies have investigated growth disturbances in children and youths with Crohn's disease and the role of nutritional therapy in growth restoration and improvement in nutritional status (Kelts et al., 1979; Kirschner, Klich, Kalman, deFavaro, Rosenberg, 1981; Layden, Rosenberg, Newchausky, Elsou, & Rosenberg, 1976; Motil et al., 1982; Strobel, Byrne, & Ament 1979). The therapeutic approaches have included intravenous hyperalimentation, combined parenteral and oral intake, and oral nutritional supplementation alone. Kelts et al. (1979) studied seven Crohn's patients ($\bar{x}$ 13.7 years) with severe growth failure, before, during, and after the use of parenteral nutrition as a supplement to oral intake. The patients received approximately eight weeks of combined oral and parenteral nutrition, achieving a minimum of 75 kcal/kg/day. Nutritional therapy demonstrated a marked increase in total body weight and lean body mass. There was also a dramatic and sustained growth acceleration: growth velocity increased significantly and continued at an increased rate for at least six months following therapy. The patients responded as chronically malnourished individuals who resumed growth in response to adequate caloric repletion, leading the authors to conclude that the growth failure of Crohn's disease is a failure of chronic inadequate nutritional intake and not a primary function of the pathophysiology of the disease.

Strobel et al. (1979) also demonstrated promising results in 17 patients (ages 9–20) with severe symptomatic Crohn's disease using home parenteral nutrition. All 17 showed a marked improvement in disease symptoms and weight gain while receiving home parenteral nutrition. Ten patients demonstrated catch-up growth, while four others showed an increase in height.

Parenteral nutrition has limitations, including expense and risk of infection. An alternative that has had documented benefits is oral nutritional supplementation. Using this method, Kirschner et al. (1981) recently demonstrated reversal in growth failure among seven adolescents with mild to severe Crohn's disease. Prior to intervention, caloric intake ranged from 1000 to 2000 kcal/day in subjects, with the average energy intake being only 56 percent of the RDA. Oral nutritional supplements (Ensure® [Ross], Vivonex® [Norwich-Eaton]) were initially added to the regular diet, providing an additional 600–1200 calories until daily energy goals were met with food alone. Oral supplementation was used for up to one year. With supplementation, the mean caloric intake was 2493 calories or about 91 percent of the RDA. The majority of these patients demonstrated catch-up growth. Linear growth velocity increased from an average of 1.8 cm/year in the first year after intervention. During the four-year observation period, six of the seven subjects returned to within 5 percent of their preillness growth curve.

Oral caloric supplementation, if started at the time growth retardation is first evident, may be sufficient to prevent serious growth impairment. If oral nutritional supplementation fails, parenteral nutrition offers a feasible adjunct with which to ensure adequate caloric intake (Kelts et al., 1979). The potential for growth restoration is dependent on the patient's age, the duration of caloric deprivation, and the timing and extent of nutritional replacement. The longer the period of deprivation and the closer the patient to puberty, the lower the potential is for growth recovery (Kelts et al., 1979).

The role of diet in the treatment of chronic IBD continues to be controversial. Recommendations for diet therapy have included avoidance of certain foods, spices, and fiber, since these substances are presumed to exacerbate gastrointestinal symptoms. The basis for most of these dietary restrictions is questionable; currently, there are more myths than facts concerning dietary therapy for IBD. No uniform dietary management can be prescribed for all individuals with IBD; rather, treatment plans should be individualized (Davidson, 1982; Grand, 1981). During periods of active illness, a low-residue, low-fiber diet is often helpful, and vitamin and mineral supplementation may be warranted. However, during stable periods there is little reason to adhere to such a diet. Overly restrictive diets often lead to suboptimal calorie and nutrient intake and take the joy out of eating.

While the occasional IBD patient may have an acquired lactase deficiency that requires milk restriction, in the vast majority it is unnecessary. It fact, its liberal use should be encouraged in those who are underweight. While many physicians and nutritionists recommend a time-limited trial of milk restriction in all newly diagnosed patients to rule out lactose intolerance, the hypothesis of a milk-protein allergy has been weakened, and it is no longer considered a cause of the disease by most authorities (Krieger, 1982).

Since dietary intake among teenagers with IBD has been repeatedly documented as poor, patients should be encouraged to eat whatever they desire in order to help maintain good intake and nutritional health. Monitoring of nutritional status is essential. Emphasis should be placed on the consumption of a balanced and nutritious diet that is acceptable to the teenager. In those who are underweight or who have growth retardation, high caloric nutritional supplementation should be used.

Malnutrition in Adolescents with Cancer

Cancer frequently has a markedly deleterious effect on the nutritional status of individuals. Malnutrition is not uncommon, especially in children and adolescents with active disease, those who have suffered a relapse, or those who are undergoing aggressive chemotherapy. The incidence of malnutrition varies widely among cancer patients; the degree is generally associated with the extent of the malignancy (van Eys, 1982). Van Eys (1979) reported overt malnutrition in 17.5 percent of a group of newly diagnosed children with abdominal or pelvic tumors and 37.5 percent among those with metastatic disease. Not only does severe malnutrition occur with greater frequency among patients with advanced neoplasia, but it appears more frequently in conjunction with certain malignancies, such as Ewing's sarcoma and Wilms' tumor, than in others, such as osteosarcoma (Rickard, Grosfeld, Kirksey, Ballantine, & Baehner, 1979; van Eys, 1979).

The causes of malnutrition are complex and multifactorial. Malnutrition may result from anorexia; involvement of the gastrointestinal tract by tumor; hypercatabolism induced by the disease; increased energy needs due to sepsis; nutrient trapping by the tumor at the expense of the host;

and cancer therapy, surgery, radiation therapy, and chemotherapy (Jaffe, 1981). Reduction in caloric intake is the most significant contributor to the development of malnutrition. Anorexia is a common consequence of cancer and may be due to progression of the disease, treatment effects, or psychological factors. Early satiety, despite feelings of hunger prior to a meal, is also frequently reported among cancer patients. The incidence and degree of anorexia and early satiety increase with progression of cancer (Theologides, 1977). Alterations in taste and smell and development of food aversion may be associated with decreased food intake. While this does not occur in all cancer patients, an elevated threshold for sweetness and lowered threshold for bitterness develop in some with progressive disease. Common food aversions include meat and chocolate. The mechanisms responsbile for gustatory and olfactory alterations are not known. In addition to a distorted taste, conditioned aversion to eating may develop in patients who experience nausea, distress, or vomiting during or after a meal. Emotional stress may also significantly interfere with intake. Patients experiencing anorexia and early satiety should be advised to eat small, frequent meals and should be encouraged to eat what they desire, when they feel like eating it. Well-meaning parents should be cautioned against trying to coerce adolescents into eating and developing an eat-a-little-more syndrome (Theologides, 1977).

A food intake inadequate for caloric demands leads to malnutrition, which in turn decreases tolerance for chemotherapy, surgery, or radiation therapy, and reduces immunocompetence with increased risk for infection. This is especially true with opportunistic microorganisms. Inadequate caloric ingestion further complicates treatment of the disease, thus threatening survival. Furthermore, malnutrition causes malaise and listlessness, and it reduces the quality of life. It should not be ignored, as it is frequently the cause of death. Shils (1979) has observed that many physicians act as if malnutrition were an inevitable sequela of cancer, and little is done to treat, much less to prevent, the condition. The severe form of protein–energy malnutrition, cachexia, is commonly observed in cancer patients who have active disease or who are undergoing therapy (Rickard et al., 1979, van Eys, 1979; van Eys, 1982). The ideal approach is prevention rather than rehabilitation of a malnourished patient; malnutrition is not inevitable. Every patient should have early and periodic assessment of his or her nutritional status to identify those at risk for nutritional depletion and deprivation as well as those who are already malnourished. Such a nutritional assessment should be part of the admission evaluation (Shils, 1979).

The importance of early nutritional evaluation was underscored recently by Donaldson and co-workers, (1981) who conducted a retrospective chart review of 244 children and youths with a variety of cancers to investigate the relationship of nutritional status at time of first diagnosis to various measurements of disease and survival. Nutritional status (measured by the ratio of weight and height compared with an age-adjusted standard) was directly related to freedom from relapse in children with solid tumors, whether they had localized or metastatic disease. In addition, improved survival was related to good nutritional status in children with localized lymphomas or solid tumors, although such a relationship was not evident in those with advanced disease.

Severe malnutrition demands intensive therapy. Attempts to prevent the cachexia of cancer with regular diets have been largely unsuccessful (Rickard et al., 1979). A rapid, safe, and efficacious approach to improving nutritional status of the cachectic cancer patient is total parenteral nutrition (TPN). Such hyperalimentation provides all essential amino acids, vitamins, minerals, and calories needed to promote weight gain, sustain a positive nitrogen balance, and maintain anabolism. At present there are no scientific data to support the belief that intravenous nutritional support will stimulate tumor growth (Jaffe, 1979).

In general, when weight falls 10 percent below ideal weight, nutritional support should be considered (Filler, Dietz, Suskin, Haffe, & Cassady, 1979; Mauer, 1979). Several studies have indicated that malnutrition associated with cancer and its treatment can be reversed or prevented by TPN (Filler et al., 1979). Rickard et al. (1979) investigated the effectiveness of enteral and parenteral nutrition in maintaining adequate nutritional states or reversing energy malnutrition in 28 children and youths with advanced neoplastic disease. Despite a concerted effort to prevent nutritional depletion by oral supplementation during the intense stage of cancer treatment, patients were unable to ingest sufficient calories to meet their needs, and dramatic weight loss ensued in 80 percent of them. Most of the patients were meeting only 50 percent of the RDA for energy. When administered for 28 or more days, TPN was highly effective in nutritionally replenishing patients. This was demonstrated by improved weight, skinfold measurements, albumin and transferrin levels, and in most cases, skin test reactivity. This and other studies have found that TPN of less than 14 days' duration is ineffective and is not sufficient to restore weight, fat reserves, and albumin concentrations of severely malnourished children and adolescents. The preceding study also found that improved nutritional status was maintained with enteral nutrition when children had finished the initial and most aggressive phase of cancer therapy and had no evidence of disease. Other studies in children and adolescents have found that TPN not only increased body weight and renewed strength and energy, but it also improved outlook and general behavior (Filler et al., 1979).

Data are still not available on the effect of TPN and improved nutritional health on tumor response or long-term cure rate in adolescents who have cancer. However, several researchers have reported that TPN in adult patients hastens postoperative recovery, improves tolerance to chemotherapy and reduces its side effects, allows continuation of cancer therapy, improves tumor response, and restores cellular immunity (Rickard et al., 1979).

Malnutrition and the Hospitalized Patient

Recent surveys have shown that malnutrition among hospitalized adults, adolescents, and children is far more common than previously recognized. Bistrian and co-workers (1974, 1976) reported that 44 percent of adult patients on a general medical service and 50 percent of adult surgical patients had protein–calorie malnutrition as evidenced by anthropometric and laboratory measurements. An association between nutritional status and length of hospital stay has been demonstrated. One recent report (Weinser, Hunker, Krumdieck, & Butterworth, 1979) revealed that on admission to a general medical service, 48 percent of adult patients were judged according to eight nutrition-related parameters to have a high likelihood of malnutrition. A malnourished state correlated with a longer hospital stay (20 days versus 12 days for patients with a low likelihood of malnutrition) and an increased mortality rate (13 percent versus 4 percent). Nutritional status progressively declined with hospitalization in 69 percent of the patients.

Surveys conducted on nutritional status of hospitalized pediatric patients have revealed results similar to those reported in adults. Merritt and Suskind's (1979) survey of hospitalized pediatric patients conducted in a large urban children's hospital found that one third of patients showed evidence of acute malnutrition. Hospitalization for more than 14 days was associated with significantly lower values for all anthropometric measurements except height for age. Parsons, Francoewe, Howland, Spengler, & Pencharz, (1980) reported the nutritional status of 182 patients in a pediatric referral center upon admission and after two weeks' hospitalization. Biochemical and anthropometric measurements were taken on all patients. Subnormal anthropometric measurements were found in 20 percent of the sample. Among the various pediatric age groups, adolescent surgical patients had the highest incidence of abnormal biochemical measurements. Folate deficiency, as assessed by red blood cell folate levels, was found in 29 percent of adolescent surgical patients, while 22 percent had reduced calcium and phosphorus levels. Since only a small proportion (6.6 percent) of the total sample remained in the hospital for two or more weeks, little could be concluded about the effect of hospitalization on the nutritional status of a patient, however, a significant decrease in skinfold thickness was noted over time.

It appears that a sizable proportion of pediatric patients enter the hospital in a suboptimal nutritional state and others become malnourished in the course of hospitalization. Patients with protein–calorie malnutrition do not tolerate illness well. They tend to have delayed wound healing, greater susceptibility to infection, and other complications (Butterworth & Weinser, 1980). The health care team needs to be aware not only of the normal nutritional needs of youths but also the impact of illness, infection, and surgery on nutritional and energy needs. This knowledge and attentiveness to inappropriate practices that can adversely affect nutritional health (as outlined by Butterworth & Weinser, 1980), coupled with routine nutrition assessments, can help prevent hospital-induced malnutrition and improve nutritional status. Clearly, nutritional evaluation and support are essential for good patient care.

Drug–Nutrition Interaction

Drug–nutrition interaction should be considered whenever any medication is prescribed. Health care providers should be alert to the possibilities of nutrient imbalances or deficiencies caused by drugs, so that undesirable effects can be minimized or prevented. Numerous drugs have the potential for affecting nutritional status. Drugs can alter food intake indirectly by producing side effects, such as anorexia, nausea, diarrhea, alterations in taste, vomiting, and dry mouth. Drugs may also interact with nutrients to decrease absorption, utilization, and metabolism of nutrients, to inhibit nutrient synthesis, or to increase excretion of nutrients (March, 1978). Conversely, nutrients and nonnutrient constituents of food or the relative composition of the diet can interact with drugs to influence drug absorption, metabolism, and overall drug action.

With drugs that have the potential to cause nutritional deficiencies, the actual occurrence of deficiencies is dependent on several factors, such as prior nutritional status and nutrient reserves, adequacy of diet, duration of drug use, physiological stress, and preexisting disease. Drug-induced nutrient deficiency generally develops slowly, reflecting a gradual nutrient store depletion, which indicates that the increased nutrient requirement imposed by the drugs is not being met by dietary intake (Roe, 1976). Vulnerability to drug-induced nutritional deficiency is greatest in children, adolescents, the elderly, the chronically ill, and those who have marginal or inadequate dietary intakes. In general, drug-induced malnutrition is most likely to be found in those indviduals who are on multiple-drug regimens and in those who are using drugs for long-term treatment of chronic illness.

Effect of Drugs on Appetite and Taste

Anorexia, which consequently results in decreased food intake, is a frequent side effect of many drugs. Stimulant drugs, frequently used in the treatment of attention-deficit disorders, are known for their appetite-depressant effects. These stimulant drugs reportedly suppress growth, which is generally believed to result from diminished food intake caused by the anorexia (Roe, 1979; Silverstone, 1968). When medication is discontinued during the summer months, catch-up growth occurs (Safer, Allen, & Barr, 1975). It is believed that growth rebound is associated with an increase in food intake (Roe, 1979). Cancer chemotherapeutic drugs may cause anorexia as well as nausea and vomiting. Aversion to specific foods may also be associated with the chemotherapy.

Certain drugs may affect appetite by altering taste sensation. Examples include the antifungal agent, griseofulvin; penicillamine, used in Wilson's disease, heavy metal poisoning, and rheumatoid arthritis; and lincomycin, used to treat systemic infection. Penicillamine may cause loss of taste, due perhaps to a zinc or copper deficiency induced by the drug (Roe, 1976, 1979). Medications that contain potassium, iodide, or potassium bromide produce a salty, bitter taste in the mouth. Other drugs, including potassium chloride, liquid chloral hydrate, paraldehyde, and liquid vitamin B complex are so unpleasant tasting that they may cause appetite suppression.

There are also drugs with side effects that stimulate appetite and, consequently, weight gain. These include insulin, sulfonylureas, barbiturates, corticosteroids, and oral contraceptives. Psychotropic drugs, such as thorazine, librium, valium, and tricyclate antidepressants, also have appetite-promoting effects.

Effect of Drugs on Nutrients

Drugs can induce malabsorption by affecting the intestinal lumen or the motility of the gastrointestinal tract or by impairing the integrity of the mucosa (Roe, 1976). Secondary malnutrition can also be induced by interference with the absorption, disposition, or metabolism of a specific nutrient (Roe, 1979). By interfering with gastrointestinal motility, some drugs, such as laxatives and cathartics, may result in loss of electrolytes, steatorrhea, and decreased uptake of glucose (Hartshorn, 1977). Mineral oil dissolves fat-soluble vitamins and decreases their absorption and should only be used for a short duration in adolescents. Certain antibiotics, particularly neomycin, bind fatty acids and bile acids and may cause steatorrhea; they may also decrease absorption of folic acid, vitamin B_{12}, and D-xylose. Antacids that contain aluminum (Maalox® [Rorer], Mylanta® [Stuart], Gelusil® [Parke-Davis]) may decrease absorption of phosphate, fluoride, and vitamin A.

Drugs may also adversely affect metabolism of various nutrients. Vitamin B_6 deficiency can result from treatment with isoniazid or cycloserine (antituberculous agents) and penicillamine by forming a complex with the vitamin and rendering it inactive. Folic acid antagonists, such as methotrexate and aminopterin, used in the treatment of neoplasms, interfere with folate metabolism and thus impair DNA synthesis. Hydrocortisone and its analogues may cause a breakdown of glycogen to glucose, resulting in hyperglycemia, increased protein catabolism, and negative nitrogen balance (Hartshorn, 1977; March, 1978).

Anticonvulsants, such as diphenylhydantoin and phenobarbital, can induce deficiencies in folate, vitamin D, and possibly B_{12}, and can cause abnormalities in bone metabolism (Roe, 1976). Reports of rickets and osteomalacia in patients on anticonvulsant medication are not uncommon (Borgstedt, 1972; Lifshitz & MacLaren, 1973; Medilinsky, 1974). The interference with vitamin D metabolism appears to occur at a stage of hepatic conversion from cholecalciferol to 25-hydroxycholecalciferol (Roe, 1976). The incidence of abnormalities appears to increase with the duration of therapy, and deficiencies are more severe if phenytoin (Dilantin® [Parke-Davis] and phenobarbital are given together (Roe, 1976). Since many children and youths who are on anticonvulsant medications have been found to have significant derangement of mineral metabolism, many authorities recommend vitamin D supplements for such patients (Hahn, 1976; Silver, Davies, Kupersmitt, Orme, Petrie, & Vajda, 1974).

The mechanism that causes folate deficiency in patients on anticonvulsants is still unknown, although many hypotheses have been proposed, including interference with conjugates, displacement of folate from protein carriers, enzyme induction leading to folate destruction, and increased metabolism of folic acid. The prevalence of megaloblastic anemia in persons taking anticonvulsants has been found to vary from 1 to 7/1000 (Roe, 1976). The number of patients with deficient folate levels is, however, much greater. The administration of folacin and vitamin B_{12} to individuals on anticonvulsant therapy has been recommended; however, folacin supplementation should not be given routinely since experimental and clinical studies have found it to have potent convulsant properties (A.D.A., 1981).

Numerous researchers have studied the effects of oral contraceptives on nutritional status (Margen & King, 1975; Newman, Lopez, & Cole, 1978; Smith, Goldsmith, & Lawrence, 1975; Weininger, Hunker, Krumdieck, & Butterworth, 1977). Low serum levels of pyridoxine, folic acid, riboflavin, vitamin B_{12}, and zinc have been detected in women taking oral contraceptives. Blood levels of vitamin A and niacin have been reported to increase, as have those of serum triglyceride. Although oral contraceptives cause many metabolic alterations, overt nutritional deficiencies are not common. The nutritional needs of an adolescent who uses oral contraceptives should be met by diet alone with no need for supplementation, unless the diet is grossly inadequate and the patient is not motivated to make dietary modifications. In such cases, a maintenance multivitamin supplement may be necessary.

Effect of Food on Drug Absorption

The influence of food and dietary patterns on drug absorption and bioavailability is complex. Absorption of drugs may be increased or decreased by the presence of food in the gastrointestinal tract. Therefore, whether a drug is taken in a fed or fasting state, as well as specific food components that may interfere with a drug's effectiveness, must be considered. Drugs that should be taken on an empty stomach—about one hour before meals or three hours after meals—include penicillin, sulfonamides, and tetracycline. With penicillin, food slows the rate of gastric emptying, permitting the drug to be exposed for a longer time to acid, which then destroys the antibiotic. Tetracycline is chelated by calcium or iron in foods, and thus, its absorption is decreased when given with meals, especially with dairy products or iron supplements (Hartshorn, 1977). Timing becomes of clinical importance in adolescents who are taking tetracycline for the treatment of acne concomitantly with iron supplementation for iron deficiency anemia. Drugs such as anticholinergic agents are given shortly before a meal to reduce gastric acid secretion and gut motility. Drugs that are irritating to the gastrointestinal tract, such as nitrofurantoin (used in urinary tract infections); phenylbutazone, an analgesic; and aminosalicylic acid, an antitubercular agent, should be administered with, or immediately after, meals to buffer the irritating effect (Hartshorn, 1977).

Pharmacological doses of single nutrients can interfere with drug therapy. Megadoses of folic acid or vitamin B_6 given to patients who are receiving diphenylhydantoin or phenobarbital for seizure disorders may reduce serum levels of these drugs and thereby reduce their therapeutic action (Roe, 1979). Large doses of vitamin K enhance blood clotting, thus blocking the effect of anticoagulants (Roe, 1979). The current popularity of megadosing with vitamin and mineral supplements makes it essential that clinicians inquire about the use of these preparations.

NUTRITIONAL ASSESSMENT OF ADOLESCENTS

Adolescents as a group are at risk for nutritional problems both from a physiological and a psychosocial standpoint. Since the presence of chronic disease or disability may seriously interfere with adequate nutrition, adolescents who have a chronic illness or disability are at particularly high nutritional risk. Given the risk, nutritional assessment should be an essential component in the evaluation of all adolescents with chronic and handicapping conditions so as to identify

1. Those who are clinically malnourished and need nutritional support
2. Those with limited nutrient stores or exceptionally high nutrient needs who are at high risk for becoming overtly malnourished without nutritional intervention
3. Those who have adequate stores and reserves, are in good nutritional health, and require no special nutritional support (Gray & Gray, 1980).

The results and interpretation of the nutritional assessment not only serve to identify the nature and degree of any nutritional problem, but also are instrumental in developing a nutrition care plan.

There is no single measurement or test that can give an accurate picture of a person's nutritional status. A complete nutritional assessment requires the evaluation of the following: dietary assessment, anthropometric measurement, clinical evaluation, and biochemical and immunological testing.

Dietary Assessment

Fundamental to all nutritional assessments is the evaluation of dietary intake. The dietary assessment should not only evaluate the nutritional adequacy of the diet but also should be aimed at identifying adolescents who may be at nutritional risk. When conducting the dietary assessment, both qualitative and quantitative dietary data are useful. Information on intake can be obtained by a number of methods, including 24-hour food recall, dietary history, records of food consumed over a three–seven day period, and a food-frequency questionnaire. The method chosen depends upon the specificity desired, the individual obtaining the nutritional data, the time available, and the cooperation of the adolescent or caretaker. Although a dietary history will yield the most data, a 24-hour food recall and a food-frequency questionnaire tend to be the most useful for non-nutritionists since they require less professional time and are easier to administer (Alton, 1982). A major limitation of using the 24-hour food recall is that it may not be representative of a typical diet. This is especially true for adolescents, since their diets generally are not consistent. For this reason, a food-frequency questionnaire should be used in addition to the 24-hour food recall. Furthermore, when taking 24-hour food recalls, patients should be asked whether the foods represent a typical daily food pattern. Inexpensive cardboard food models as well as three-dimensional plastic models are available to help assess quantities of food eaten.

Food intake can be compared with the recommended food guide for adolescents to establish dietary adequacy.* Suspected deficiency or excesses of quantitative dietary information can be translated into nutrient data and then compared to the RDA. Numerous computer programs, some of which can be patient operated, are currently available for nutrient analysis of diets.

Additional information that is valuable in the dietary assessment of the adolescent includes meal and snack patterns, identification of cultural food habits, consumption of unusual food or pica, use of snacks, use of vitamin or mineral supplements, adherence to fad diets or unorthodox dietary regimens, exercise and activity patterns, substance use, food preferences, and attitudes and beliefs about food. Other relevant information includes cooking and storing facilities, food availability in the home, food budget, living situation and life style, and the primary person responsible for shopping and preparing of the food. All of these variables have bearing on the adequacy of the adolescent's diet and will aid in identifying any nutritional problems that may exist.

Anthropometric Measurements

Anthropometric measurements, such as height, weight, skinfold measurements, and arm circumference, are used to assess growth patterns, protein and energy reserves, undernutrition and overnutrition, and the proportion of muscle mass to body fat.

Height and weight measurements remain important indices of nutritional status and assessment of growth (Fomon, 1976). The recommended standards for assessing growth are the National Center for Health Statistics (NCHS) growth charts, which contain the heights and weights of children and adolescents ages 2–18 years and the percentiles for each group. Serial height and weight measurements should be used in evaluating growth status. Deviations in growth may be indicative of nutritional problems. Weight-for-age values of more than two standard deviations above or below those for height for age may be indicative of overweight or underweight problems (Alton, 1982). As noted previously, while short stature is associated with many chronic diseases, it is often secondary to undernutrition rather than to the disease itself (Merritt & Blackburn, 1981). Height tends to be indicative of long-standing nutritional status, while changes in weight reflect short-term nutritional adequacy. During the nutritional assessment, one needs to document recent weight changes. Blackburn and Thornton

---

*The basic recommended daily food pattern for adolescents is four servings of milk or dairy products, two servings of meat or protein equivalent, four servings of fruits or vegetables (one serving of which is high in vitamin C), and four servings of whole grain or enriched breads and cereals.

(1979) note that an excellent clue to impending protein–calorie malnutrition is a recent involuntary weight loss of ten percent or more of total body weight. Since weight measurements alone do not express relative body composition changes in terms of fat and lean body mass, additional anthropometric measurements, such as skinfold measurements and arm circumference, need to be performed.

Skinfold measurements are an indirect measurement of body fatness or calorie storage and consist of measuring a double layer of skin and subcutaneous fat at a specific body site with skinfold calipers. Skinfold thickness has been correlated with other estimates of body fat such as those derived from radiographic, densitometric, isotope dilution, and K40 counting methods, and it is considered a good index of overall body fatness (Gray & Gray, 1980). There is general agreement that the tricep skinfold area is the best single site to use, particularly for adolescents. The correlation coefficient can be increased only slightly by adding additional skinfold measurements, except for those with atypical fat distribution in whom multiple sites are useful.

Skinfold measurements are susceptable to error, and a standardized procedure is essential for reliable results. Proper methods for anthropometric measurements are described by Jelliffe (1966); the Committee on Nutritional Anthropometry (1956); and Owen (1982). The two major instruments available for measuring skinfolds are the Lange (Cambridge Scientific Industries, Inc.) and Harpenden (H.E. Morse Co.) calipers. Various inexpensive plastic calipers are also currently available, although they are less accurate.

Mid-upper arm circumference is a measure of calorie and protein stores. Arm circumference and triceps skinfold can be used to calculate both the arm muscle circumference and the arm muscle area, both of which are sensitive indices of body protein reserves. Both measures are commonly depressed with protein—calorie malnutrition (Grant 1979). These measurements can be calculated by either formula* or with the use of nomograms (Gurney & Jelliffe, 1973).

When interpreting anthropometric measurements, percentiles rather than percentages of a standard should be used. Percentiles indicate the position of a patient's measurements within a normal population rather than comparing them with standards considered to be ideal (Gray & Gray, 1980). Percentile tables for triceps skinfold, arm muscle circumference,

---

*Arm muscle circumference = Mid-arm circumference - [π x triceps skinfold]

    (mm)   (mm)   (mm)

Arm muscle area = $\dfrac{\text{Arm muscle circumference (mm)}^2}{4 \times \pi}$

  (mm²)

and arm muscle measurements for children and adolescents are currently available (Frisancho, 1974; Owen, 1982). Measurements below the 5th percentile constitute evidence of depletion, while patients whose measurements are between the 5th and 15th percentiles can be considered at risk for becoming depleted (Gray & Gray, 1980). Skinfold measurements are useful in the follow-up and monitoring of adolescents who are identified as having a potential or an existing problem of obesity. Minimum triceps skinfold thicknesses suggestive of obesity have been published by Seltzer and Mayer (1965).

Biochemical Assessment

Biochemical determination of nutritional status may consist of measuring circulating levels of nutrients in biological fluids, such as blood or urine, utilizing tests of functional enzymes or accumulation of precursors, and taking measurement of body composition. The prime objective in using laboratory tests in evaluating nutritional status is to detect marginal deficiencies, or risk of deficiency, before overt clinical signs of disease appear. Laboratory test should be ordered on an individual basis to confirm any suspicious clinical or dietary findings or dietary practices that may cause nutrient deficiencies or toxicities. They should also be selected on the basis of knowledge of the illness, medications, or treatments that may cause nutritional abnormalities. The interpretation of laboratory data is often difficult and does not always correlate with either clinical or dietary findings. Reproducibility is often poor due to technical problems. Results may also be affected by factors other than nutrition, such as infection, dehydration, drug therapies, circadian rhythms, or hepatic and renal disease. Furthermore, appropriate norms for adolescence are often lacking (Zerfas, Shorr, Newman, 1977). Caution must be used when interpreting test results. Biochemical tests of nutritional status are particularly valuable when used in combination with anthropometric indices and dietary and clinical findings. Table 7-2 lists nutritional biochemical norms for adolescents.

There are a number of biochemical parameters that are frequently used as indices for protein–calorie malnutrition. These include serum albumin, total lymphocyte count, creatinine height index, total iron-binding capacity of transferrin, and delayed hypersensitivity skin testing. As with anthropometric measurements, a single biochemical test should not be considered a definitive statement of nutritional status and should be used cautiously. For further information on the application of these tests in the nutritional assessment of hospitalized or chronically ill adolescents, the reader is referred to Merritt and Blackburn (1981), Cooper and Heird (1982), and Reimer, Michener, & Steiger (1980).

Table 7-2

Laboratory Assessment of Nutritional Status in Adolescents

Test	Age	Deficient	Acceptable
Serum protein (g/dl)	6–16	—	6.0+
	16+	6.0–6.4	6.5+
Serum albumin (g/dl)	6+	<2.8	3.5+
Hemoglobin (g/dl)	13–16 M	<12	13.0+
	13–16 F	<10	11.5+
	16+ M	<12	14.0+
	16+ F	<10	12.0+
Hematocrit (%)	13–16 M	<37	40.0+
	13–16 F	<31	36.0+
	16+ M	<37	44.0+
	16+ F	<31	38.0+
Serum iron (μg/dl)	6–12	<50	50.0+
	12+ M	<60	60.0+
	12+ F	<40	40.0+
Transferrin saturation (%)	12+ M	<20	20.0+
	12+ F	<15	15.0+
Serum ferritin (ng/ml)	12+	<10	>10
Urinary thiamine (μg/g creatinine)	10–15	<55	150+
	16+	<27	65+
RBC transketolase*	All ages	25+	<15
Urinary riboflavin (μg/g creatinine)	10–16	<70	200+
	16+	<27	80+
Urinary n'methyl nicotinamide (mg/g creatinine)	Adults	<0.5	1.6+
Red cell folate (ng/ml)	All ages	<140	160+
Serum folate* (ng/ml)	All ages	<3	6+
Serum vitamin B_6* (pg/ml)	All ages	<100	100+
Serum ascorbin acid (mg/100 ml)	All ages	<0.1	0.2+
Plasma vitamin A (μg/100ml)	All ages	<10	20+
Plasma carotene (μg/100ml)	All ages	<20	40+
Serum vitamin E (mg/dl)*	All ages	<0.5	0.7+
Red cell hemolysis in* H_2O_2	All ages	>20	<10

Adapted from Christakis, G. (Ed.). Nutritional Assessment in Health Programs. *American Journal of Public Health,* 1973, *63;* and Grant, A., *Nutritional Assessment Guidelines* (2nd ed.). Seattle, WA: 1979. With permission.
* Criteria may vary with different methodology

Table 7-3
Physical Signs Indicative or Suggestive of Malnutrition

Body area	Normal appearance	Signs associated with malnutrition
Hair	Shiny; firm; not easily plucked	Lack of natural shine; hair dull and dry; thin and sparse; hair fine, silky and straight; color changes (flag sign); can be easily plucked.
Face	Skin color uniform; smooth, pink, healthy appearance; not swollen	Skin color loss (depigmentation); skin dark over cheeks and under eyes (malar and supra-orbital pigmentation); lumpiness or flakiness of skin of nose and mouth; swollen face; enlarged parotid glands; scaling of skin around nostrils (nasolabial seborrhea)
Eyes	Bright, clear, shiny; no sores at corners of eyelids; membranes a healthy pink and are moist. No prominent blood vessels or mound of tissue or sclera	Eye membranes are pale (pale conjunctivae); redness of membranes (conjunctival injection); Bitot's spots; redness and fissuring of eyelid corners (angular palpebritis); dryness of eye membranes (conjunctival xerosis); cornea has dull appearance (corneal xerosis); cornea is soft (keratomalacia); scar on cornea; ring of fine blood vessels around corner (circumcorneal injection)
Lips	Smooth, not chapped or swollen	Redness and swelling of mouth or lips (cheilosis); especially at corners of mouth (angular fissures and scars)
Tongue	Deep red in appearance; not swollen or smooth	Swelling; scarlet and raw tongue; magenta (purplish color) of tongue; smooth tongue; swollen sores; hyperemic and hypertrophic papillae; and atrophic papillae
Teeth	No cavities; no pain; bright	May be missing or erupting abnormally; gray or black spots (fluorosis); cavities (caries)
Gums	Healthy; red; do not bleed; not swollen	"Spongy" and bleed easily; recession of gums
Glands	Face not swollen	Thyroid enlargement (front of neck); parotid enlargement (cheeks become swollen)

Skin	No signs of rashes, swellings, dark or light spots	Dryness of skin (xerosis); sandpaper feel of skin (follicular hyperkeratosis); flakiness of skin; skin swollen and dark; red swollen pigmentation of exposed areas (pellagrous dermatosis); excessive lightness or darkness of skin (dyspigmentation); black and blue marks due to skin bleeding (petechiae); lack of fat under skin
Nails	Firm, pink	Nails are spoon-shape (koilonychia); brittle, ridged nails
Muscular and skeletal systems	Good muscle tone; some fat under skin; can walk or run without pain	Muscles have "wasted" appearance; baby's skull bones are thin and soft (craniotabes); round swelling of front and side of head (frontal and parietal bossing); swelling of ends of bones (epiphyseal enlargement); small bumps on both sides of chest wall (on ribs)—beading of ribs; baby's soft spot on head does not harden at proper time (persistently open anterior fontanelle); knock-knees or bowlegs; bleeding into muscle (musculoskeletal hemorrhages); person cannot get up or walk properly
Internal Systems:		
Cardiovascular	Normal heart rate and rhythm; no murmurs or abnormal rhythms; normal blood pressure for age	Rapid heart rate (above 100 tachycardia); enlarged heart; abnormal rhythm; elevated blood pressure
Gastrointestinal	No palpable organs or masses (in children, however, liver edge may be palpable)	Liver enlargement; enlargement of spleen (usually indicates other associated diseases)
Nervous	Psychological stability; normal reflexes	Mental irritability and confusion; burning and tingling of hands and feet (paresthesia); loss of position and vibratory sense; weakness and tenderness of muscles (may result in inability to walk); decrease and loss of ankle and knee reflexes

Adapted from Christakis, G. (Ed.). Nutritional Assessment in Health Programs. *American Journal of Public Health*, 63, 1973. With permission.

Clinical Evaluation

A clinical examination is essential in nutritional screening in order to detect nutritional deficiencies and signs of malnutrition. Areas of body that exhibit abnormalities due to malnutrition are the skin, eyes, tongue, mucous membranes of the mouth and eyes, nail beds, palm surfaces, hair, skeleton, and the nervous system. Table 7-3 lists physical signs indicative or suggestive of malnutrition.

Physical signs and symptoms of malnutrition usually occur in the latter stages of nutrient depletion. It should be emphasized, however, that the signs of malnutrition are nonspecific; they may be related to nonnutritional factors, such as poor hygiene or excessive exposure to the sun, cold, or wind, or they may reflect multiple nutrient deficiencies. In view of the multiple factors that may present as malnutrition, physical findings that suggest a nutritional abnormality should be regarded as clues rather than diagnostic signs and should be confirmed by other clinical, laboratory, and dietary findings.[99]

Color slides* are available to assist the health professional in identifying and standardizing physical signs of nutritional deficiency. Although nonphysicians can be trained to detect and recognize the major signs of nutritional abnormalities, they should alert the physician to any findings so that he or she can conduct a more thorough examination.

REFERENCES

Abitol, C.L. Effect of energy and nitrogen intake upon urea production in children with uremia and undernutrition. *Clinical Nephrology*, 1978, *10*, 9.

Altman, K., Bondy, A., & Hirsch, B. Behavioral treatment of obesity in patients with Prader-Willi syndrome. *Journal of Behavioral Medicine*, 1978, *1*(4), 403.

Alton, I. Nutritional needs and assessments. In R.W. Blum (Ed.) *Adolescent health care; clinical issues*. New York:Academic Press, 1982.

American Dietetic Association. Infant and child nutrition: concerns regarding the developmentally disabled. *Journal of the American Dietetic Association*, 1981, *78*(5).

Baer, M.T. *A manual for State Title V Programs*. No. MCT–00167–01–0. Nutrition services for children with handicaps: December, 1982, 1–44.

Bistrian, B.R., Blackburn, G.L., Hallowell, E., & Heddle, R. Protein status of general surgical patients. *Journal of the American Medical Association*, 1974 *230*, 858.

Bistrian, B.R., Blackburn, G.L., Vitale, J., Cochran, D., & Nayler, J. Prevalence of malnutrition in general medical patients. *Journal of the American Medical Association* 1976, *235*, 1567.

---

*For color slides contact Sandstead, Carter, & Darby. How to diagnose nutritional deficiencies in daily practice. *Nutrition Today* (5). 1140 Connecticut Avenue N.W., Washington, D.C. 20036.

Bistrian, B.R., Blackburn, G.L., & Stanbury, J.B. Metabolic aspects of a protein-sparing modified fast in the dietary management of Prader-Willi obesity. *New England Journal of Medicine*, 1977, *296*, 774–779.

Blackburn, G.L., & Thornton, P.A. Nutritional assessment of the hospitalized patient. *Medical Clinics of North America*, 1979, *63*(5), 1103.

Borgstedt, A.D., Bryson, M., Young, L.W., & Forbes, G.B. Long-term administration of anti-epileptic drugs and the development of rickets. *Journal of Pediatrics*, 1972, *81*, 9.

Butterworth, C.E., & Weinser, R.L. Malnutrition in hospital patients: assessment, In R.S. Goodhart, & M.E. Shils (Eds.) *Modern nutrition in health and disease*. Philadelphia: Lea & Febiger, 1980.

Calvert, S., & Davies, F. Nutrition of children with handicapping conditions. *Public Health Currents*, Jan.–Feb., 1978.

Chase, H.P., Long, M.A., & Lavin, M.H. Cystic fibrosis and malnutrition. *Journal of Pediatrics*, 1979, *95*, 337.

Christakis, G. (Ed.). Nutritional assessment in health programs. *American Journal of Public Health*, 1973, *63* (Suppl.), 1082.

Committee on Nutrition Anthropometry. Recommendations concerning body measurements for the characterization of nutritional status. *Human Biology*, 1956, *28*, 111.

Cooper, A., & Heird, W.C. Nutritional assessment of the pediatric patient including the low birth weight infant. *American Journal of Clinical Nutrition*, 1982, *35*, 1132.

Coplin, S.S., Hine, J., & Germican, A. Out-patient dietary management in the Prader-Willi syndrome. *Journal of the American Dietetic Association*, 1976, *68*(4), 330.

Davidson, M. Nutrition in adolescents with inflammatory bowel disease. In M. Winick (Ed.), *Adolescent nutrition*. New York: John Wiley & Sons, 1982.

Donaldson, S.S., Wesley, M.N., DeWys, W.D., Suskind, R.M., Jaffe, N., & Van Eys, J. A study of the nutritional status of pediatric cancer patients. *American Journal of Diseases of Children* 1981, *135*(12), 1107.

Dwyer, J. Nutritional requirements of adolescence. *Nutrition Reviews* 1981, *39*, 56.

Eddy, T.P., Nicholson, A.L., & Wheeler, E.F. Energy expenditures and dietary intakes in cerebral palsy. *Neurology*, 1965, *7*, 377.

Filler, R.M., Dietz, W., Suskind, R.M., Haffe, H., & Cassady, J.R. Parenteral feeding in the management of children with cancer. *Cancer*, 1979, *43*(5), 2117.

Frisancho, A.R. Triceps skinfold and upper arm muscle size norms for assessment of nutritional status. *American Journal of Clinical Nutrition*, 1974, *27*, 1052.

Grand, R.J. Model for the treatment of growth failure in children with inflammatory bowel disease. In R.M. Suskind (Ed.), *Textbook of pediatric nutrition*. New York: Raven Press, 1981.

Grant, A. *Nutritional assessment guidelines* (2nd ed.). Seattle, WA: 1979.

Gray, G.E., & Gray, L.K. Anthropometric measurements and their interpretation: principles, practices and problems. *Journal of the American Dietetic Association*, 1980, 77, 534.

Gurney, J. and Jelliffe, D. Arm anthropometry in nutritional assessment; nomogram for rapid calculation of arm muscle circumference and cross-sectional muscle and fat areas. *American Journal of Clinical Nutrition*, 1973, *26*, 912.

Hahn, T.J. Bone complications and anticonvulsants. *Drugs*, 1976 *12*, 201.

Hartshorn, E.A. Food and drug interactions. *Journal of the American Dietetic Association*, 1977, *70*(1), 15.

Hayes-Allen, M.C., & Tring, F.C. Obesity: another hazard for spina bifida children. *British Journal of Preventative Social Medicine*, 1973, *27*, 192.

Heald, F.P. The adolescent. In D.B. Jelliffe and E.F.D. Jelliffe (Eds.), *Nutrition and growth*. New York:Plenum Press, 1979, 239–252.

Hegsted, D.M. Current knowledge of energy, fat, protein and amino acid needs of adolescents. In J.I. McKigney, & H.N. Munro (Eds.), *Nutrient requirements in adolescence*. Cambridge:MIT Press, 1976.

Hubbard, V.S., & Mangrum, P.J. Energy intake and nutrition counseling in cystic fibrosis. *Journal of the American Dietetic Association*, 1982, *80*, 127.

Jaffe, N. Nutrition and childhood malignancy. In R.M. Suskind (Ed.), *Textbook of pediatric nutrition*. New York: Raven Press, 1981.

Jelliffe, D.G. *The assessment of nutritional status of the community*. (WHO monograph, No. 53) Washington, D.C.: U.S. Government Printing Office, 1966.

Kelts, D.G., Grand, R.J., Shen, G., Watkins, J.B., Werlin, S.E., & Boehme, C. Nutritional basis of growth failure in children and adults with Crohn's disease. *Gastroenterology*, 1979, *76*, 720.

Kirschner, B.S., Klich, J.R., Kalman, S.S., deFavaro, M., & Rosenberg, I.H. Reversal of growth retardation in Crohn's disease with therapy emphasizing oral nutritional restriction. *Gastroenterology*, 1981, *80*, 10.

Kraemer, R., Rudeberg, A., Hadorn, B., & Rossi, E. Relative underweight in cystic fibrosis and its prognostic value. *Acta Paediatrica Scandinavica*, 1978, *67*, 33.

Krieger, I. *Pediatric disorders of feeding, nutrition and metabolism*. New York:John Wiley & Sons, 1982.

Lapey, A., Kattwinkel, J. DiSant' Agnese, P.A., & Laster, L. Steatorrhea and azotorrhea and their relation to growth and nutrition in adolescents and young adults with cystic fibrosis. *Journal of Pediatrics*, 1974, *84*, 328.

Layden, T., Rosenberg, J. Newchausky, B., Elsou, C., & Rosenberg, I. Reversal of growth arrest in adolescents with Crohn's disease after parenteral alimentation: *Gastroenterology*, 1976, *70*, 1017.

Lifshitz, F., & MacLaren, N.K. Vitamin D-dependent rickets in institutionalized mentally retarded children receiving long-term anticonvulsant therapy. I. A survey of 288 patients. *Journal of Pediatrics*, 1973, *83*, 612.

Lucas, B. Nutrition and the adolescent. In P.L. Pipes (Ed.), *Nutrition in infancy and childhood*. St.Louis: V.C. Mosby Co., 1981.

March, D.C. *Handbook: Interactions of selected drugs with nutritional status in man*. Chicago: American Dietetic Association, 1978.

Margen, S., & King, J.D. Effect of oral contraceptive agents on the metabolism of some trace minerals. *American Journal of Clinical Nutrition*, 1975, *28*, 392.

Marino, D.D., & King, J.C. Nutritional concerns during adolescence. *Pediatric Clinics of North America*, 1980, *27*(1), 125.

Mauer, A.M. *Nutritional problems of the child with cancer*. (Pediatric nutrition handbook). Evanston, IL: American Academy of Pediatrics, 1979.

McCaffery, T.D., Nasor, K., Lawrence, A.M., & Kirsner, J.D. Severe growth retardation in children with inflammatory bowel disease. *Pediatrics*, 1970, *45*, 386.

McGanity, W. *Nutrient requirements in adolescents*. Cambridge: MIT Press, 1976.

Merritt, R.J., & Blackburn, G.L. Nutritional assessment and metabolic response to illness of the hospitalized child. In R.M. Suskind (Ed.), *Textbook of pediatric nutrition*, New York:Raven Press, 1981.

Motil, K.J., Grand, R.J., Matthews, D.E., Bier, D.M., Maletskos, C.J., & Young, V.R. Whole body leucine metabolism in adolescents with Crohn's disease and growth failure during nutritional supplementation. *Gastroenterology*, 1982, *82*, 1359.

Newman, L.J., Lopez, R., Cole, H.S., & et al. Riboflavin deficiency in women taking oral contraceptive agents. *American Journal of Clinical Nutrition*, 1978, *31*, 247.

Owen, G.M. Measurement recording and assessment of skinfold thickness in childhood and adolescence: report of a small meeting. *American Journal of Clinical Nutrition*, 1982, *35*, 629.

Parsons, H.G., Francoewe, T.E., Howland, P., Spengler, R.F., & Pencharz, P.B. The nutritional status of hospitalized children. *American Journal of Clinical Nutrition* 1980, *33*, 1140

Phelps, W.M. Dietary requirements in cerebral palsy. *Journal of the American Dietetic Association*, 1951, *27*, 869.

Reimer, S.L., Michener, W.M., & Steiger, E. Nutritional support of the critically ill child. *Pediatric Clinics of North America*, 1980, *27*(3), 647.

Rickard, K. Brady, M.S., & Gresham, E.L. Nutritional management of the chronically ill child. *Pediatric Clinics of North America*, 1977, *24*(1), 157.

Rickard, K.A., Brady, M.S., Hempel, J., & Gresham, E. Care of children with conditions characterized by high risk. *Journal of the American Dietetic Association*, 1976, *68*, 546.

Rickard, K.A. Grosfeld, J.L., Kirksey, A. Ballantine, T.V.N., & Baehner, R.L. Reversal of protein-energy malnutrition during treatment of advanced neoplastic disease. *Annals of Surgery*, 1979, *190*(6), 771.

Robinson, M.J., & Norman, A.P. Life tables for cystic fibrosis. *Archives of Diseases of Childhood*, 1975, *50*, 962.

Roe, D.A. *Drug-induced nutritional deficiencies.* Westport: Avi Publ. Co., 1976.

Roe, D.A. Interactions between drugs and nutrients. *Medical Clinics of North America* 1979, *63*(5), 985.

Ruby, D.O., & Matheny, W.D. Comments on growth of cerebral palsied children. *Journal of the American Dietetic Association*, 1962, *40*(6), 525.

Sandstead, H.H. Zinc deficiency in Crohn's disease. *Nutrition Review*, 1982a, *40*(4), 109.

Sandstead, H.H. *Nutritional role of zinc and effects of deficiency.* In M. Winick (Ed.), New York: John Wiley & Sons, 1982b.

Safer, D.J., Allen, R.P., & Barr, E. Growth rebound after termination of stimulant drugs. *Journal of Pediatrics*, 1975, *86*, 113.

Seltzer, C, & Mayer, J. A simple criterion of obesity. *Postgraduate Medicine* 1965, *38*, A101.

Shepherd, R., Cooksley, W.G.E., & Domville Cook, W.D. Improved growth and clinical, nutritional and respiratory changes in response to nutritional therapy in cystic fibrosis. *Journal of Pediatrics*, 1980, *97*(3), 351.

Shils, M.E. Principles of nutritional therapy. *Cancer*, 1979, *43*(5), 2093.

Shwachman, H. Nutritional considerations in the treatment of children with cystic fibrosis. In R.M. Suskind (Ed.), *Textbook of Pediatric Nutrition.* New York: Raven Press, 1981.

Silver, J., Davies, T.J., Kupersmitt, E. Orme, M., Petrie, A., & Vajda, F. Prevalence and treatment of vitamin D deficiency in children on anti-convulsant drugs. *Archives of Diseases of Childhood*, 1974, *49*, 344.

Silverstone, J.T., & Stunkard, A.J. The anorectic effects of dextroamphetamine sulfate. *British Journal of Pharmacology*, 1968, *33*, 513.

Smith, J.L., Goldsmith, G.A., & Lawrence, J.D. Effects of oral contraceptive steroids on vitamin and lipid levels in the serum. *American Journal of Clinical Nutrition*, 1975, *28*, 371.

Solomons, N.W., Wagonfeld, J.B., Rieger, C., Jacob, R.A., Bolt, M., Horst, J., Rothberg, R., & Sandstead, H. Some biochemical indices of nutrition in treated cystic fibrosis patients. *American Journal of Clinical Nutrition*, 1981, *34*(4), 462.

Sproul, A., & Huang, N. Growth patterns in children with cystic fibrosis. *Journal of Pediatrics*, 1964, *65*, 664.

Strobel, C.T., Byrne, W.J., & Ament, M.E. Home parenteral nutrition in children with Crohn's disease: an effective management alternative. *Gastroenterology*, 1979, *77*, 272.

Suskin, R.M. The nutritional support service: an organized approach to the nutritional care of the hospitalized and ambulatory pediatric patient. In R.M. Suskind (Ed.), *Textbook of pediatric nutrition.* New York: Raven Press, 1981.

Tanner, J.M. Growth at adolescence (2nd Ed.). Oxford:Blackwell Scientific Publishers, 1962.

Theologides, A. Nutritional management of the patient with advanced cancer. *Postgraduate Medicine*, 1977, *61*(2), 97.

Van Eys, J. Malnutrition in children with cancer. *Cancer*, 1979, *43*(5), 2030.

Van Eys, J. Nutrition and meoplasia. *Nutrition Reviews*, 1982, *40*(12), 353.

Weininger, J., & Briggs, G.M. Nutrition update. *Journal of Nutritional Education*, 1977, *9*, 173.

Weinser, R.L., Hunker, E.M., Krumdieck, C.L., & Butterworth, D.E. Hospital malnutrition. A prospective evaluation of general medical patients during the course of hospitalization. *American Journal of Clinical Nutrition*, 1979, *32*(2), 418.

Zerfas, A.J., Shorr, I.J., & Newman, C.G. Office assessment of nutritional status. *Pediatric Clinics of North America*, 1977, *24*(1), 253.

Robert Wm. Blum

8

Sexual Health Needs of Physically and Intellectually Impaired Adolescents

While extensive literature exists on most chronic conditions, physical disabilities, and mental handicapping conditions of childhood and adolescence, remarkably little research has been published on one of the central concerns faced by disabled teenagers and their families—sexuality.

Historically, these populations have tended to be sheltered socially (Bidgood, 1974) while carrying out their daily living in a "fishbowl existence." The consequences of this have included limited contact with same and opposite sex peers (Dorner, 1977), delays in learning gender-appropriate and socially appropriate behavior, and concerns that their behavior is hypersexual (Johnson & Johnson, 1982).

This chapter will explore the issues related to the development of emerging sexuality in disabled youths; the issues faced by their parents, as well as themselves; and their current contraceptive needs, alternatives, and controversies.

SEXUALITY AND NORMAL BEHAVIOR

It is essential, not only for the purposes of this chapter but for working with all youths and their families, that the concepts of sexuality be expanded far beyond the boundaries of genital sex to include issues such as sex-role socialization; physical maturation and body image; social relationships with the same and the opposite sex; and future plans, including the possibilities of marriage, childbearing, and child rearing. Fundamental assumptions that underlie this discussion will include the conviction that all human beings, even the most severely disabled, are sexual from birth till death (Calderone, 1982). Second, despite variations in the onset and timing of puberty that might differentiate certain disabled youths from their able-bodied peers, the tasks of sexual maturation are essentially the same for all teenagers (Morgenstern, 1973). Third, due to the paucity of research, there is very little understanding of how the multiplicity of disabling conditions of childhood interfere with or inhibit the process of healthy sexual development. At best, only glimpses into that dynamic are available, and only for some conditions. The risk is to extrapolate from what is known to the universe of handicapping conditions.

Talking in terms of *normal* sexual behavior entails the risk of confounding notions of moral, social, statistical, clinical, and subjective norms (Johnson and Kempton, 1981). The discussion is further complicated because social and cultural norms surrounding sexual expression are rapidly changing as reflected through the media, dress, and premarital and extramarital relationships (Blos and Finch, 1974).

Far more useful than talking of the normalcy of a given behavior is focusing upon the context within which the behavior occurs. It is the context more than the behavior itself that will determine the consequences of that behavior. On the most self-evident level, the exposure of one's genitals at home and masturbating in the privacy of one's bedroom carry with them far different consequences than does the public display of the same behavior. Social attitudes vary more according to the setting of a behavior than according to the behavior itself. Mitchell, Doctor, & Butler (1978) surveyed the attitudes of 117 staff members of three residential facilities regarding a range of heterosexual and homosexual behavior. Their data indicate that the acceptability of all behavior varied primarily on the basis of the degree of privacy of the act and to a lesser extent on the act itself. However, the members of the staffs of these institutions did, overall, have clear notions of what was legitimate or acceptable sexual behavior for institutionalized, mentally retarded adults—the more intimate the sexual contact, the more unacceptable the behavior was considered under any circumstance. The need is to focus less on whether behavior conforms to one's concept of normalcy and more on the consequences of a given behavior (Johnson & Johnson, 1982). The underlying question is whether the behavior enhances, hinders, or has little impact on healthy sexual development.

ADOLESCENT SEXUAL DEVELOPMENT AND DISABILITIES

The normal age range for the onset of puberty in able-bodied teenagers is between 8 and 16 years for females (with menarche at 12.5 years) and a year later for males. Chronic illnesses and disabilities can alter this pattern.

Early pubertal development is associated with a host of acute and chronic conditions. Central nervous system (CNS) tumors, such as optic and hypothalamic gliomas, both of which are associated with neurofibromatosis (Fienman & Yakovac, 1970); astrocytomas, ependymomas, and germinomas in males (in females these tumors are associated with delayed puberty); hypothalamic teratomas; and hormone-secreting hamartomas are all associated with true sexual precocity. So, too, are McCune-Albright syndrome (polyostotic fibrous dysplasia), which is associated with irregularly edged cafe-au-lait spots, fibrous dysplasia, and bone cysts (Benedict, 1966) and von Recklinghausen's disease (neurofibromatosis) that has associated smooth-bordered cafe-au-lait spots, axillary freckles, and subcutaneous and internal masses (neurofibromas). Seizures, visual defects, and mental retardation may be associated with pubertal delay as well. Neural tube defects are associated with precocious puberty: females with spina bifida, for example, experience menarche, on an average, more than a year prior to their able-bodied peers.

Conversely, delayed pubertal development is associated with at least as extensive a list of chronic and disabling conditions as is precocious development. Gonadotropin deficiency of multiple etiologies is the primary cause of pubertal delay. The most common type of CNS mass leading to sexual infantilism is craniopharyngiomas, which have their peak incidence between 6 and 15 years of age. Other extracellular masses encroaching on the hypothalamus can also result in delayed sexual development: germinomas, hypothalamic and optic gliomas, astrocytomas, and rarely, chromophobe adenomas. Congenital CNS lesions, ranging from septo-optic dysplasia and holoprosencephaly to cleft palate or lip, may be associated with hypothalamic dysfunction (Yen & Jaffe, 1978). Syndromes and chronic illnesses with concomitant pubertal delay are numerous. Females with Down's syndrome, for example, average menarche at 18 years 4 months, or about six years behind their healthy peers (Johnson & Johnson, 1982). There are also some data to support the observation of later onset of menstruation, and irregular cycling, in mentally retarded females whose deficiencies are prenatal and organic in nature (Meyerwitz, 1971; Philips, 1967).

While the variation in rate of physiological maturation is great in the chronically ill and disabled teenager, there is little evidence that the patterns and rates of physical sexual maturation for the majority of patients with mentally handicapping conditions are other than normal (Hammer, Wright, & Jensen, 1967; Mosier, Grossman and Dingman, 1962). Furthermore, the chronically ill and physically and mentally disabled are confronted with the same difficulties of sexual adjustment as all other adolescents (Hall, Morris, & Baker, 1973). As a result, despite the variance that may exist in timing of puberty, it is incumbent on health professionals and educators to view those with chronic illness or disabilities as they do those who are able-bodied and of normal intelligence. As Paradowski (1977) noted, "It is clear that neither the limitations of physical disability nor the prospect of long hospitalization invalidates the sex drive."

SEX EDUCATION

"The mentally retarded [physically disabled and chronically ill] do indeed tend to be retarded with respect to sex education and this is one of the characteristics they share most fully with the brilliant and so-called normal" (Johnson, 1975). Sex education for what? That is the first and most critical question. What are the assumptions that underlie sex education of disabled or chronically ill? How does one take into consideration the fact that life expectancy is limited for many? For some, physical limitations restrict normal sexual response, and for others, childbearing and child rearing pose problems of enormous proportions. As Hamilton (1976) notes, "Sex education for normal children is designed under the (possibly mistaken) assumption that eventually these young people will form relationships leading to marriage." But what about the retarded? The teenager with chronic renal disease or cystic fibrosis? The wheelchair bound? What are the assumptions that govern the approaches to these youths?

Johnson and Johnson (1982) note three philosophical approaches to dealing with sex education. The traditional approach equates sex with procreation and holds that other sexual activity is inappropriate. Certainly, such an orientation poses significant problems in working with adolescents for whom future procreation is either unlikely or highly undesirable.

The tolerant philosophy acknowledges that sexuality of disabled populations is a reality "to be dealt with rationally, knowledgeably, and humanistically" (Johnson & Johnson, 1982). The focus of this philosophy is on the context of behavior more than on the inherent appropriateness of a given activity. The third position, cultivation of sexual enjoyment, holds that sexual gratification should be encouraged and taught, much like tennis or chess. While not the orientation of the majority, this concept is especially provocative when one thinks of an individual whose avenues of sexual experimentation are severely restricted due to physical limitations. The chance that he or she will stumble upon ways of self-pleasuring or responding sexually to others is markedly less than it is for their able-bodied peers. Human beings learn their responses through observation. With few role models available, deliberate education may be the only route for learning sexual expression.

Parents often feel ill-equipped to teach the multiple aspects of sex education. Goodman, Budner, and Lesh (1971) found that among parents of mentally retarded youth, there was a high degree of concern that their teenagers obtain sex education, but they did not see themselves as the primary educators. Hammer, Wright and Jensen (1967) found that while parents of retarded girls often taught them about menstruation, discussions rarely were extended to other aspects of sexuality. Turner (1970) found that only one third of the parents of disabled youths surveyed discussed sex education and the majority limited discussion to the birthing process. Turchin (1974) had similar findings in his interviews of trainably mentally retarded (TMR) youths; he found that mothers believed that teachers were more qualified to give sex education than parents, doctors, or social workers. Almost three-fourths of the mothers responded that their children had never asked them any questions about sex, dating, marriage, or the birth process. Based upon responses to his interviews, Turner established a priority list for sex education programs for the disabled:

1. Personal hygiene
2. Menstruation
3. Venereal disease
4. Birth control
5. Marriage
6. Masturbation
7. Pre-marital sex

In a study of learning disabled youths, Rothenberg, Franzblau, & Greer (1979) found markedly incomplete knowledge or erroneous information regarding body parts, reproduction, sexual development, birth control, and venereal disease. Most of the study adolescents were totally ignorant of birth control, and many were unable to distinguish basic body parts. Other studies validate these findings among physically and emotionally disabled youths (Bloom, 1969).

Not only is a knowledge base critical for healthy sexual development—a knowledge base that is not currently being provided in the home—but so, too, is the opportunity to learn and practice heterosexual social skills. While Turchin (1974) notes the lack of opportunity for the practice of such social skills by TMR youths, the same observations have been made for young people who are wheelchair bound (see Strax, Chapter 4 of this edition), have spina bifida (Blum, 1983), or are paraplegic (Sparks, 1981). Needed is the teaching of appropriate touch, affection, and love (Kempton, 1978). It is also necessary to teach and role model appropriate interpersonal responses in same-sex and heterosexual settings, so as to affirm positive and avoid potentially abusive situations (Craft & Craft, 1978). Problems arise when the burden of this education falls upon the shoulders of parents, many of whom avoid sex-related language and topics. For successful learning, it may be necessary for the educator (parent, teacher, or health professional) to "simplify, repeat, demonstrate and/or role play sex-related concepts (Johnson & Johnson, 1982)." This is a great deal to expect of most parents, who fear their disabled child's emerging sexuality with all the questions and uncertainty associated with it.

PARENT AND ADOLESCENT ATTITUDES

Studies have repeatedly shown that parental discomfort in dealing with issues of sexuality relating to their disabled children extends beyond sex education. Egyeda and Bentley (1981) found that parents of mentally retarded youths expressed difficulty in seeing them as sexual beings. Turchin (1974) in his study of TMR adolescents and their parents, found that 40 percent of mothers surveyed believed their teenagers would never be able to date. In the same study, while over half of the mothers believed their retarded children were able to feel romantic love, only one fifth believed their children might someday have the ability to marry.

For parents, awareness of the emerging sexuality of their disabled adolescent raises many new and threatening issues. Implicit in this awareness is the change of status from child to adult, and with it a shift toward greater autonomy. Parents for whom "managing" the disabled child has been a life's focus over the preceding 15 or 20 years are now faced with shifting their own life goals and purposes. Likewise, for those whose offspring have sustained inherited disabilities, parental supervision has been a vehicle to assuage misdirected guilt. Now comes a time for dealing with their sense of responsibility for having "caused" the illness or disability.

Frequently, many unanswered questions persist for parents vis-a-vis their teenager's emerging sexuality: What are reasonable expectations for the teenager's social and sexual future? What are the genetic implications for their children? What is the teenager's maximal level of anticipated sexual functioning? How and where does one learn heterosexual social skills? What are the physiological risks of childbearing for the teenager? How competent a parent might he or she be?

The disabled teenager is in no better position to answer the myriad of social and sexual questions that face his or her family than are the parents. Rather, encumbered by limited social contacts and perhaps diminished cognitive capacity, the disabled adolescent has less information on human sexuality and body functioning than do able-bodied age-matched peers (Dorner, 1977). Furthermore, of the information obtained, such a teenager is in a compromised position for sorting fact from fantasy (Craft & Craft, 1978; Egydea & Bentley, 1981; Morgenstern, 1973). Rothenberg et al. (1979) found that among a population of learning-disabled youth many were unable to correctly identify body parts; over half had incomplete knowledge of menstruation, reproduction, and pregnancy; and most were totally ignorant of venereal disease and birth control. Hall et al. (1973) found that among a population of educable retarded youth, most failed more than half of the knowledge-based questions, especially in areas concerning conception, contraception, and venereal disease. These findings are consistent with those of Bloom (1969) who found that physically and emotionally disabled youths were functionally ignorant of pubertal changes and reproduction. To what extent this deficiency of knowledge is a function of social isolation, as compared with other causes limiting access to information, is only speculative. The consequence is that their inadequate knowledge, coupled with deficient social skills, make the disabled especially unprepared for assuming sexual responsibility (Rothenberg, et al., 1979) and vulnerable to sexual exploitation (Gordon, 1971).

The risk of assault and socially unacceptable sexual behavior is increased when combined with attitudes of liberal sexual behavior. While Edgerton (1971) indicated that retarded youths avowed traditional and conservative attitudes toward sex, such was not the finding of Hall, et al. (1973). In that study, EMR youths indicated a more liberal attitude and less rigid interpretation of sexual rules than their parents would have predicted.

Sex education for the physically and mentally disabled needs a three-pronged approach. Evidently, there is great need for information that is appropriate developmentally and cognitively, information that takes into consideration physiological limitations. To be useful, such information must initially acknowledge the inherent sexuality of all individuals and then progress through human structure and reproductive functioning (including pregnancy and menstruation) to include discussions of contraception, venereal disease, and sexual assault.

Secondly, there is a need within sex education to teach the role that context plays in defining the appropriateness of a behavior. Given that most children and young adolescents are concrete learners (Piaget, 1958), the notion that appropriateness depends less on the act and more on the situation is difficult at best. For those with intellectual limitations, the concept is even more problematic; however, it is the understanding of this concept that will allow for a balance between sexual pleasure and social deviance.

Finally, a core issue of sex education for those with disabilities is the understanding that sex is more than genital union. Social skills with the same and opposite sex, with disabled and able-bodied youths, has been repeatedly shown to deserve focus in sex education planning. For those with disabilities, as well as for their able-bodied counterparts, there is a need to learn that the ability to perform does not build a solid relationship.

> Absence of sensation does not mean absence of feelings. Inability to move does not mean inability to please. The presence of deformities does not mean the absence of desire. Inability to perform does not mean inability to enjoy. Loss of genitals does not mean loss of sexuality (Sparks, 1981).

The author concurs with Carparulo and Kempton (1981) in stressing the following points:

1. Accurate and useful sex education is a necessary component in the education of mentally retarded and physically disabled youths.
2. The mentally retarded, chronically ill, and physically disabled have a right to express their sexuality in an appropriate manner.
3. Caution must be taken to prevent policies that are too restrictive from being established.
4. Sex education that emphasizes the crisis aspects of sexual expression (the *don't* approach) should not be offered.
5. The danger is not too much information but, rather, not enough information.
6. Normal psychosexual development is suppressed by long periods of institutionalization and hospitalization. Behavior upon reentry into the mainstream may be inappropriate. However, education and good socialization programs can assist the patient in a smooth transition into the community.
7. In all instances, the rights of the mentally retarded, chronically ill, and physically disabled should be taken into account and never violated.

DETERMINING CONTRACEPTIVE NEEDS

While a detailed discussion of contraceptive needs and precautions is beyond the scope of this chapter, there are some generic issues and some disease-specific concerns worthy of emphasis. There is first a question of whether contraception is needed before determining the strength and liabilities of individual methods.

The most self-evident initial question is whether the patient is currently having sexual intercourse or is planning to in the near future. While seemingly straightforward, this issue can be especially complex for chronically ill and disabled youth. Not only may there not be a knowledge base or intellectual functioning sufficient for a language between practitioner and patient, but the individual's desires to view himself or herself as sexually active may lead to the request for contraceptive services. Conversely, the fear of their daughter's pregnancy or their son's impregnating others may lead parents to prematurely seek contraceptives for their child, when education and counseling would be more appropriate.

Even if the individual is not currently sexually active, it may be misguided to dismiss the need for contraception. Many parents seek contraception for their disabled children because they fear that due either to physical or intellectual limitations, their children are at special risk for sexual assault. Under such circumstances, it is necessary to understand the social settings in which the youths interact with members of the same and opposite sex; the times they are unescorted and in public, and thus potentially at risk for assault; the types of adult supervision at school and in social settings; and the individual's personality—whether seductive or aggressive, passive or assertive. If risk exists, contraceptive prophylaxis may be warranted.

On the other hand, if the adolescent is currently sexually active, there are a number of questions that, much like the sexual history for any another client, are essential knowledge before one can assist the individual in contraceptive decision making. If the client is male, the contraceptive alternatives are currently restricted to condoms and vasectomy, which will be discussed under Sterilization. Condoms have a higher than average fail rate in the hands of adolescents (Hatcher, 1982) in general; and if they represent the primary contraceptive method of certain disabled populations, e.g., those with mental limitations, it would appear that the risk increases (Sparks, 1981). Conversely, Arnold and Cogswell (1981) indicated that teenagers can be educated to use condoms efficiently; especially when combined with vaginal contraceptive foam or cream, this method can be highly effective. The key issues in its use appropriateness appear to be: intellectual functioning of the client, frequency of intercourse, and number of partners. The individual in a steady relationship, who is frequently having intercourse, has needs that are significantly different from those of an individual in multiple relationships and those who have intercourse sporadically. Contraceptive alternatives should be recommended accordingly.

For females, the contraceptive options (as well as the burden of responsibility) are greater than for their male counterparts. A number of questions should guide the clinician in assisting the sexually active, disabled female in selecting contraception.

Carparulo and Kempton (1981) suggest that questions for candidates for oral contraception should include the following:

1. Does the individual assume responsibility for any act on a regular daily basis?
2. Is she able to monitor the side effects of the pill and seek refills when needed? Or is there someone with whom she lives who can serve in those capacities?
3. Does she take medications or have an underlying condition that may be incompatible with oral contraception or that may limit the pill's effectiveness?

Likewise, if an intrauterine device (IUD) is being considered, certain prior information is critical:

1. Is the individual in a regular relationship, or does she have multiple partners? The risk of uterine infection is increased with the IUD, and it rises significantly when multiple partners are involved.
2. Does she have an underlying condition or take medications that increase the risk of complications from menorrhagia associated with the IUD?
3. Does she have the capability to monitor and report the major side effects of the IUD? Does she know the side effects?
4. Is this an individual who is not afraid, or can be taught, to tough her genitalia so as to check the string of the IUD?

If the answer to one or more of the above questions is negative, alternatives need to be considered. If barrier methods (e.g., diaphragm, foam and condoms, the sponge) are not appropriate because of physical limitations or use effectiveness, two primary alternatives remain: medroxyprogesterone acetate and sterilization.

Medroxyprogesterone Acetate

While injectable progestogens have not gained widespread acceptance in the United States, they have broad-based acceptance throughout the world. The most commonly used forms are medroxyprogesterone acetate (Depo-Provera® [Upjohn]) and norethindrone enanthate. Either drug is used at a dose of 150 mg IM every three months.

Despite their wide usage, the FDA has refused to approve injectable progestogens for contraceptive use in the United States. The argument focuses on carcenogenic potential since mammary hyperplasia has been demonstrated in the laboratory in beagles; possible teratogenicity; and possible complications as a result of irregular bleeding, which may require other medications for control (Maine, 1978). Based upon these observations, the FDA concluded that there is no demonstrated need for the drug.

Others disagree. The Committee on Drugs of the American Academy of Pediatrics (1980) while acknowledging the potential side effects, after reviewing all the available data concluded that "there is no conclusive evidence that Depo-Provera is harmful to humans." Based upon its analysis, the Committee concluded that there are two primary adolescent populations who would benefit from this form of contraception:

The first group comprises those with significant intellectual impairment or major emotional disturbances. For these individuals, injectable progestogens would provide two avantages over other noninvasive contraceptives. As an injectable form, its effectiveness is independent of compliance, and thus, its use and theoretical effectiveness are synonymous at .3/100 woman years—comparable to oral contraception (Hatcher, 1982). Because the shot provides protection for at least one, and probably two months, beyond the recommended three month-return, the margin of effectiveness safety is quite substantial.

A second benefit of a progestogen-only contraceptive for the mentally impaired adolescent is the cessation of menstruation that often results. Rosenfield (1974) noted ammenorrhea to be 23 percent at one month of use and 69 percent after two years of consecutive use of Depo-Provera. As the Academy of Pediatrics (1980) notes:

> Menstrual flow creates a major emotional disturbance or hygienic problem for a small number of intellectually impaired adolescents (or their caretakers) and the cessation of menstrual function . . . may be a desirable side effect.

The second adolescent population possibly to benefit from injectable progestogens are those sexually active females who, because of their underlying pathological condition, are precluded from using either estrogen-containing contraceptives or an IUD. These conditions can include blood dyscrasias such as sickle cell disease (Perkins, 1971), cardiac anomalies, (Kaplan, 1979) and perhaps paraplegia.

Despite the benefits and effectiveness of this contraceptive modality, its use remains controversial. Some (e.g., Greydanus & McAnarney, 1980) note that since the drug is not approved for contraceptive use by the FDA, they do not recommend it for adolescent clients. Others argue that it is abusive to use an unapproved modality on a population from whom informed consent is at best incomplete.

Sterilization

The request for sterilization rarely comes directly from the patient but most typically from the parents, whose primary concerns may include the threat of sexual assault, fears about their child's present or potential sexual activity, concerns regarding masturbation and other self-stimulatory behavior, and problems in management of menstrual hygiene. While the appropriate response to these issues is not necessarily sterilization, when sterilization is considered the problem is complicated by legal and ethical constraints.

In 1973, due to alleged and documented abuse, the federal government established a moritorium on federally funded sterilization of the mentally retarded under the age of 21 (Holder, 1977). The problem is further complicated in that almost half of all states have neither enabling nor prohibitive legislation to guide the clinician or the courts (Perrin, Sands, & Tinker, 1976). The consequence is that physicians, hospitals, and courts tend to avoid making decisions concerning sterilization and turn to more reversible options whenever feasible (Paul & Scofield, 1979).

The central ethical issue is that of informed consent—the assurance that alternative methods and options have been explained and understood, as have the medical risks of the sterilization process were it to be undertaken (Duncan, 1979). Given the generally irreversible nature of the procedure, it is critical that the patient understand its permanence.

On the other hand, because the assurance of such an understanding is difficult, and at times impossible, it is unwise to extrapolate that sterilization is thus inappropriate and should not be performed in problem situations. The benefits to the individual patient (Wheeless, 1975), as well as patient acceptance (Perrin, et al., 1976) have been previously documented. The ethical issues have also been reviewed (Gaylin, 1978). Wheeless (1975) showed benefits to include elimination of menses; provision of contraception, and reduction of occult pelvic pathology. To totally restrict access to this treatment modality disregards the needs of some patients. On the other hand, the task of safeguarding patients from the misapplication of sterilization technologies remains.

The *Consent Handbook* (1977) of the American Association on Mental Deficiency provides a guide to obtaining informed consent. Carparulo and Kempton (1981) outline ten points to consider:

1. Give the patient a full explanation of the procedure.
2. Explain its purpose.
3. Describe what will occur in a clear manner.
4. Describe the benefits of the procedure.
5. Describe the disadvantages of the procedure, including its permanence.
6. Review alternatives.

7. Answer all questions fully.
8. Determine that the individual is going through the procedure voluntarily.
9. Advise him or her of the right to withdraw consent prior to the procedure.
10. Ascertain that all legal obligations have been met.

So as to safeguard the rights of the individual patient and his or her parents and potential offspring, Perrin et al., (1976) proposed a protocol involving a health team of physician, nurse practitioner, family-planning counselor, social worker, and psychologist. While it is possible to combine roles so as to reduce the cost of such an approach, the core principle remains sound. The physician (perhaps in conjunction with a nurse-clinician) would obtain the medical and genetic history, complete the physical examination and perform all necessary laboratory studies. The psychologist, under this system, would administer intelligence and social-maturity testing and would evaluate the patient's sexual knowledge and understanding; the latter components perhaps being done in conjunction with a family-planning counselor. And when appropriate, further family evaluation would be completed by the psychologist or social workers. This approach closely parallels that of Smiley (1975). The benefits of such an approach lie in the planned manner in which the physical, intellectual, social, and sexual issues are taken into consideration in planning for sterilization. Such an approach may result in what Paul and Scofield (1979) call an informed request. If the patient has an IQ of greater than 70, most authorities believe he or she is the responsible legal agent to make the request and to give consent (Kreutner, 1981).

There are four primary techniques for the performance of sterilization in females and one in males. Each has its advocates. While a detailed discussion of techniques is available elsewhere, the alternatives for females are laparoscopic tubal fulguration, postpartum tubal ligation, total abdominal hysterectomy, and vaginal hysterectomy; the method for males is vasectomy.

SUMMARY

Far more central to the issue of sterilization than the method selected is the involvement of the adolescent in the decision-making process. The goal in sterilization, as in all forms of contraception, is not to arrest sexual development and not to encumber sexual expression of the physically or intellectually disabled, but, rather, to assist the patient in obtaining maximal sexual health while respecting the concerns of his or her primary care givers as well as the rights of potential offspring.

REFERENCES

Arnold, C. & Cogswell, B. A Condom Distribution Program for Adolescents: The findings of a feasibility study, *American Journal of Public Health,* 1971, *61*:739.

Benedict, P.H. Sex precocity and polyostotic fibrous dysplasia. *American Journal Diseases of Children,* 1966, *3,* 429–432.

Bidgood, F.E. Sexuality and the handicapped: SIECUS Report. *Journal for Special Education of the Mentally Retarded,* 1974, *11,* 199–208.

Bloom, J.L. Sex education for the handicapped adolescents. *Journal of School Health,* 1969, *39,* 363–367.

Blos, P., & Finch, S. Sexuality and the handicapped adolescent. In J.A. Downey, & N.L. Low, (Eds.), *The child with disabling illness.* Philadelphia: W.B. Saunders, 1974, 521–540.

Blum, R. The adolescent with spina bifida. *Clinical Pediatrics,* 1983, *22,*(5), 331–335.

Calderone, M. Sexuality: A continuum from childhood through adolescence. In R. Blum (Ed.), *Adolescent health care.* New York: Academic Press, 1982.

Carparulo, F., & Kempton, W. Sexual health needs of the mentally retarded adolescent female. *Issues in Health Care of Women,* 1981, *3,* 35–46.

Committee Report on Drugs. AAP, Medroxyprogesterone acetate (Depo-Provera) *Pediatrics,* 1980, *65*(3), 648.

Craft, A., & Craft, M. *Sex education for the mentally handicapped.* Boston: Routledge & Kegan Paul, Ltd., 1978.

Dorner, S. Problems of teenagers. *Physiotherapy,* 1977, *63*(6), 190.

Duncan, S. Ethical problems in advising contraception and sterilization. *The Practitioner,* 1979, *223,* 237–242.

Edgerton, R. *Sexual behavior and the mentally retarded.* Paper presented at the NICHD Symposium on Human Sexuality and the Mentally Retarded. Hot Springs, AK, November 1971 as quoted in Hall, J. et al., 1973.

The American Association on Mental Deficiency. *The consent handbook,* Washington, D.C., 1977.

Egyeda, C., & Bentley, P. Developing sexuality: A model for intervention with mentally retarded adolescents. In Sampson J. ed., *Childhood and Sexuality.* Montreal: Editions Etudes Vivant, 1981.

Fienman, N., & Yakovac, W. Neurofibrotosis in childhood. *Journal of Pediatrics,* 1970, *76,* 339–347.

Gaylin, W. The ethics of sterilization. *Hastings Center Report,* 1978, *8*(3), 28–33.

Goodman, L., Budner, S., & Lesh, B. The parent's role in sex education for the retarded. *Mental Retardation,* 1971, *9*(1), 43–46.

Gordon, S. Missing in special education: Sex. *Journal of Special Education,* 1971, *5,* 351–354.

Greydanus, D., & McAnarney, E. Contraception in the adolescent. *Current Concepts for the Pediatrician,* 1980, *65*(1), 1–11.

Hall, J. E., Morris, H.L., & Baker, H.R. Sexual knowledge and attitudes of mentally retarded adolescents. *American Journal of Mental Deficiencies,* 1973, *77*(6), 706–709.

Hamilton, J. The retarded adolescent: a parent's view. *Family Planning Perspectives,* 1976, *8*(6), 271.

Hammer, S., Wright, L., & Jensen, D. Sex education for the retarded adolescent: A survey of parental attitudes and methods of management in 50 adolescent retardates. *Clinical Pediatrics,* 1967, *6,* 621–627.

Hatcher, R. *Contraceptive technology: 1982–83.* New York: Irvington, 1982.

Holder, A. *Legal Issues in Pediatrics and Adolescent Medicine.* New York: John Wiley & Sons, 1977.

Johnson, D., & Johnson, W. Sexuality and the mentally retarded adolescent. *Pediatric Annals,* 1982, *11*(10), 847–853.

Johnson, W.R., & Kempton, W. *Sex education and counseling of special groups: The mentally and physically disabled, ill and elderly.* Springfield: Charles C. Thomas, Pub., 1981.

Johnson, W. *Sex education and counseling of special groups.* Springfield: Charles C. Thomas, Pub., 1975.

Kaplan, S. The adolescent with operated or unoperated congenital heart disease. *Postgraduate Medicine,* 1974, *56,* 147–152.

Kempton, W. Sex education for the mentally handicapped. *Sexuality and Disability,* 1978, *1,* 137–146.

Kreutner, A.K. Sexuality, fertility and the problems of menstruation in mentally retarded adolescents. *Pediatric Clinics of North America,* 1981, *28*(2), 475–480.

Maine, D. Depo: the debate continues. *Family Planning Perspectives,* 1978, *10,* 343–347.

Meyerwitz, J. Sex and the mentally retarded. *Medical Aspects of Human Sexuality,* 1971, 95–118.

Mitchell, L., Doctor, R., & Butler, D. Attitudes of caretakers toward the sexual behavior of mentally retarded persons. *American Journal Mental Deficiencies* 1978, *83*(3), 289–296.

Morgenstern, M. The psychosocial development of the retarded. In F. de la Cruz, & G. La Veck, *Human sexuality and the mentally retarded.* Bruner: Mazel, 1973, 15–28.

Mosier, H.D., Grossman, H.J., & Dingman, H.F. Secondary sex development and mentally deficient individuals. *Child Development,* 1962, *33,* 273–286.

Paradowski, W. Socialization patterns and sexual problems of the institutionalized, chronically ill and physically disabled. *Archives of Physical Medicine and Rehabilitation* 1977, *58,* 53–59.

Paul, E., & Scofield, F. Informed consent for fertility control services. *Family Planning Perspectives,* 1979, *11*(3), 159–168.

Perkins, R. Contraception for sicklers. *New England Journal of Medicine,* 1971, *285,* 296–299.

Perrin, J., Sands, C., & Tinker, D., A considered approach to sterilization of mentally retarded youth. *American Journal Diseases of Children,* 1976, *130,* 288–290.

Piaget, J. *The growth of logical thinking from childhood to adolescence.* New York: Basic Books, 1958.

Philips, J. Psychopathology and mental retardation. *American Journal of Psychiatry,* 1967, *124,* 29.

Rosenfield, A. Injectable long-acting progestogin contraception: A neglected modality. *American Journal of Obstetrics and Gynecology.* 1974, *120,* 537–541.

Rothenberg, G. S., Franzblau, S. H., & Greer, J.H. Educating the learning disabled adolescent about sexuality. *Journal of Learning Disabilities,* 1979, *12*(9), 10–14.

Smiley, C. Sterilization and therapeutic abortion counseling for the mentally retarded. *Illinois Medical Journal,* 1975, *147,* 291–293.

Sparks, B.L. Sexual counseling of the family. *South African Medical Journal,* 1981, (Feb. 28), 291–293.

Turchin, G. Sexual attitudes of mothers of retarded children. *Journal of School Health,* 1974, *44,* 490.

Turner, E. Attitudes of parents of deficient children toward their child's sexual behavior. *Journal of School Health,* 1970, *40,* 548–550.

Wheeless, C. Abdominal hysterectomy for surgical sterilization in the mentally retarded. *American Journal of Obstetrics and Gynecology,* 1975, *122,* 872–878.

Yen, S., & Jaffe, R.B. *Reproductive endocrinology.* Philadelphia: W.B. Saunders Company, 1978.

Robert Wm. Blum

9

Compliance with Therapeutic Regimens Among Children and Youths

Among clinicians, adolescents have an image of being chronic noncompliers with therapeutic regimens. Often factors such as emerging independence from family, rebelliousness, and peer pressure are blamed.

While adolescent-specific data only recently have begun to emerge, an extensive literature currently exists that explores the extent of noncompliance in the general population. The consensus of these studies is that 25–50 percent of the general population fail to comply with one or another aspect of the medical regimen (Becker, 1974; Bowen, Rich, & Schlatfield, 1961; Gordis & Markowitz, 1971; Kellaway & McCrae, 1979; Martens, Frazier, Hirt, Meskin, & Prosheck, 1973). While data on the pediatric population are less extensive, numerous studies document poor compliance in this group as well (Haggerty & Roghman, 1972; Ruley, 1978).

Interest in the subject derives from the self-evident observation that unless complied with, the therapeutic agent or intervention cannot work (Feinstein, 1976). Becker and Maiman (1975) note that despite extensive documentation of the phenomenon, compliance remains one of the most poorly understood of health behaviors. This chapter will first address the definition of terms and complexity of the problems of compliance behavior from both clinical and methodological perspectives. The dimensions of the problem of noncompliance in children and youths will subsequently be explored, and those factors that appear to influence compliance in the pediatric population will be identified. Finally, the health-belief model will be reviewed as a framework for understanding compliance and noncompliance.

CHRONIC ILLNESS AND DISABILITIES IN CHILDHOOD AND ADOLESCENCE   ISBN 0-8089-1635-1

DEFINITION OF COMPLIANCE

The predominant definition of compliance is that espoused by the McMaster University Symposium on Compliance:

> The extent to which the patient's behavior (in terms of taking medication, following diets or executing other life-style changes) coincides with the clinical prescription.

Clinical prescriptions, however, are usually of two types: additive and restrictive (Gordis, 1976). The former adds medications and procedures, such as bronchial drainage, to the daily routine; the latter, asks the patient to restrict certain activities, such as high-carbohydrate diets, contact sports, and foods containing phenylalanine. Noncompliance, then, allows for a wide range of behaviors from omission to errors in dosage to commission, such as taking unprescribed or additional medications (Christensen, 1978).

Hulka, Casell, Kupper, & Burdett (1976) divide drug-taking failures into scheduling misconceptions, defined as lack of the appropriate medication schedule, and schedule noncompliance, defined as correct knowledge but faulty behavior.

Certainly, for the pediatric population, parents represent a critical variable regarding the extent and nature of noncompliance (Mattar & Yaffe, 1974). The role of the parent was reemphasized by Irwin, Millstein, & Shafer (1981) who found parental involvement to be the key determinant of adolescent appointment-keeping behavior. On the other hand, as teenagers increasingly have access to health services on their own, their dependence on parental controls for adherence to medical regimens continues to decline.

THE MEASURES OF COMPLIANCE

While individuals tend to be viewed as either compliant or noncompliant, the problem is far more complex than that dichotomy allows. An individual, for example, may rigorously comply with prescribed medications, intermittently comply with the therapy, such as bronchial drainage, and ignore some of the prescriptive life-style changes, such as the avoidance of smoking cigarettes or marijuana. Any measure of compliance must consider these multiple dimensions. Sackett proposes a four-dimensional model:

1. Appointment-keeping behavior
2. Short-term medication compliance

3. Long-term medication compliance
4. Adherence to diet prescriptions and other therapeutic regimens

Some investigators (e.g. Marston, 1970) propose a composite score of compliance that takes into account both the degree of complexity of the regimen and the extent of compliance with the multiple therapies. While such a score may be of theoretical interest, it is of limited clinical utility, for it fails to take into consideration both qualitative issues (which components of the regimen are being followed and which rejected), and quantitative concerns (the extent of compliance with each of the component therapies, from rigorous adherence to total rejection).

Compliance behavior is a multidimensional interactional model; however, as was previously noted, most research dichotomizes the population. Gordis (1976) notes that research on the topic tends to use either a statistically derived or an arbitrary cutoff point to distinguish compliers from noncompliers. Occasionally, researchers avoid the dichotomy by viewing compliance along a continuum of appointment keeping, drug taking, and other therapeutic behavior.

Once the definitional hurdles are cleared, both the researcher and the clinician face another complex problem—how to measure the phenomenon. There are numerous methodological considerations (Leonard, 1982):

1. A lack of definitional consistency, which limits comparative studies.
2. Sampling problems that include the randomness of sample frame and lack of follow-up of non–appointment keepers (assuming them to be noncompliers).
3. Problems with control groups (to withhold accepted therapies is highly unethical; however, to have no outcome baseline along a continuum of use of a given therapy limits the accuracy of clinical observations).
4. Problems inherent in cross-sectional studies (to define an individual's compliance behavior at one point in time says little about past or future performance).

Direct Measures

Analysis of body fluids (most frequently serum, urine, and more recently, saliva) have advantages over other measures of compliance. Using this technique, either drug levels, a metabolite, or biological marker is analyzed as to its presence and body fluid level. Such measurements can provide either qualitative or quantitative data; however, quantitative information is more time-consuming and expensive to obtain. While the direct method is inherently appealing, there are numerous problems that limit its practical usefulness:

1. The measured body fluid level may be more a function of the timing of the test than compliance.
2. The bioavailability of drug, and thus body fluid levels, may vary depending on route of administration, interaction with other drugs, or diminished absorption due to foods.
3. The invasive nature of the method (e.g., venipuncture or urine analysis) may engender resentment and noncompliance.
4. Results may vary depending on the setting (e.g., home versus office or clinic).

Indirect Measures

Indirect measures of compliance have included outcome measures, patient self-assessment, physician assessment, and pill counts.

Outcome Measures

One major assumption underlying outcome as a measure of intervention is that the therapy is the critical variable in determining the outcome of a patient. Korsch, et al. (1978) studied children who underwent renal transplants and found an association between noncompliance and weight loss, change in renal function, and reduction of cushingoid features. As a generalization, such associations may be valid, but applying such generalizations to individuals is risky, for numerous external variables interact to affect therapeutic outcome, independent of patient compliance.

Patient Self-Assessment

A second indirect measure of patient compliance is the self-report. This approach has been used in a number of studies in the general population (Gordis, 1976; Marston, 1970) as well as the pediatric age groups (Feinstein, 1959; Francis, Korsch, & Morris, 1969; Gordis, Markowitz, & Lilienfield, 1969). Consensus is that such a method results in significant overestimation of compliance. On the other hand, there are few data to indicate that "complying patients misrepresent themselves as noncompliers, nor is there evidence that those who profess noncompliance at interview are lying" (Leonard, 1982). This is to say that if, at interview, a patient reports noncompliance, there is little reason to distrust that report. The converse, however, does not hold. As Litt and Cuskey (1980) note, there are a number of limitations to this method, including the skill of the interviewer, the patient's recall ability, and the patient's fear of repercussions.

Physician Assessment

An alternative to the self-report is the physician report; there are few data that support physician accuracy is better than chance. Davis (1968) found medical students better able to predict compliance behavior than staff physicians. Caron and Roth (1968) asked 27 ward residents to predict compliance behavior for antacid use in patients. They found physician error to be 32 percent with 22 of 27 physicians overestimating compliance. Other studies (Blackwell, 1979; Charney, 1967) confirm the observations of Caron and Roth that physician predictive skills regarding compliance behavior are not much better than chance alone.

One frequently overlooked aspect of prescriptive drug compliance is whether the prescription has been dispensed and received. National data indicate that 3 percent of all prescriptions remain unfilled after ten days. Factors such as financial status and medical and pharmaceutical insurance will affect this measure, and thus it may be a poor measure of overall compliance behavior.

Pill Counts

The pill-count method of measurement was compared with patient self-reports in a pediatric outpatient clinic (Francis et al., 1969), and it was found that pill counts more accurately reflected noncompliance than did self-reports. On the other hand, in Bergman's study (1963) of pediatric patients' compliance with penicillin for streptococcal pharyngitis, pill count was a significantly less-sensitive measure of noncompliance than was urine analysis for levels of antibiotic excretion.

While pill counts assume that missing pills were consumed by the identified patient, this is not always the case. Furthermore, other problems of this measure of compliance include the setting in which the pill count occurs (home versus clinic), the degree of surprise in effecting the pill count, and the patient's desire to appear socially acceptable (through pill discard prior to a clinic visit). In addition, the pill-count method fails to indicate the pattern of medication use (e.g., whether the prescribed medications were taken at the prescribed times (Christensen, 1978).

One problem in the measurement of compliance is that we may be searching for a single measure for what is a complex and interrelated phenomenon. As Leonard (1982) notes, "There is little evidence that various forms of compliance (appointment keeping, short- and long-term medication compliance, diet, and life-style changes) are more than modestly related to each other, or that compliance in any one area is stable over time." On the other hand, there is evidence that the complexity of the medical regimen does negatively influence compliance outcomes.

EXTENT OF NONCOMPLIANCE AMONG CHILDREN
AND YOUTHS

Because of the numerous methodological, conceptual, and definitional problems discussed earlier, estimates of noncompliance in both the pediatric and the general populations are woefully inaccurate. Haynes (1976) estimated that 50 percent of patients fail to fully comply with prescribed regimens. Other estimates range from 20–80 percent (Litt & Cuskey, 1980). Mattan and Yaffe (1974) report that noncompliance may be higher in the pediatric population than in adults. They estimated the range of pediatric noncompliance to be between 34 percent and 82 percent. While there is wide discrepancy as to specific percentages, there is general agreement that noncompliance is a problem of major proportions in pediatrics (Haggerty & Roghmann, 1972; Ruley, 1978; Wilson, 1973).

There is less agreement as to the extent and impact of adolescent noncompliance. While Korsch (1978) and Smith, Rosen, Trueworthy & Lowman (1979) found teenagers to be more noncompliant than their disease-matched younger peers, Litt and Cuskey (1981) did not find this to be the case. Others (Irwin et al., 1981) have found factors other than age to be major determinants of compliance behavior during the adolescent years.

FACTORS THAT INFLUENCE COMPLIANCE

Both Becker (1976) and Caplan (1976) have commented on the vast, diffuse, unsystematic data that have been generated to explain compliant behavior. In the end, however, data are often contradictory, noncomparative in nature, and noncontributory to understanding of a problem. Here some of the key factors that have been associated with pediatric therapeutic compliance will be reviewed. These include demographic variables, disease factors, the health care setting patient–therapist relationship, and family variables.

Demographic Factors

While many studies have explored characteristics such as age, sex, race, and education, few have shown any association of these with compliance behavior. In a study on pediatric compliance with penicillin therapy in a private-practice setting, Charney (1967) found no association between age and compliance. Such was also the conclusion of Wilson (1973) who found little association between age and medication errors, adherence, and antacid consumption. For the adolescent population, Litt and Cuskey

(1981) as noted previously, found no difference in younger patients in a sample of youths with juvenile rheumatoid arthritis. Korsch (1978) did find age to be a factor influencing compliance behavior, with teenagers less compliant than younger renal transplant patients.

Much like age factors, sex seems to be a weak distinguisher between compliers and noncompliers. The belief that males are less likely to follow through with medical regimens is not supported in the literature; rather, there is a hint that adult males may follow through on long-term medical treatments more rigorously than females do (Marston, 1970).

Socioeconomic status and parental education levels are associated in indirect ways. There is some evidence that the larger the economic gap between the provider and the patient, the less likely they are to be talking a common language (Nir & Cutler, 1978). Second, the intervening variable between socioeconomic status and compliance may be access to health services (Haynes, 1976). Kegeles (1963) found a direct association between income and frequency of dental visits. Whether the same association exists for medical visits, however, is uncertain due to the difference in reimbursement mechanisms for medical and dental visits. It would seem more plausible to hypothesize a bimodal distribution of utilization in association with income, with those in the low–middle income range (the medically indigent) least likely to access services.

Individual and Parental Factors

Beyond socioeconomic status, a number of familial variables have been investigated as to their contribution to understanding compliance behaviors. Numerous studies have developed profiles of compliers, frequently describing such individuals as responsible, mature, stable, articulate, or responsive. The uncomfortable feeling arises that these adjectives may more reflect the interviewers' image of themselves than an objective description of those who comply with therapeutic regimens.

Other studies have developed psychological profiles of compliers as having fewer psychological problems, a more positive body image, or greater self-esteem than those who fail treatment. When one looks at these findings in the light of those by Kellerman, Zeltzer, Ellenberg, Dawh, & Rigler (1981) and Offer et al. (see Chapter 5), there is little reason to believe that the majority of children and youths with a wide range of chronic diseases suffer serious injury to body image or self-esteem. Perhaps it is the disease itself that determines the psychological and social implications for the individual and thus the impact on compliance as well (vida infra, p. *151*).

While intelligence may be correlated with the ability to articulate an understanding of the disease and the need for medicine (Becker, Radius,

Rosenstock, Drachman, Shuberth, & Teets, 1978), there is little to support its association with compliance (Schmidt, 1977). Watkins, Williams & Martin (1967), using outcome measures in a group of diabetic patients, found an inverse relationship between intelligence and degree of control. In a study of patients with cystic fibrosis, Meyers, Dolan, & Mueller (1975) found no difference in disease knowledge between mothers whose children were considered to be compliant and those whose children were not.

Other familial factors that have been positively correlated with compliance include family supportiveness (Litt & Cuskey, 1981; Heinzelmann & Bagley, 1970); family communications (Korsch, 1978); and family expectations for successful completions of the therapeutic regimen (Oakes, 1970). Family involvement has proved to be controversial, with some investigators (e.g., Irwin, 1981) indicating improved adolescent appointment-keeping behavior with parental involvement and others (e.g., Litt & Cuskey, 1981) finding the converse to be true.

Patient–Provider Factors and the Role of the Setting

As with many other variables that have been studied regarding compliance behavior, the data regarding the physician–patient relationship is confusing and contrary to expectation. Davis (1968) found noncompliant patients to express more negative feelings toward their physicians, and Korsch et al. (1978) found compliance to increase with positive feelings of the patient toward the care provider. Becker, Drachman, & Kirsch (1974) also found that consistency of the physician was associated with appointment keeping in an acute pediatric setting.

On the other hand, it may be a faulty extrapolation from positive patient–physician relationship to therapeutic compliance. Meyers et al. (1975) found no relationship between affection for care provider and compliance in patients with cystic fibrosis; and Charney (1967) found that drug-taking behavior of patients with acute illness (pharyngitis and otitis media) was better when the duration of the patient–physician relationship was less than four years.

Characteristics of the setting that have been linked with noncompliance include expense and inconvenience (Alpert, 1964), extended waiting time (Haynes, 1976), and public clinics (Litt & Cuskey, 1980).

Disease and Therapeutic Factors

Marston's (1970) finding of a positive association between severity of illness and compliance conflicts with Davis' (1968) finding of a negative association. The duration of illness, however, and the complexity of the therapeutic regimen have both been associated with noncompliance (Sackett, 1976). Furthermore, the degree of change demanded of the individual appears to significantly affect compliance. Haynes (1976) has indicated a ranking of life changes with diminishing compliance behavior:

1. Acquire new habits (e.g., take medications)
2. Alter old habits (e.g., change dietary behaviors)
3. Alter personal habits (e.g., discontinue smoking)

Furthermore, it is reasonable to postulate that those medications or procedures for which there is a rapid positive or negative response through either compliance or omission would be most highly correlated with compliance. Examples would include pancreatic enzymes for the cystic fibrosis patient (omission rapidly results in bloating and abdominal discomfort) and bronchodilators (use rapidly results in relief of acute asthmatic symptoms). Conversely, those therapies for which response is symptomatically undiscernable would be at greatest risk for noncompliance. Insulin use for diabetes and the last few days of antimicrobial therapy for otitis media (once symptomatic relief had been obtained) are but two examples.

It would also be reasonable to assume that the severity of the disease process would be positively associated with compliance, but as has been shown, the association is tenuous. It is known, however, that there is only a weak correlation between medically diagnosed severity and patient-perceived severity of illness. The relationship between perceived severity of illness and compliance has been confirmed in multiple studies (Becker, Maiman, Kirscht, Haefner & Drachman, 1977; Meyers et al., 1975). The extent of perceived illness is directly linked with the sense of personal vulnerability.

Sackett (1976) noted five specific factors associated with noncompliance that summarize the previous discussion. They are as follows:

1. Disease: psychiatric diagnosis
2. Regimen: complexity, degree of behavioral change, duration
3. Therapeutic source: inefficient and inconvenient clinics
4. Patient–therapist interaction: inadequate monitoring, patient dissatisfaction
5. Patient: inappropriate health beliefs, previous or present noncompliance with other regimens, family instability

THE HEALTH-BELIEF MODEL

Expanding on the notion of the patient's perceived vulnerability, Becker (1974) elaborated a model called the *health-belief model* to explain health promotion (Roenstock, 1966) and compliance behavior (Becker &

Maiman, 1975). Over the past decade, the model has been extensively used in the study of compliance behavior in children and youths (Becker Drachman and Kirsch 1974; Becker, Maiman, Kirscht, Haefner, & Drachman, 1977; Maiman & Becker, 1974; Becker et al., 1978).

First developed by Rosenstock in 1966, the health-belief model was developed to explain preventive health behavior. To avoid disease-stimulating behavior, Rosenstock argued, an individual would need:

1. A sense of personal susceptibility
2. An awareness that the disease was of at least moderate severity
3. A belief that the action would be beneficial to reduce the risk of disease

Furthermore, to assume disease-avoiding behavior, the barriers of cost, convenience, pain, and embarrassment must be overcome. Finally, there would need to be a cue or event that would serve as a call-to-action stimulating behavior change.

The model is based upon Lewins *value–expectancy* theory, (1944) which assumes behavior change will occur depending on the value an individual places on a particular outcome (e.g., the eradication of an infection, or a normal blood glucose level) and the expectation that the proposed action will result in the outcome desired (Rosenstock, 1924). Applying this model to health behavior, Maiman and Becker (1974) note that the degree to which an individual complies with a health-promoting behavior is relative to the subjective desire to reduce susceptibility or severity.

Becker's application of the value–expectancy model, as depicted in Figure 9-1, reflects the interaction of motivation-ascribed value to illness, and thus illness reduction, and the probability that the new behavior or therapy will reduce the threat.

Research has tested the empirical value of this model (Kirscht & Rosenstock, 1977; Radius, Becker, Rosenstock, Drachman, Shuberth, & Teets, et al.; 1978, Kasl, 1974) and confirms the following:

1. The predictive value of the model
2. The gap between patient knowledge of the disease and therapies and therapeutic compliance
3. That compliance with one aspect of therapy increases the likelihood of compliance with other aspects
4. That family support and stability increases the likelihood of compliance

Becker et al. (1977) expanded the model for the pediatric setting, based upon the assumption that the mother is the gatekeeper of the child's compliance. This adaptation looks at compliant behaviors as stemming from a readiness to undertake recommended compliance behavior, filtered

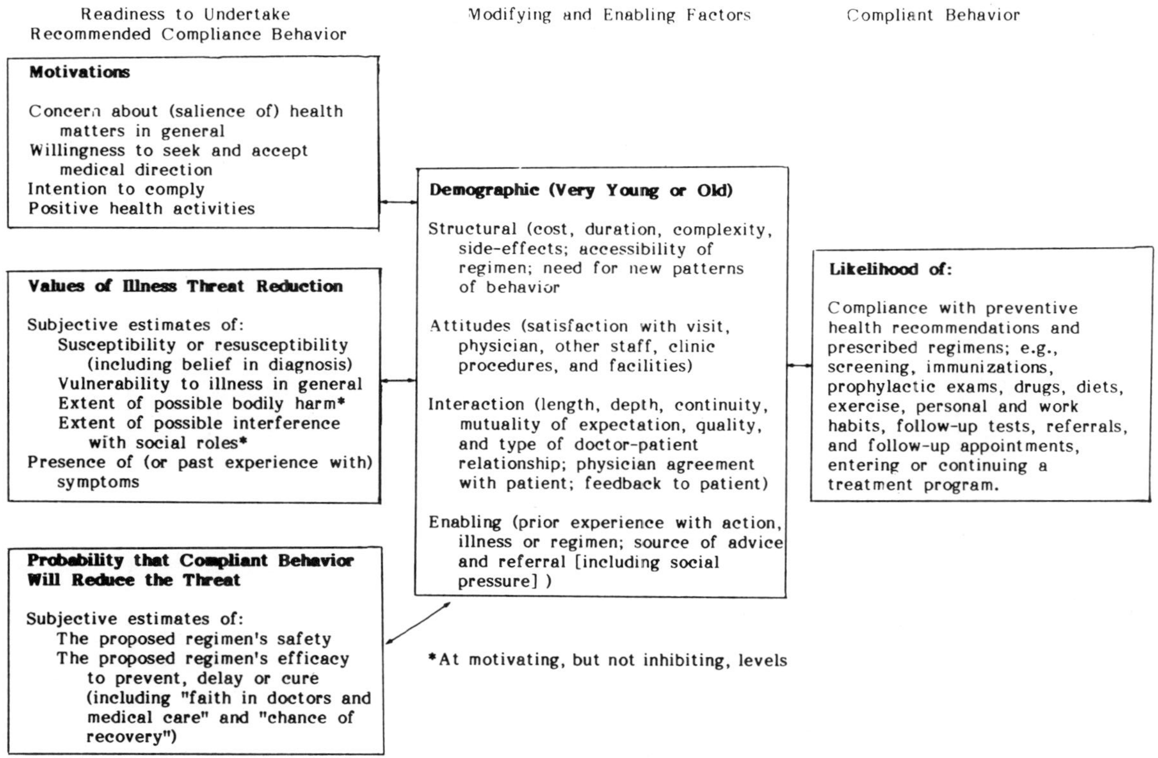

Readiness to Undertake Recommended Compliance Behavior
Modifying and Enabling Factors
Compliant Behavior
Motivations
Concern about (salience of) health matters in general
Willingness to seek and accept medical direction
Intention to comply
Positive health activities
Values of Illness Threat Reduction
Subjective estimates of:
Susceptibility or resusceptibility (including belief in diagnosis)
Vulnerability to illness in general
Extent of possible bodily harm*
Extent of possible interference with social roles*
Presence of (or past experience with) symptoms
Probability that Compliant Behavior Will Reduce the Threat
Subjective estimates of:
The proposed regimen's safety
The proposed regimen's efficacy to prevent, delay or cure (including "faith in doctors and medical care" and "chance of recovery")
Demographic (Very Young or Old)
Structural (cost, duration, complexity, side-effects; accessibility of regimen; need for new patterns of behavior
Attitudes (satisfaction with visit, physician, other staff, clinic procedures, and facilities)
Interaction (length, depth, continuity, mutuality of expectation, quality, and type of doctor-patient relationship; physician agreement with patient; feedback to patient)
Enabling (prior experience with action, illness or regimen; source of advice and referral [including social pressure])
*At motivating, but not inhibiting, levels
Likelihood of:
Compliance with preventive health recommendations and prescribed regimens; e.g., screening, immunizations, prophylactic exams, drugs, diets, exercise, personal and work habits, follow-up tests, referrals, and follow-up appointments, entering or continuing a treatment program.

Figure 9-1. A model of compliance behavior. (Reprinted from Becker, M. et al., The Health Belief Model and Prediction of Dietary Compliance: A Field Experiment, *Journal of Health and Social Behavior,* 1977, *18,* 348. With permission.)

through modifying and enabling factors. Much like the adult model from which it is derived, readiness has three components: motivations (e.g., concern for the child's health and fear that he or she will get sick); perceived threat (e.g., perceived vulnerability to illness, susceptibility, potential seriousness or severity of the problem; and perceived probability that compliance will reduce threat (e.g., faith in therapist and therapy, feelings of control over the problem). Likewise, modifying and enabling factors are divided into three component parts: demographic–social variables; structural factors (such as cost, safety, and duration of the regimen); and enabling factors (including degree of family functioning and past experiences with the problem and regimen).

During the late 1970s, Becker extensively tested this model in a study of treatment for otitis media (Becker, et al., 1974), compliance with dietary regimens (Becker, et al.,1977), and compliance with asthma regimens (Becker, et al., 1978). What emerged from those studies was that the mother's general health concerns for her child and her perceived sense of the child's vulnerability to illness were most closely associated with compliant behavior.

While the model is useful for understanding general aspects of compliance behavior, much remains unexplained. Where the adolescent model fits between the adult and pediatric models depends on many factors, such as age, cognitive and developmental functioning, chronicity of illness, past experiences with the condition, degree of family functioning, and extrafamilial support systems.

RECOMMENDATIONS FOR IMPROVING
COMPLIANCE IN CHILDREN AND YOUTHS

While the compliance literature is frequently contradictory and confusing, the bottom line is that clinicians must still act. They must develop therapeutic regimens and assist their patients in fulfilling the therapeutic contract. It is in that spirit that the following recommendations are offered:

1. Simplicity: data indicate that compliance diminishes as treatment plans become increasingly complex; therefore, it is critical to make the plan as unencumbered as possible.
2. Return control to the patient (or the family). Becker has noted that a sense of control is a key aspect of readiness for compliance. Control can be returned to the patient (or family) by using explicit therapeutic contracts and negotiating those aspects that require life-style changes. Examples would be (Bernarde and Mayerson, 1978) diet management, exercise regimens, and frequency of taking medications. The goal of

this approach is that the treatment be tailored to the individual's life-style. As duration of therapy continues, such contracting becomes increasingly important.

3. Make explicit outcome expectations; whether the therapeutic inter-vention is curative, rehabilitative, or maintenance in nature, it is crit-ical that the therapist and patient–family expectations be parallel. Likewise, it is essential to discuss what visable or symptomatic changes, if any, can be expected from the therapy; i.e., can the in-dividual be expected to feel better as a result of the intervention?

4. If few visible or symptomatic improvements are derived from the therapy (e.g., insulin therapy for diabetes or chemotherapy prophy-laxis for those with a Mantoux positive skin test), frequent monitoring is warranted. If the therapeutic intervention makes the individual feel worse (as is the case, at times, with oral theophylline preparations or tumor chemotherapy), close and consistent physician follow-up is even more essential.

5. The risk for clinicians is to overestimate the compliance of those most like themselves and to underestimate the compliance of those who are most different. The trap can be avoided in part by combining clin-ical observations and outcome measures with self-report and bio-chemical measures whenever cost and invasiveness do not preclude their use. In evaluating compliance, it is wise to measure not only appointment-keeping or drug-taking compliance, but behavior changes as well.

6. Fear is at best a short-term motivator, for it is impossible to chronically maintain a high level of anxiety. Messages that create a positive ap-peal—stimulate a desire to participate in the activity—appear to be most effective.

7. Education and knowledge are not the handmaidens of compliance; thus, while it is important for adolescent patients to understand their disease and therapeutic process up to their capacity, it is faulty thinking to assume that compliance will be the by-product of that understand-ing.

8. Patient acceptability of therapeutic services improves compliance. Acceptability can be enhanced by reducing waiting time for appoint-ments, ensuring confidentiality when appropriate, providing for phy-sician and other therapist continuity, and decreasing access barriers to therapy (e.g., cost of medications and transportation limitations).

REFERENCES

Alpert, J. J. Broken appointments. *Pediatrics,* 1964, *34,* 127–132.

Becker, M.H., Drachman, R.H., & Kirsch, J.P. A new approach to explaining sick-role behavior in low income populations. *American Journal of Public Health,* 1974, *64,* 205–216.

Becker, M.H., Maiman, L.A., Kirscht, J.P., Haefner, D.P., & Drachman, R.H. The health belief model and prediction of dietary compliance: A field experiment. *Journal of Health and Social Behavior,* 1977, *18,* 348–365.

Becker, M.H., & Maiman, L.A. Sociobehavioral determinants of compliance with health and medical care recommendations. *Medical Care,* 1975, *13*(1), 10–24.

Becker, M.H., Radius, S.M., Rosenstock, I.M., Drachman, R.H., Shuberth, K., & Teets, K.C. Compliance with a medical regimen for asthma: A test of the health belief model. *Public Health Reports,* 1978, *93*(3), 268–277.

Benarde, M.A., & Mayerson, E.W. Patient–physician negotiation. *Journal of the American Medical Association,* 1978, *239*(14), 1413–1415.

Bergman, A., & Werner, R. Failure of children to receive penicillin by mouth. *New England Journal of Medicine,* 1963, *268,* 1334.

Blackwell, B. Treatment adherence: A contemporary overview. *Psychosomatics,* 1979, *20*(1), 27–35.

Bowen, R.G., Rich, R., and Schlotfeldt, R.: Effects of Organized Instruction for Patients with the Diagnosis of Diabetes Mellitus, *Nursing Research,* 1961, *10:*15–9.

Caplan, R.D. *Adhering to medical regimens:* The University of Michigan: Pilot Experiments in Patient Education and Social Support. 1976, Ann Arbor, Mich.

Caron, H.S., & Roth, H.P. Patients' cooperation with a medical regimen. *Journal of the American Medical Association* 1968, *203,* 922–926.

Christensen, D.B. Drug-taking compliance: A review and synthesis. *Health Services Research,* 1978, *13*(2), 171–187.

Charney, E., Bynum, R., Eldredge, D., Frank, D., MacWhinney, J.B., McNabb, N., Scheiner, A., Sumpter, E., & Iker, H. How well do patients take oral penicillin? A collaborative study in private practice. *Pediatrics* 1967, *40,* 188–195.

Davis, M., & Eichhorn, R.L. Compliance with medical regimens: A panel study. *Journal of Health and Human Behavior,* 1963, *4,* 240–249.

Davis, M.S. Physiologic, psychologic, and demographic factors in compliance with doctor's orders. *Medical Care,* 1968, *6,* 115–122.

Feinstein, A.R. Compliance bias and the interpretation of therapeutic trials. In D. L. Sackett & R.B. Haynes (Eds.), *Compliance with therapeutic regimens.* Baltimore, Maryland: John Hopkins University Press, 1976.

Francis, V., Korsch, B., & Morris, M. Gaps in doctor–patient communication: Patients' response to medical advice. *New England Journal of Medicine,* 1969, *280,* 535–540.

Gordis, L. Methodological issues in the measurement of patient compliance. In D.L. Sackett, R.B. Haynes, (Eds.), *Compliance with therapeutic regimens.* Baltimore, Maryland: Johns Hopkins University Press, 1976.

Gordis, L., & Markowitz, M. Evaluation of the effectiveness of comprehensive and continuous pediatric care. II. Effectiveness of continuous care in influencing patient compliance. *Pediatrics,* 1971, *48,* 766–776.

Gordis, L., Markowitz, M., & Lilienfield, A.M. The inaccuracy of using interviews to estimate patient reliability in taking medications at home. *Medical Care,* 1969, *7,* 49–54.

Haggerty, R.J., & Roghmann, K.J. Noncompliance and self-medication: Two neglected aspects of pediatric pharmacology. Pediatric Clinics of North America, 1972, *19,* 101–116.

Haynes, R.B., Gibson, E.S., Hackett, B.C., Johnson, A.L., Sackett, D.S., Taylor, D.W., & Roberts, R.S. Improvement of medication compliance in uncontrolled hypertension. *Lancet,* 1976, *1*(7972) 1265–1268.

Heinzelman, F., & Bagley, R. Response to physical activity programs and their effects on health behavior. *Public Health Reports,* 1970, *85* 73–81.

Hulka, B.S., Casell, J.C., Kupper, L.L., & Burdette, J.A. Communication, compliance, and concordance between physicians and patients with prescribed medication. *American Journal of Public Health,* 1976, *66*(9), 847–853.

Irwin, C., Millstein, S., & Shafer, M. Appointment keeping behavior in adolescence. *Journal of Pediatrics,* 1981, *99*(5), 799–802.

Kasl, S.V. The health belief model and behavior related to chronic illness. In M.H. Becker (Ed.), *The health belief model and personal health behavior.* New Jersey: Charles B. Slack, 1974.

Kegeles S.S. Why people seek dental care; a test of a conceptual formulation. *Journal of Health and Human Behavior,* 1963, *4,* 166–173.

Kellaway, G.S.M. & McCrae, E. The effect of counseling on compliance-failure in patient drug use therapy, *New Zealand Medical Journal,* 1979, *89(630):* 161–164.

Kellerman, J., Zeltzer, L., Ellenberg, L., Dash, J., Rigler, D. Psychological effects of illness in adolescence, *Journal of Pediatrics,* 1980, *97:* 126–131.

Kirscht, J.P., & Rosenstock, I.M. Patient adherence to antihypertensive medical regimens. *Journal of Community Health,* 1977, *3*(2),, 115–124.

Korsch, B.M., Fine, R.N., & Negrete, V.G. Noncompliance in children with renal transplants. *Pediatrics,* 1978, *61,* 872–876.

Lewin, K., Dembo, T., Festinger, L., and Sears, P. Level of aspiration. In J. McV Hunt (Ed.), *Personality and the behavior disorders.* New York: Ronald Press, 1944.

Leonard, B. *Compliance with medical regimens: A review and critique.* Unpublished paper, University of Minnesota 1982.

Litt, I., & Cuskey, W.R. Compliance with medical regimens during adolescence. *Pediatric Clinics of North America,* 1980, *27,* 3–15.

Litt, I.F. & Cuskey, W.R. Compliance with salicylate therapy in adolescence with juvenile rheumatoid arthritis. *American Journal Diseases of Childhood,* 1981, *135,* 434–436.

Maiman, L.A., & Becker, M.H. The health belief model: Origins and correlates in psychological theory. *Health Education Monograph,* 1974, *2,* 336–353.

Marston, M. Compliance with medical regimens: A review of the literature. *Nursing Research,* 1970, *19.*

Martens, L.V., Frazier,P.J., Hirt, K., Meskin, K.H., & Prosheck, J. Developing brushing performance in second graders through behavior modification. *Health Services Reports,* 1973, *88,* 818–823.

Mattar, M.G., & Yaffe, S.J. Compliance of pediatric patients with therapeutic regimens. *Pediatrics,* 1974, *54.*

Meyers A., Dolan, T.F., & Mueller, D. Compliance and self medication in cystic fibrosis. *American Journal of Disabilities in Children,* 1975, *129,* 1011–1013.

Nir, Y., & Cutler, R. The Unmotivated Patient syndrome: survey of therapeutic interventions, *American Journal of Psychiatry, 135*(4): 442.

Oakes, T.W., Ward, J., Gray, R., Klavker, M., & Moody, P. Family expectations and arthritis patient compliance to a hand resting splint regimen. *Journal of Chronic Diseases,* 1970, *22,* 757–764.

Radius, S.M., Becker, M.H., Rosenstock, I.M., Drachman, R.H., Shuberth, K.C., & Teets, K.C. Factors influencing mothers' compliance with a medication regimen for asthmatic children. *Journal of Asthma Research,* 1978, *15*(3),, 133–149.

Rosenstock, I.M. Historical origins of the health belief model. In M.H Becker (Ed.), *The health belief model and personal health behavior.* New Jersey: Charles B. Slack, Inc., 1974.

Rosenstock, I.M. Why people use health services. *Milbank Memorial Fund Quarterly,* 1966, *44,* 94–127.

Ruley, E.J. Compliance in young hypertensive patients. *Pediatric Clinics of North America,* 1978, *25,* 175–182.

Sackett, D.L. The magnitude of compliance and noncompliance. In D. L. Sackett, & R.B. Haynes (Eds.), *Compliance with therapeutic regimens*. Baltimore, Maryland: Johns Hopkins University Press, 1976.

Schmidt, D.D. Patient compliance: The effect of the doctor as a therapeutic agent. *Journal of Family Practice*, 1977, *4*, 853–856.

Smith, S.C., Rosen, D., Trueworthy, R & Lowman, J.: A reliable method for evaluating drug compliance in children with cancer. *Cancer*, 1979, *43*, 169–173.

Watkins, J.D., Williams, T., & Martin, D., A study of diabetic patients at home, *American Journal of Public Health*, 1967, *57:* 452–459.

Wilson, J.T. Compliance with instructions in the evaluation of therapeutic efficacy. *Clinical Pediatrics*, 1973, *12*.

Robert Wm. Blum

10

The Dying Adolescent

Adolescence is a time measured by firsts—new experiences that bring the developing teenager into contact with his or her emerging potential. It is a time when expanding capability is apparent in a new appearance. It is a time when the world is seen as boundless and one's potential equally without limit (Konopka, 1968).

Terminal illness conflicts with the normal developmental tasks of adolescence. One can no longer maintain a myth of invulnerability and omnipotence. Desire for independence conflicts with the increasing dependence on others to meet the tasks of daily living. Social isolation restricts social role experimentation, and thus, social development is limited.

This chapter will review the emergence of an understanding of death from childhood through adolescence. The stages of death awareness will be explored, as will the interrelationships among cognitive and social development and death awareness. Finally, implications for clinical practice will be identified.

STAGES OF DEATH AWARENESS

Infancy and Young Children

While cognitively unaware of boundaries between self and others, the infant under the age of one does appear to have a somatic response to separation. In 1946, Spitz published his classic paper on anaclitic depression, in which he observed failure to thrive in infants who were denied nurturance through separation from their parents. Initially, these children developed weepy behavior, when previously they had been happy and outgoing. Weepiness gave way to withdrawal, which was accompanied by weight loss, and frequently, insomnia. By their first birthday, failure to thrive was marked.

Mauer (1966) indicated that infants, wavering between sleep and wakefulness, are beginning to experience the difference between being and nonbeing. By three months of age they are playing *peek-a-boo,** alternating terror with delight. The dependency of infancy heightens the separation anxiety at about eight months of age, when the infant begins to realize that he or she and the mother are indeed two people and not one. The difference between being and nonbeing and between self and others are major distinctions that the infant makes during the first year of life. At this stage the primary focus of the seriously ill infant is the attendant pain and separation from parents entailed by the illness; rejection of the nurturance of others may stem from the rejection experienced by the failure of significant others to make the pain subside (Vore, 1974).

Ages One to Five Years

Long before the child reaches kindergarten, he or she is regularly confronted with loss, separation, and death. Kilman (1968) described a survey from a nursery school of 16 children wherein the children reported having the following experiences in a random two-week period of time: a tonsillectomy, injury of a relative in an automobile accident, the hospitalization of a sibling in the middle of the night, a brother's surgery, death of a grandparent, extended absence of a parent due to an oversea's trip, death of a turtle and cat, and the recent discovery of the death of an uncle during the preceding month. Rochlin (1967) has shown that children between the ages of three and five years are fully aware of death. Nagy showed that at this age, death represents a departure, separation, and sleep. Some deny its existence; others cannot separate death from life and therefore, view it as a transient, reversible process. Rochlin (1967) concludes, "At a very early age, well-developed mental faculties are functioning to defend oneself against the realization that life may end."

Nagy (1948) concurs that even at this early age children do not accept

---

* Peek-a-boo in medieval English means *alive and dead.*

death: "To die means the same as living, under changed circumstances."
Nagy (1948) sees the three-year-old's perceptions as active denial of death:

What endeavor brings about the identification of death with the departure or with sleep? In early infancy, that is, under five, its desires guide the child even at the price of modifying the reality. Opposition to death is so strong that the child denies death, as emotionally it cannot accept it.

Much like the younger child, the child below the age of five plays numerous games experimenting with being and nonbeing. Hide-and-seek replaces peek-a-boo. By three years of age, holsters are strapped to the toddler's side, and games of war become afternoon entertainment. Fairy tales and fables, such as *Hansel and Gretel* and *Snow White,* serve to reinforce three predominant themes of death: death is abandonment, the dead can return to life, and death is the reward of evil.

The Five- to Ten-Year-Old

In the first major study of children's attitudes toward death, Schilder and Wechsler (1934) studied hospitalized children from 5 to 15 years of age. Through the use of questionnaires, and subsequently through the use of eight provocative drawings, they found that children of this age dealt matter-of-factly and realistically with death. While not categorized by age, the authors found that children distinguish between what they observe and what they have been told. If they see disagreement, they have little need to reconcile the contradiction. Schilder and Waechter (1934) conclude that the fear of death is rare in childhood. Similar findings have not been substantiated in more recent studies. Alexander and Alderstein (1959) found that words associated with death elicited an increased emotional response in all ages of children and adolescents. In this study, death anxiety seemed to be heightened in children from 5 to 8 years of age, and in youths from 13 to 16. Under ten years of age, images of violence, fears of physical injury, and mutilation represent the major concerns regarding death for the healthy child.

Nagy (1948) found that between the ages of five and nine years, death was personified either as a separate person or as the return of the dead. As the former, "[Death] puts on a white coat and a death face . . . I know it's just a man who has put on a death-face. He was in the circus once." As a spirit: "Death can't be seen, like the angels can't be seen because they are spirits. I imagine death is a bad man's skeleton brought to life." In this age group death is a distinct personality. Compared with earlier age groups, children from five to nine see death as dinstinct from life. It is imagined as a negative external force, which is not inevitable but is rather the result of misdeeds. Death is not reversible in a physical sense, but life persists as a spirit (Swain, 1979).

On the other hand, Spinetta, Rigler, and Karon (1974) have shown that children six to ten years old are acutely aware of their own impending death. Through the use of three-dimensional hospital room replicas, Spinetta measured personal space in leukemic children from six to ten years of age and found that the distance they placed four significant figures (mother, father, nurse, and doctor) from the bed in the replica widened as death neared. This increasing distance was not noted in frequently hospitalized youths who had nonprogressive chronic illnesses.

These findings ran contrary to much of the early research in children's death anxiety. There are two concurrent themes of that research: What are childrens' changing images of death? And what is their perception of their own death? There has been far greater concordance in the former than in the latter area. As Spinetta notes, many have held to the notion that due to limited intellectual ability, the child under ten experiences little death anxiety (Deboskey, 1970; Ingalls, 1971; Sigler, 1970). On the other hand, researchers and clinicians have noted that children under ten who are faced with their own impending death are aware that something very serious is occurring (Binger, 1969; Kastenbaum, 1970; Schowalter, 1970). While healthy children in this age group are concerned with mutilation and the physical harm associated with death, Waechler (1971) found that fatally ill children more frequently verbalize their concerns and fears of dying (Waechler, 1971). These findings, together with those of Spinetta, et al. (1973), indicate that even at a very young age, children in the United States have the awareness and language to discuss their personal concerns in facing death.

The Preadolescent and Adolescent Years

Nagy (1948) found that by the age of ten most children endorsed the notion that death is the cessation of corporeal life. At that age, death is viewed as a universal experience separate from life. Much like those a few years younger than themselves, most adolescents in Swain's study (1979) saw death as a transition from physical capability to spiritual life. Approximately 25 percent of youths endorsed the notion that death represented the total, complete, and irreversible cessation of life—a belief held by 17 percent of 2–16-year-old children. Not only is it an end to corporeal life as we know it, it is inevitable both for others and self. Furthermore, it represents the consequence of physical life and is viewed by youths as an event either occurring in the remote future (40 percent) or by chance (53 percent).

In a study of midwestern children and youths, McIntire, Angle, &

Struempler (1972) found that 20 percent of 13- to 16-year olds viewed death as total cessation, while 60 percent envisioned spiritual continuation, and 20 percent believed in continued cognizance postmortem. Through studying the metaphors used by adolescents to describe death, Farley (1979) found that for males between 15 and 16 years of age (10th grade), death was pictured as more violent (*grinning butcher, threatening father*) than for either their age-matched female counterparts or males two years their senior (12th grade). For the latter two groups, death was viewed in less threatening metaphors (*last adventure, end of a song, misty abyss*). This age discrepancy is consistent with the findings of Alexander and Alderstein (1959), that stimulation of youths 13 to 16 years of age by words associated with death provoked increased emotional responses and anxiety. In only one other age group (five- to eight-year-olds) was there a similar response. The authors conclude that because the ego is developing in early adolescence and is unstable, it is more threatened by death than at other developmental periods.

The Limits of a Maturational View of Death Awareness

To summarize, the stage-based theory of death awareness represents an expansion and reaffirmation of Nagy's (1948) original work on postwar Hungarian children, in whom she found three predominant stages: death as departure or sleep, death as an inevitable negative event that is the consequence of misdeeds, and death as a universal experience representing the end of corporeal life. While this thesis has been supported by further research (Kliman, 1968; Zeligs, 1967), others contend that it is both historically and culturally bound. Swain (1979) and McIntire, et al. (1972) found far fewer images of fantasy and personification of death and more focus on organic decomposition compared with Nagy's (1948) study. Furthermore, Rochlin (1967) found significant variations with relation to socioeconomic status. Children of lower-income parents tended to cite violent images of death, while middle-class children viewed death as a function of old age.

Another limitation of the developmental model is that it assumes greater differences among and between age groups than may in fact exist. Bluebond-Langner (1979) notes that many of the major differences between the child and the adult are frequently more linguistic than conceptual. To substantiate this perspective she points to the work of Kubler-Ross (1969) who found that many adults speak of death in terms of separation and life elsewhere—descriptions that, according to the maturational theorists, are extinguished by seven to ten years of age.

While few children under five years of age in Swain's (1979) study

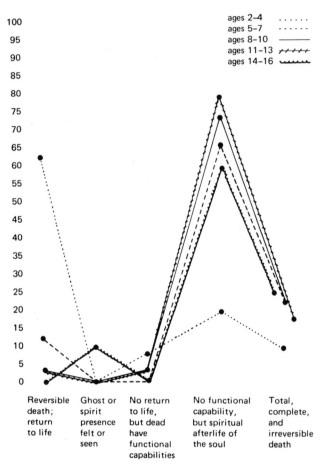

100   ages 2–4   . . . . . .
       ages 5–7   - - - - - -
95   ages 8–10   ————
       ages 11–13   ⟋⟋⟋⟋
90   ages 14–16   ⌣⌣⌣⌣

Reversible	Ghost or	No return	No functional	Total,
death;	spirit	to life,	capability,	complete,
return	presence	but dead	but spiritual	and
to life	felt or	have	afterlife of	irreversible
	seen	functional	the soul	death
		capabilities		

Figure 10-1. Concept of finality of death: percentage of children in each age level responding to each category of the concept. (Reprinted from Swain, H. Childhood views of death. *Death Education*, 1979, 2, 341–358. With permission.)

endorsed the concept that death was the irreversible end of life, only 17 percent of her oldest population 13–16-year-olds held to that belief. When comparing the concepts of death's finality and inevitability, Swain found a significant degree of concordance in all ages over two (Fig. 10-1–10-3). Finally, implicit in a maturational perspective is the assumption of a final outcome—a common end-point—that constitutes the sole adult perspective. It implies a natural linear toward the correct understanding of one's mortality. There is substantial evidence, however, to indicate multiple adult perceptions of death. As Kastenbaum (1967) notes: "[Regarding death] we lack a truly convincing idea of the 'goal' or 'maturational' outcome that the process of growth is moving toward."

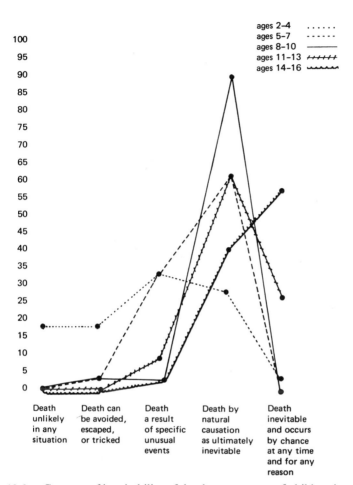

Figure 10-2. Concept of inevitability of death: percentage of children in each age level responding to each category of the concept. (Reprinted from Swain, H. Childhood views of death. *Death Education,* 1979, *2,* 341–358. With permission.)

ADOLESCENT DEVELOPMENT AND THE CRISIS OF DYING

While the perceptions of death awareness do not appear to parallel the physiological, cognitive, and social changes from childhood through adolescence, those changes do have an impact on the perceptions of one's own mortality. Likewise, to face the limits of one's existence at an early age has a significant impact on development.

From a physiological perspective, the hallmark of adolescence is an increase in the rate of development. For many with life-limiting illnesses,

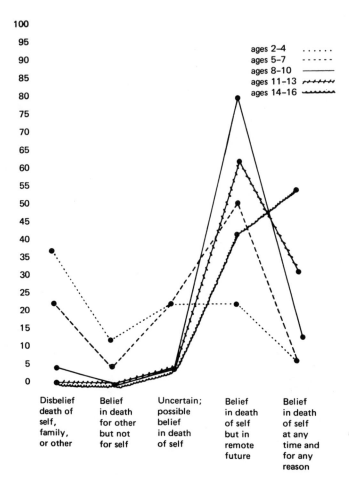

Figure 10-3. Concept of death as a personal event: percentage of children in each age level responding to each category of the concept. (Reprinted from Swain, H. Childhood views of death. *Death Education,* 1979, *2,* 341–358. With permission.)

physical maturation is delayed. The teenager with Crohn's disease, end-stage renal failure, or cystic fibrosis, because of growth failure will enter puberty later than his or her peers. Consequently, chronically or terminally ill teenagers often appear years younger than their chronological or developmental age and thus are treated more like a young child than a maturing adolescent. Such maturational discrepancies, coupled with the exigencies of therapy, serve to reinforce differences from peers, further isolating the chronically ill teenager (Blum, 1981).

Such isolation becomes problematic, not only because of the loneliness that ensues but also in its developmental impact. Erikson (1963) notes that during adolescence peers serve as multiple mirrors, reflecting

back onto the individual interpretations and reactions to actions and behaviors. It is through the process of initiating an action and then observing
the multiple responses of significant others that the individual learns the
social skills of perspective-taking and anticipation of others' reactions.
Furthermore, this process is critical for teenagers in learning to shift from
viewing themselves as controlled by others to having impact on their own
and others' lives. Social isolation inhibits this process. Frequent hospitalizations reinforce both the feelings of being different and the social isolation experienced by youths with serious illness. In the face of intermittent
and unpredictable hospitalizations, friends are constantly unsure of how
close to become. As a result, at an age when there is usually a shift of
attention from parents to peers, the shift is slow for youths which chronic
and terminal illness, resulting in prolonged dependence on parents. This
dependence is reinforced, not only as a result of their relative isolation
from their peers but also by the demands of treatment and by parental
pull. Fatal illness frequently has its origin during childhood, at which time
parents closely supervise drug regimens, special diets, and physical therapy
as if the disease were their own. This objective need for supervision during
childhood is frequently coupled with a sense of parental guilt. The relationship between parent and child during the first decade of life, coupled
with the parents' feelings of responsibility, makes the adolescent's transition from dependence through independence to interdependence most
difficult. Added to this dynamic is the social isolation from peers that
results in a teenager with little impetus to move from the security (and
frustration) of dependence on parents.

The consequence of delayed physical maturity, social isolation, and
increased parental dependence is delayed social development (Coupey,
1980). Such social retardation may limit educational and counseling efforts
of health care providers.

Associated with physical and social development during the teenage
years is a cognitive shift from concrete to abstract reasoning. One component of this shift is the development of the capacity to extrapolate, or
draw upon old experiences to solve new problems not previously encountered. Adolescence is commonly viewed as a period of experimentation, of seeking new experiences. From a developmental perspective,
such experimentation becomes the substrate for cognitive growth. The
more restricted one's range of experiences, the fewer resources one has
to draw upon for problem solving. Such a capacity is predicated upon the
individual's being exposed to multiple new experiences throughout the
preadolescent and adolescent years (Inhelder & Piaget, 1958). Those with
chronic and terminal illness have decidedly fewer such experiences than
their healthy peers; as a result, they lack the experiential substrate for
healthy cognitive growth (Coupey, 1980). Brewster (1982) found that chil-

dren's understanding of their disease process, their need for treatment, and the role of medical personnel was primarily determined by their cognitive maturation.

For the healthy adolescent, one psychological device that allows youths to sample life's experiences more broadly is the myth of invulnerability. Such a belief is not denial, but is rather a perspective of one who has interpreted the new competencies associated with the physiological changes of puberty as limitless potential (Elkind, 1967). Such a belief in one's invincibility is denied those with chronic illness. Family, peers, health providers, and personal fear conspire to increasingly constrict the world of experiences for those with a potentially fatal illness. It is from experimentation that the boundaries of one's potential are learned (Blum, 1982). Such is the nature of reality testing. Denied new and varied experiences against which to establish boundaries between reality and fantasy, the adolescent with a life-limiting disease may have more difficulty in distinguishing real possibilities from desired outcomes.

Another hallmark of the newly emerging cognitive skills of adolescents is the pondering and rumination so often associated with that stage of life (Freud, 1971; Hankoff, 1975). One aspect of this reflective thought, as Erikson (1959) points out, is the focus on various dimensions of time. From childhood through adolescence, three intersecting understandings of time develop: time as an abstraction (as in *my life is but a drop in the vast ocean of time),* a historic understanding of time (as in *there was a time before me, and life will continue after I am gone),* and a personal sense of time (as in *I have a future as well as a past).*

Initially, the child learns from his or her own past, i.e., what life was like as an infant and a young child. As a concrete learner, there are many landmarks for the recent past, such as photographs, mementos, and adult recollections. There are few comparable markers for the future. It is late in childhood and throughout adolescence that one begins to understand time as an abstract concept that is artificially structured. Not only is the abstraction understood, but the teenager begins to perceive himself or herself as one who will live in the future as well as the past (Coleman, 1972).

Erikson (1959) labels the temporal confusion an adolescent may experience in maintaining perspective and expectancy as time diffusion. Hankoff (1975) notes that under such conditions of time diffusion, the adolescent may either excessively structure every present moment to meet preconceived notions of the future or may go to the other extreme and reject future possibilities altogether in favor of short-term gratification. Kastenbaum (1959), studying the phenomenon of time and dying among adolescents, found a rejection of future possibilities and a hostility when the interviewer asked about future goals. Without a guiding sense of expectancy, it is reasonable to anticipate that the adolescent faced with terminal illness will experience time diffusion. Certainly, one of the most problematic areas for the clinician working with chronically ill children and youths is in describing the course of illness over time. Without the cognitive understanding of the future or the capacity to project into the future, the teenager with a life-threatening illness reasonably may turn to present-moment gratification. This problem is compounded by Kastenbaum's (1959) finding that references to future events provoke resentment and anger in adolescents who sense that theirs is not the future of their able-bodied peers.

The developmental differences faced by those youths with life-threatening illnesses do not imply that they represent a psychopathological population. On the contrary, studies by Tavormina, Kastner, Slater, & Watt (1976), Zelter, Kellerman, Ellenberg, Dash, & Rigler, (1980) and Kellerman, Zeltzer, Ellenberg, Rigler (1980) found that those who demonstrated the greatest psychological stress showed the least overt signs of disability. This seemingly paradoxical finding has been confirmed by others, with the implication being that it is the perception of illness far more than the physiological manifestations that affect one's functioning.

CLINICAL ISSUES

For health professionals to successfully work with dying adolescents they must first confront their own mortality (Farrow, 1980). The tendency is to keep a distance from those who have come to be the most dependent. This is true physically (Sigler, 1970; Sudnow, 1967) as well as through death-denying euphemisms (Kastenbaum, 1972). The myth that children should be immune to death prevails; as Kastenbaum notes:

> The kingdom where nobody dies, as Edna St. Vincent Millay once described childhood, is the fantasy of grown-ups. We want our children to be immortal—at least temporarily (Kastenbaum, 1972).

A second myth to which many professionals subscribe is that there is a normative sequence through which those facing death not only do but must pass and that it is the clinician's task to faciliatate that passage. Bowlby (1961) describes a three-step sequence:

1. *Separation–protest phase.* This stage is characterized by the urge to recover the lost love object.
2. *Disorganization phase.* During this stage, the individual exhibits feelings of worthlessness, wide mood swings, and impulsive behavior.
3. *Reorganization phase.* It is during this phase that there is an accommodation to death and a shift back and forth to a prior impulsive stage.

Kubler-Ross (1969) describes a five-stage sequence that progresses from denial to acceptance:

1. *Denial and Isolation.* This represents the initial stage that buffers the shock of the news; it allows the individual to slowly incorporate new information.
2. *Anger.* Anger is frequently displayed randomly, making this stage difficult for both family and clinician. It results from the loss of control one has assumed one has had over life.
3. *Bargaining.* With the illness viewed as a punishment, the patient at this stage attempts to strike a bargain for longer life.
4. *Depression.* With the realization that a bargain is not possible, depression becomes a tool to prepare for the impending loss of all the love objects.
5. *Acceptance.* This is not a happy stage; rather, it is almost void of feelings. It is a stage of detachment and of living one day at a time.

What Bowlby (1961), Kubler-Ross (1969) and others indicate is that the dying trajectory is not a linear downward slope; rather, it is more like a wave with peaks and valleys. It is at times of disease exacerbation or extreme physical discomfort that adolescents tend to wrestle with the fatal consequences of their illness, at other times they act as if they are healthy (Blum, 1981). The terminally ill adolescent is not always terminally ill; however, he or she is always a teenager. Adults often have normative expectations of those who are dying, and for the adolescent to behave otherwise represents denial. Likewise, health professionals tend to have normative expectations of the pace at which youths should progress from one stage to the next. Especially true is the expectation that the stage of anger should give way to acceptance; as the agonal phase of the illness approaches, frustration and the sense of failure increase when one is faced with a teenager whose anger or denial persists. The critical issue is that as with many events during life, how one dies and the degree of insight one has into that experience are not dependent upon the affect displayed. While Kubler-Ross speaks of acceptance, the poet disagrees:

> Do not go gentle into that good night
> Rage, rage against the dying of the light.
>
> (D. Thomas, 1957)

Related to the health professional's expectation of a normative (and rapid) passage through the stages of dying to the phase of acceptance is the belief that the health professional must be *honest*. What being honest involves is rarely explicated. If the findings of Spinetta, Rigler, and Karon (1974) are valid, it is reasonable to believe that children who are dying have an awareness of an enormous impending event, even at a very young age, and even though it is never articulated. They frequently gain their awareness through the nonverbal messages projected by family and hospital personnel. As one 14-year-old boy said, "I know the game's up now. Dr. S. doesn't come 'round as he used to on a daily basis." Teenagers tend to orient to the nonverbal at least as much, if not more than, the verbal messages: "We listen to the music more than the words." While it is feasible to maintain a conspiracy of silence in order to avoid discussing the consequences of terminal illness, the silence itself reveals the truth.

On the other hand, honesty must be viewed within the context of the individual adolescent's cognitive and psychological development, and discussions should be oriented to meet his or her needs. Specifically, most youths are concrete thinkers, and as such, their concern is less on death (the abstraction) and more on the process of dying (the concrete) (Coupey, 1980). Likewise, for the teenager who is present-time oriented, honesty does not mean playing out the course of the illness or the treatment plan to its time-extended conclusion. Rather, there is a need—if understanding is going to occur—for discussions to focus on the present and the short-term future and on the immediate impact of both the illness and the treatment. Finally, honesty means listening to the questions being asked and answering them directly, rather than answering the questions that may have been expected. Much like adults, teenagers reveal how much information they wish to have. To tell them more than they wish to know is as dishonest as to withhold desired information. The issue is not whether to tell or not tell a teenager his or her diagnosis; rather, the important question is how much information to verbally share. The answer is in the questions that are asked. A final component of honesty is the sharing with patients of anxiety and concerns from a human, as well as a professional, perspective (Silber, 1981). As Gabriel (1979) said:

> Physicians are not trained to share their own feelings with their patients about death. I think it can be entirely appropriate with adolescents to let them know what you are feeling. Open communication is a two-way street. That's part of the honesty.

Adolescent Concerns

Based upon a weekly support group for youths with overwhelming chronic illness (Blum & Chang 1981), a number of primary concerns emerge:

Reintegration Into Peer Groups

While isolating the patient from peers and family, the hospital provides a degree of comfort and security in a setting in which one need not explain or justify differences. Appearances and behavior rarely need explanation.

The thought of returning home and starting school after a prolonged hospitalization is frequently anxiety-provoking. Central to this anxiety is the teenagers' felt need to explain their absence (and thus illness) to peers. On the other hand, many youths have long ago ceased trying to explain:

> I don't try to tell them [friends] anymore. I'd have to get into what it [cystic fibrosis] is doing to my body; they couldn't handle it. It happened a lot before when I told people what was going on with me; then they couldn't look or talk to me anymore.

The need to *pass,* or to be inconspicuous, often results in practices detrimental to health, such as eating inappropriate foods, suppressing a cough, or taking unwarranted risks. On the other hand, social distance from peers is not always experienced as a negative. Because of the physical limitations imposed by serious chronic illness, many youths do not have the capacity to run with peers at a pace comparable to their healthy friends, thereby necessitating choices. A 14-year-old boy reflected on this as one of the advantages of his illness:

> Before I was sick I used to run with my friends and do everything they did, but now I can't. Because I don't have so much energy, I have to watch what they do, then pick and choose. You know, some things they do are real silly, and I'm glad I don't have to join them.

Conflicts Concerning Health Maintenance

Both in the hospital and at home, conflicts frequently arise among and between the chronically ill teenager and parents, health care providers, and other adults around the "ownership" of illness issues, such as personal control and management of therapeutic regimens. Feelings of frustration and resentment and disruption of life routines due to illness and hospitalization tend to underlie conflicts between teenage patient and adults. The cycle of frustration leading to compliance failure, followed by acute relapse or recurrent illness and then hospitalization, is seen many times.

Parent–adolescent conflicts frequently center on issues of parental infantilization of their teenage children that disallows the new competencies of adolescence that the chronically ill teenager is striving to realize. Management of diet, drugs, or level of activity becomes a focus of conflict and "acting out" or noncompliant behavior results. For the adolescent with terminal illness—more than all other youths—their world is outside their control. If they are to be active participants in their own health care plan, it is critical that they be empowered by those managing their illness to make basic decisions over their health care. Such an empowerment is inherent in a contract approach to managing chronic illness. For teenagers to use their illness as a weapon against others through noncompliance, they must view that illness as belonging more to (and being more the responsibility of) others than themselves. Active planning is needed to draw them into their disease management, to reverse the process and return the ownership of the illness to the patients themselves.

Normal Developmental Needs

Normal development needs appear rarely to be acknowledged by physicians who work with seriously ill youths. As a result, the teenager is left ill informed and frustrated. Special areas of concern include:

1. Life planning and future goals
2. Sexuality: sterility, sexual potency, and physical attractiveness
3. The relationship of stress to illness
4. Limits and risks of physical exertion
5. Modification of medical regimens based on life-style

One of the most isolating of all stigmas is the label *terminally ill,* which is borne by many with serious chronic illness. Such a label limits future life planning and sets boundaries on relationships. Irrespective of the projected duration of one's life, all people have goals they wish to attain. For those whose life span is shortened by illness, the care giver's task is to assist him or her to establish short-term goals that are realistic and achievable.

Death and Dying

For the adolescent, the terminableness of life due to illness comes in glimpses; for instance, when friends with a similar illness die or when the individual is feeling weak or debilitated. Terminal illness is not a single progressive event but one that fluctuates with one's sense of well-being. It is at times when the teenager feels most ill that he or she deals with the issue of dying. Adolescent concerns focus more on the concrete issues of how one dies than on the greater abstractions about the nature of death.

OBSERVATIONS AND RECOMMENDATIONS

In childhood, management of chronic illness is frequently supervised by parents. It is, in a real sense, the parents' problem. The task in adolescence is shifting responsibility for the illness so that it becomes the patient's problem and no longer that of the parents. This shift requires working with both the adolescent and the parents.

Chronically ill teenagers have the same developmental needs as all other youths. They need opportunities to develop peer relationships and to experiment with different personalities and styles. Seriously ill youths need help in expanding their horizons, for there are numerous forces conspiring to limit their options.

At a period of life when it is most difficult to be different, seriously ill adolescents are always seen as different. One role of the health care team is to modify the medical, dietary, and exercise regimens so as to minimize differences and improve the fit between disease management and life-style.

The assumption that an informed patient is a well-adjusted patient needs to be examined (Brewster, 1982). Both verbally and nonverbally, teenage patients will reveal the extent of the information they wish to be given. Honesty entails being sensitive to their cues and thus neither withholding nor overproviding information.

The assumptions that clinicians need to correct teenagers' distorted ideas and deal with their denial system or magical thinking need to be reevaluated. If these serve as defense mechanisms, the staff needs to proceed carefully, lest they break down defenses without providing alternatives to take their place (Brewster, 1982).

The assumption that there is a linear, stepwise progression toward the acceptance of death is a generalization fraught with problems when applied to a specific individual. There is no normative way to die. In working with youths who are dying, health-care providers need to sort their own fears from those of the patients and their own needs from what the patients are requesting. Second, they need to meet those needs based upon an understanding of the cognitive and social structures of the adolescents.

When a teenager faces death, he or she will frequently select one person with whom to share feelings. To be selected is a gift from that individual. Knowing what to say is less important than being able to be there. If you are afraid—say so. If you don't know what to say—say that. If you don't want to talk—that's all right. As long as you want to be there, you can't "blow it" (Timmons, 1976). You can't take away another's illness or pain, but you can help them live as fully as possible within their limitations.

REFERENCES

Alexander, I., & Alderstein, A. Death and religion, In H. Feifel (Ed.), *The meaning of death.* New York: McGraw-Hill & Co., 1959.

Binger, C., Ablin, A., Feuerstein, R., Kushner, J., Zoger, S., & Mikkelsen, C. Childhood leukemia: emotional impact on patient and family. *New England Journal of Medicine,* 1969, *280,* 414–418.

Bluebond-Langner, M. Meanings of death to children. In H. Feifel (Ed.), *New meanings of death.* New York: McGraw-Hill & Co., 1979.

Blum, R., & Chang, P. A group for adolescents facing chronic and terminal illness. *Journal of Current Adolescent Medicine,* 1981, *3*(6), 7–12.

Blum, R., & Resnick, M. Sexual decision-making. *Pediatric Annals,* 1982, *11*(10), 797–805.

Blum, R. Chronic and handicapping conditions: Implications for diagnosis and treatment. *Compendium of Resources on Adolescent Health*, DHHS, 1982.

Blum, R., & Chang, P. A group for adolescents facing chronic and terminal illness. *Journal of Current Adolescent Medicine*, 1981, 7–12.

Bowlby, J. Processing of mourning. *International Journal of Psychoanalysis*, 1961, *42*, 317.

Brewster, A. Chronically ill hospitalized children's concepts of their illness. *Pediatrics*, 1982, *69*(3), 355–363.

Coleman, J. Identity in adolescence: present and future self concepts. *Human Development*, 1972, *15*, 1.

Coupey, S., & Cohen, M. A developmental approach to the chronically ill adolescent. *Feelings*, 1980, *22*(2), 1.

Deboskey, M. *The chronically ill child and his family*. Springfield, IL: Charles C. Thomas, 1970.

Elkind, D. Egocentrism in adolescents. *Child Development*, 1967, *38*, 1028–1031.

Erikson, E. *Childhood and society*. New York: W. W. Norton & Co., 1963.

Erikson, E. *Identity and the life cycle*. New York: International University Press, 1959.

Farley, F. The hypostatization of death in adolescence. *Adolescence*, 1979, *14*(54), 341–350.

Farrow, J. Dealing with severely ill adolescents. *Journal of Current Adolescent Medicine*, 1980, *April*, 15.

Freud, A. *The ego and the mechanism of defense*. New York: International Universities Press, 1971.

Gabriel, G. Death and the dying adolescent. *Transitions*, 1979, *2*(5), 16.

Hankoff, L. Adolescence and the crisis of dying. *Adolescence*, 1975, *10*(39), 373–389.

Ingalls, A., & Salerno, M. *Maternal and child health nursing*. St. Louis: Mosby, 1971.

Inhelder, B., & Piaget, J. *The growth of logical thinking: From childhood to adolescence*. New York: Basic Books, 1958.

Kastenbaum, R., & Aisenberg, R. *The psychology of death*. New York: Springer, 1970.

Kastenbaum, R. The child's understanding of death: How does it develop? In E. Grollman (Ed.), *Explaining death to children*. Boston: Beacon Press, 1967.

Kastenbaum, R. Time and death in adolescence. In H. Feifel (Ed.), *The meaning of death*. New York: McGraw Hill, 1959.

Kastenbaum, R. The kingdom where nobody dies. *Saturday Review*, 1972, (Dec. 23), 38.

Kellerman, Zeltzer, L., Ellenberg, L. Dash, J. & Rigler, D. Psychological effects of illness in adolescence. I. Anxiety, self-esteem and perception of control. *Journal of Pediatrics*, 1980, *97*, 126–131.

Kliman, G. *Psychological emergencies of childhood*. New York: Grune & Stratton, 1968.

Konopka, G. Requirements for healthy development of adolescent youth. *Adolescence*, 1968, *7*(3):1-26.

Kubler-Ross, E. *On death and dying*. New York: Macmillan, 1969.

Mauer, A. Maturation of concepts of death. *British Journal of Medical Psychology* 1966, *39*, 35–41.

McIntire, M., Angle, C., & Struempler, L. The concept of death in Midwestern children and youth. *American Journal of Diseases of Childhood*, 1972, *123*, 527–532.

Nagy, M. The child's theories concerning death. *Journal of Genetic Psychology*, 1948, *73*, 3–28.

Piaget, J. *The growth of logical thinking from childhood to adolescence*. New York: Basic Books, 1958.

Rochlin, G. How younger children view death and themselves. In E.A. Grollman (Ed.), *Explaining death to children*. Boston: Beacon Press, 1967.

Ross, E.K. On death and dying. New York: MacMillan, 1969.

Schilder, P., & Wechler, D. The attitudes of children toward death. *Journal of Genetic Psychology,* 1934, *45,* 406–451.

Schowalter, J. The child's reaction to his own terminal illness. In B. Schoenberg, et al. (Eds.), *Loss and grief: Psychological management in medical practice.* New York: Columbia University Press, 1970.

Sigler, A. The leukemic child and his family. In M. Deboskey (Ed.), *The chronically ill child and his family.* Springfield, IL: C.C. Thomas, 1970.

Silber, T. Physician–adolescent patient relationship, the ethical dimension *Pediatric Annals,* 1981, *10,* 408.

Spinetta, J., Rigler, D., & Karon, J. Personal space as a measure of a dying child's sense of isolation. *Journal of Consulting and Clinical Psychology.* 1974, *42*(2), 751–756.

Spinetta, J., Rigler, D., & Karon, J. Anxiety in the dying child. *Pediatrics,* 1973, *52,* 841–844.

Spitz, R. Analytic depression. *Psychoanalytical Studies of the Child,* 1946, *2,* 313–342.

Sudnow, D. *Passing on: The social organization of dying.* Englewood Cliffs: Prentice-Hall, 1967.

Swain, H. Childhood views of death. *Death Education,* 1979, *2,* 341–358.

Tavormina, J., Kastner, L., Slater, P., & Watt, S. Chronically ill children. *Journal of Abnormal Child Psychology,* 1976, *4*(2), 99–110.

Thomas, D. *Collected poems.* New York: New Directions, 1957.

Timmons, A. Leukemia! Is it so awful? *Journal of Pediatrics,* 1976, *88*(1), 147–148.

Vernick, J., & Karon M. Who's afraid of death on a leukemia ward? *American Journal of Diseases of Children,* 1965, *109,* 393–397.

Vore, D. A child's view of death. *Southern Medical Journal,* 1974, *67*(4), 383, 384.

Waechler, E. Children's awareness of fatal illness. *American Journal of Nursing,* 1971, *71,* 1168–1177.

Zeligs, R. *Children's experiences with death.* Springfield, IL: Charles C. Thomas, 1967.

Zeltzer, L., Kellerman, J., Ellenberg, L., Dash, J., & Rigler, D. Psychological effects of illness in adolescence. II. Impact of illness in adolescents—Critical issues in coping styles. *Journal of Pediatrics,* 1980, *97*(1), 132–138.

Sue N. Sauer

11
Siblings of Children Who Have Died

Coping with the loss of a child is one of the most poignant and stressful events encountered by families. Grieving for any loss is painful, but the loss of a child carries new dimensions with it. Upon the death of a child, a family suffers tremendous emotional trauma and upheaval. The seeming injustice of a child's death threatens the family's values about the meaning and value of life.

A death in a family frequently leads to profound and enduring disturbances within and between the family members. Communication within the family unit may deteriorate or may be inadequate to meet the stress; this leads to further disintegration of family ties. The stresses resulting from a child's death can activate old family conflicts, exacerbate existing tensions, and adversely affect the integrity of the family unit and the emotional well-being of individual family members.

The purpose of this chapter is to identify feelings and characteristics that are generic to siblings who experience the loss of a brother or sister. Included is a review of the family structure and its influences and the common reactions of children and adolescents to grief. This background provides information that should facilitate the understanding of siblings' reactions in a grief group.

LOSS

Grief resulting from a loss is not something to be casually exorcised, but a process to be understood. The process is more than physical, more than psychological, more than spiritual, and more than social in nature.

CHRONIC ILLNESS AND DISABILITIES IN CHILDHOOD AND ADOLESCENCE   ISBN 0-8089-1635-1
 Copyright © 1984 by Grune & Stratton.

It is a totally encompassing human experience. Its very dimensions require an enormous and challenging study.

The Family Structure and Influences

A child's reaction to death is an internal and personal process, and is also interrelated with the normal and altered family dynamics. A family, like an individual, develops its own special identity with many characteristics, attributes, and stereotypes. As a family identity grows, family similarities begin to develop. Members often display similar personality characteristics, coping skills, defense mechanisms, and even sense of humor. When a family is faced with stress, anxiety, or conflict from a child's death, the individuals tend to show common reactions; certain trends emerge that are family hallmarks. For example, families with inadequate communication patterns find it difficult to manage their relationships and their loss because each is uncertain about the feelings of the other family members. They may be fearful of hurting the others in the family. Often they carry out their feelings in either an aggressive or a passive manner; or they may hide their painful feelings instead of interacting with the family.

Families evolve many ways of dealing with the effects of anxiety and depression. Some families express these emotions through worrying and complaining. Others become locked into depression, compulsions, or obsessions relating to the death of a child. Depression has a contagious effect on the family. In some families, a parent or other member may dominate, and thus determine the emotional tone. The usual ways of dealing with disturbances are often ineffective in a grief situation. Appropriate help must be offered to a bereaved family. Counseling should begin at the same time the death occurs, before conflicts and anxieties arise that cause behavior difficulties or symptom formation. The reliability of support systems is important in maintaining the family's equilibrium.

Reactions of Adolescents to Death

Because of greater understanding and maturity, normal adolescents are better able to cope with the finality of death. Unlike younger children, they do not depend as completely upon parental figures for development and feelings. They are loosening ties to parents, and their emotional attachments are invested in the peer group or adult figures outside the family. Adolescence is, however, a period of turmoil, tension, and unpredictable behavior. Adolescents are in a state of flux; their personality goes through many changes. These adjustments are related to the numerous tasks that are involved in this developmental stage. These tasks consist of dealing with problems related to finding one's basic identity: sexual adjustment and reorganization; fears and feelings about the opposite sex; developing moral values, concepts, and principles; vocational pursuits; social demands; and establishing a self-concept and personal ideals.

Adolescents are faced with the major task of developing a philosophy of life. This task is basic to many of the major decisions they must make regarding vocational choice, sexual and moral attitudes, and life's meaning. These influences of mind and emotion also underlie the attitudes and reactions of adolescents toward death. Adolescents are idealistic, and this idealism creates anxiety about their own future, life, and death. Adolescents develop a belief in, and often a preoccupation with, immortality. Added to this is a society that floods their mind with death-defying concepts. Because the future is associated with the unknown, the tendency of the teenager is to focus on the present and to seek immediate gratification of needs. Another mechanism for coping with feelings about death and dying is denial, which allows them to feel that death is something that only happens to other people. Some adolescents react to their fear of death by taking unnecessary risks with their own life. Perhaps in tempting death, they are trying to overcome fear by confirming their control over mortality. As adolescents evolve their philosophy of life, they need to incorporate their increasing awareness of personal mortality.

It is quite obvious that young people in this society who are struggling to develop their philosophy of life will experience many conflicting emotions and feelings when a sibling dies. They experience disorganization and feel empty, worthless, and inadequate. Their judgment, perceptions, and reality testing are hindered. Having the opportunity to discuss these feelings provides a means of restoring significant adaptation in their lives. After the death of a loved one, the adolescent must face the external world with all of its turmoil. The teenager who is most apt to need special help in dealing with a sibling's death is the one who cannot talk about it when it occurs.

Adolescent mourning may be difficult to identify because depression and mood swings are normal occurrences in this age group. Adolescent reactions and ability to resolve the loss are extremely variable and unique to the individual. At the time of crisis, their ability to deal with anxiety and their adaptability can be assessed. The effect of loss on adolescents' development will be determined by their inward drive, their degree of maturity, and the quality of their external relationships.

Sibling Grief

The sources and variety of disturbances in a child's life may be numerous and difficult to disentangle because each child's relation to the death of a sibling is unique. Cain, Fast, & Erickson (1964) found the determinants of children's responses to the death of a sibling to include the following:

1. The nature of the death
2. The age of the child
3. The characteristics of the sibling who died
4. The child's degree of actual involvement in the sibling's death
5. The child's preexisting relationship to the dead sibling
6. The immediate impact of the death on the parents
7. The parents' handling of the initial reactions of the surviving child or children
8. The reactions of the community
9. The death's impact upon the family structure
10. The availability to the child and parent of various "substitutes"
11. The parents' enduring reactions to the sibling's death
12. The major concurrent stresses on the child at the time of the sibling's death

Cain et al. (1964) went on to note that developmental capacity is a critical component in determining the response of an individual to the death of a sibling. This developmental capacity includes psychosexual and ego development, with particular emphasis on cognitive capacity to understand death. The effects of death upon a child obviously are not static but undergo constant developmental transformation and evolution.

Most of the literature published to date focuses on case studies of children who are undergoing psychotherapy in order to work through the loss of a sibling; few children pursue this route. On the other hand, little research has been done on the normal adaptive process of children to a sibling's death. This chapter will focus more on normative than pathological grief responses.

THE SIBLING SUPPORT GROUP: ITS HISTORY, STRUCTURE, AND RULES

While literature on parental responses to the death of a child indicates their need for support, help for the grieving family tends to be sporadic and left to those who are untrained.

In 1972, a group therapy program was established at St. Paul Children's Hospital to assist grieving parents in their struggle to return to a more normal life after the death of a child. The program originated because of requests from parents seeking support and ways to adjust to a life without their child.

Over the ensuing years, parents would ask for ways to help their children to cope with the loss of a sibling and the subsequently emerging problems. Parents needed to find ways to answer children's questions and facilitate their grief. Because of their own overwhelming grief, parents stated that frequently they did not have sufficient emotional energy to help their children. Because of this perceived need, a sibling support group was formed in 1980.

While the sibling group meets on the same evening as the parent support group, the parents meet bimonthy, whereas the children meet only once a month. There are reasons for this difference: First, children appear to progress through their grieving process faster than adults and thus do not need to meet as often. Second, when the parents meet alone for one of their bimonthly sessions, they feel more freedom to remain and socialize with other parents after the session. The necessary constraint of having to take their children home on a school night places restrictions that limit the effectiveness of the adult group.

While the number of participants in the sibling group has ranged from 6 to 13, the goal is to keep numbers well below the maximum. At its upper limit, it is impossible for all participants to have equal ''discussion time'', it is difficult to establish group cohesiveness, and it is exhausting for the facilitator. Likewise, while the age range was extended from 6 to 19, it has been found that discussions have at times been frightening, confusing, and upsetting for those under 10. Graphic descriptions of traumatic deaths and emotional outbursts of anger or frustration are difficult for the younger child to understand. Because of these observations, the trend is toward a separate group for those under ten.

The rules of the group are simple and are aimed at relinquishing control to group participants, ensuring confidentiality, and maintaining open-ended group participation. No didactic instruction is given about the grieving process. The members do not have to make a committment to return to future group sessions. At the end of each session, general feedback is provided by the group facilitator to the parents' group. Such a summary establishes a link between the parents and their children and opens family communications. It gives parents a chance to ask questions about their child. It also provides a sense of what the group is about to parents whose children have not been sibling group members.

The Process of Grieving for a Dead Sibling

Several observations have evolved during the three-year experience of the sibling grief group. Later in the chapter, case examples will illustrate the following observations:

1. Children and adolescents proceed through their grieving more rapidly than do adults. The young person's attitude—that they need to get on with living—influences the process.

2. The group members feel an immediate bond with others in the group because of their common denominator of having lost a brother or sister. They will confirm this observation with statements to each other such as, "I feel I've known you all my life"; or, as one 16-year-old girl shared, "I would never be caught dead talking to an 11-year-old, creepy boy at school, but here in the group, you're my friend, and I feel very close to you."

3. The group discusses many topics that normally would not be discussed with parents or family. For example, they often discuss dreams, supernatural phenomena, problems at school, personal worries, worries about their parents, nuclear war, and fears about their own future and the future of their family. They also discuss issues such as body decomposition and burial fantasies that they would not discuss with their family for fear that it would be disrespectful or could hurt other family members.

4. Most children do not share their grief with other siblings in the family, no mater how close they are. They tend to share their grief and obtain support from one of their parents, a close friend, or another significant adult, such as a school counselor. They appear to feel uneasy about the prospect of opening old wounds or exacerbating raw wounds in other hurting family members.

5. All group participants express their feeling that their families have changed significantly. As one boy shared, "It used to be unique being a family of five boys. It's not so unique being a family of four boys anymore." They all desire greater communication within the family but realize that their parents are emotionally paralyzed and unable to facilitate closeness at this time of their grief.

6. All of the children have a need to share the unique happenings or characteristics of their sibling. They often bring pictures, poems written by the sibling, or model airplanes the sibling constructed. These acts help convey the uniqueness of the relationship and the specialness of the sibling.

7. All of the group members express a sadness about not having had a chance for closure, a chance to say a very special phrase to the child before he or she died, such as, "Gee, you were a neat brother" or "I liked having you for a sister."

8. Children and adolescents often exhibit adjustment problems to grief through behavioral problems at school. Problems may be exhibited by withdrawing from others or, at times, by more deviant behavior, such as exposing themselves sexually.

9. Youngsters in general can cope with more trauma and devastation than adults think they can. More open acceptance may be the result of conditioning by constant media exposure.

10. Children are sensitively aware of ways parents have of enshrining the dead child. A fairly typical example is the dead sibling who was a difficult child during life being presented as the model child in death.

11. Children protect their parents and attempt to maintain thoughts and feelings the parents cherish. They will protect and reinforce a parent's false notions about a dead sibling. They don't wish to shatter what they think is a parent's lasting vision or betray the family secrets.

12. Children and adolescents are willing, if encouraged, to write down their feelings and expressions about the dead sibling. They perform this emotional outlet in the form of poems, letters, or a nighttime diary.

13. Siblings feel grief is an extremely private and personal matter. They are inhibited when strangers or observers join the group, and even feel antagonistic toward them.

14. Children with dead siblings are more aware of threats to life and of death. They are vividly aware of nuclear war issues, car accidents, and how and where people die. They also are more frightened and affected by these threats than they were prior to the death of their sibling. The myth of immunity is no longer protective.

15. The parent's coping reactions to the loss of the sibling greatly influence the child's adjustment.

16. Adolescents, like parents who have successfully moved through the adjustment process, exhibit a need and a sense of duty to help others who are experiencing a loss.

Case Excerpts From the Sibling Group Sessions

School problems are frequently discussed and resolved in the group. The group participants frequently talk of "punching out" a schoolmate who may have said something like "Your sister was a creep anyway and I'm glad she died." Due to the frequency that such incidents are relayed, one suspects that many are unlived fantasies and expressions of anger rather than accurate reporting of events at school.

The group members advise each other about ways to handle problem schoolmates, often with statements of physical retribution such as, "If that happened to me, I would take him outside and bust him good."

Upon gaining the group trust, members often reveal long-standing problems at school that they have been dealing with alone. One girl, for example, revealed that she had to leave school every day at 2:30, sobbing, upset, and unable to attend her three remaining classes. This girl's brother had accidentally died of a gunshot wound to the head while playing Russian roulette. She shared with the group that every afternoon at school a boy would come up behind her in the hallway and quietly utter in her ear, "bang bang." In addition to being tormented, she was very frightened by this boy and consequently never told a teacher or her parents about it. Once discussed, it was easy to intervene and stop the tormenting.

A 12-year-old boy was referred to the group because he had been exposing himself at school. Counselors and his parents felt that his behavior might be related to unresolved conflicts about the death of his two sisters. The two girls had died seven years earlier in a train accident. The boy was the only remaining child. The boy's mother had done very little to resolve her grief over the seven-year period and was referred to the parent group.

Participants in the group often need to talk about the details of the sibling's death, and one evening the group asked this boy to explain how his sisters had died and whether they had suffered or been killed instantly. The boy revealed that their death had never been discussed in the family and that he had always wanted to know this information. He was asked if he felt he could now go to his parents and ask them about the details of his sisters' death because the group had asked him to share these events. In other words, the group had given him permission to express his need and a way to approach the forbidden subject with his parents. He did do this. The parents related that he was greatly relieved and that he could not wait to return to the group to share his new understanding. He also told his parents that in the group he felt accepted for himself. His problem behavior at school quickly resolved, and, from observations, family unity and communication appeared much improved as well.

There are many ways surviving children share the uniqueness of their dead brother or sister in addition to relating experiences. They frequently bring personal, artistic, or creative endeavors of the dead sibling to show to the group. A surprising number of adolescents have written wills. Many of these adolescents died suddenly without reason to suspect they were going to die. These wills may be another indication of an adolescent's preoccupation with death and his or her frequent pondering of a life beyond. Many poems that the siblings share with the group reflect the dead child's feelings about death, God, and heaven. Some are very startling, causing the family to search for meaning in the phrases and words.

Pictures are proudly shared with the group. The pictures not only show the child when he or she was well but also when sickly or with no hair. The condition or looks of the dead child do not seem to matter to the surviving sibling. There is a need to share every aspect of their brother or sister with others.

One of the 12-year-old boys in the group had been in a car accident with his mother and sister on the way to an Alanon meeting. They were hit by a drunken driver and his sister was killed instantly. The boy and his mother were comatose for three weeks and over a month, respectively. Because of their coma, the boy and mother had been deprived of the reality of the 14-year-old girl's death, and they had difficulty in adjusting. They had been receiving psychological counseling in addition to the parent and sibling support groups. As a means of assisting them in their grieving, the counselor had them obtain the scene-of-the-accident pictures from the coroner, and in a private session prior to the support group meeting, they said goodbye to the girl through picture visualization.

The boy attended the sibling group after the private session and appeared to have his attention focused elsewhere. Suddenly, in the middle of the session, he ran from the room and returned with the coroner's pictures of his sister. His desire to share these pictures with the others was strong and obvious. Having seen these pictures earlier, the facilitator was confronted with the dilemma of whether to expose the others to the very explicit, traumatic exposures of the dead girl. The boy's need, however, was great and persistent. After consultation, the boy agreed to remove the most vivid pictures and pass the others around the group face down in order to give each child the option of looking or not. Each group member chose to look at the pictures. The result of this experience ended with the sibling group members accepting the pictures simply as John's dead sister, overlooking the details of her death. This experience affirmed, once again, the realization that children accept more graphic reality than adults often feel they can.

One function of the facilitator in the group is to assist members in their understanding of events or processes occurring within their family. The siblings express their negative feelings about their parents' new overprotectiveness by complaining, "My mom's always harping at me or making me check in at nine o'clock." Their understanding can be aided by a statement from the facilitator such as, "You know why she is doing that, don't you?" It helps them to say, "Yea. She's worried that I'm gonna die, too." This reinforcement aids the realization that their parents are experiencing normal reactions and that this overprotectiveness reflects love and caring.

Other complaints from siblings center around parents comparing the dead child with the remaining siblings with comments such as, "My mom's always saying, 'your hands are just like Marie's.'" It is helpful to indicate to the sibling that such comments are intended as compliments and not negative comparisons.

The siblings also relate family incidents that reveal their understanding of their parents' need to enshrine the dead child. As one boy shared, "In memory of my sister, my parents bought a young tree, a special buckeye tree, and they put it in the backyard where they could watch it grow up to adulthood and blossom." The children accept this enshrinement and are very protective about the family's actions or expressions. Only rarely are feelings of anger expressed about such activities.

After the death of a sibling, teenagers report hating to have people touch them frequently: "I'm sick of people mauling me and saying, Oh, honey, how are you?" Aunts and uncles tend to do this most frequently, and the adolescents resent it. The only touch for which they express a desire is the occasional touch of a parent. They do not want to be forced to talk.

The surviving siblings relate that they are aware of changes and differences in their behavior. For example, they have a low threshold for teasing by peers; generally they are not in a teasing mood and therefore tend to interpret the teasing incorrectly. Furthermore, the small stresses of daily living tend to prove more irritable in relation to the major crisis they are facing.

Other feelings often discussed are those of shyness and insecurity that emerged after the death of their brother or sister. The new shyness makes them feel that they are alone and without friends. They express concern that friends abandon them because they act "different," and friends will not wait for them to get back to normal.

Most feel vulnerable and open to hurt and rejection. They attribute their vulnerability to the difficulty in sorting their mixed emotions about the dead sibling. When they feel hurt, they report that they respond by rejecting their parents, even without intending to do so. Many times the rejection is a result of parents wanting to help. They express that they wish to handle the problems by themselves: "We hurt in our own way and don't want to share it, so we reject our parents because we're getting older, and they're trying harder."

On the other hand, the family seems more important than friends; it became more important because of the death. Surviving siblings feel the family will be more important for the rest of their life. A renewed sense of importance is given to doing things with the family and spending time talking about enjoyable family happenings, particularly those that happened before the death.

Grieving adolescents do not want changes in family rules. They understand and can be tolerant when parents are strict and overprotective, however, they frequently express that "parents shouldn't take advantage of us because of the death and change the rules."

The school environment evokes many feelings and reactions, such as: "I hate having to explain to everyone that my sister died"; "I feel awful when everyone at school is talking about a funny story that happened to their sister or brother, or when they show pictures of their families"; "If I show mine, I have to talk about my sister to these kids, and I don't want to." Strong feelings are also expressed about what they feel is phoniness in their peers: "I hate it when other kids act nice to me just because I lost my brother." They dislike teachers talking to the classroom about other people dying. They feel some teachers may use their sibling's death as gossip: "I take it personally and wonder what the teacher said about me when my brother died."

Most adolescents express loneliness in school: "A lot of kids stay away from me now and I don't call them either"; "I feel like I'm more alone, more intense. Part of the reason is because I sit around more, do less, am less active, and rebel more. I hate feeling this way, but I can't help it."

Advice from Siblings to Others Experiencing a Loss

The following advice was offered as the siblings thought about how to become happier:

1. Be around someone, but it matters who you want to be around.
2. Talk with other teens who have lost someone, because they are the only ones who know what you are feeling.
3. Know that you need someone, but not just anyone.
4. Go to a support group. If you try to do it by yourself, it doesn't work, and later it gets worse.
5. It helps to know you're not the only one thinking about death.
6. Think of comforting thoughts, such as "They had a good life, they are happy, or they are with God."
7. It's a comforting thought to know you helped another kid through it.
8. Keep occupied and try to forget. This helps in some ways, but if you aren't careful, it catches up with you.
9. It helps to be around someone you view positively, like my Sea Explorer Scout Leader. It helps me to try to see myself this way in the future. It gives me direction and a feeling I'll be OK.
10. Don't think you should get better real soon. It takes a year.
11. Holidays need special preparation. It helps to think about why we can no longer watch the Muppets or the John Denver Family Christmas Show.
12. Be yourself, most of all.

CONCLUSION

After a few months of group participation, the adolescents form strong opinions about the structure and dynamics of the group. They feel the role of the participants is to listen to each other; give feedback, encouragement, and support; talk and get problems out in the open; share feelings; and be open to others. Most important is to be each other's friend.

They believe death, school, feelings, laws, future plans, drunk drivers, funerals, cemeteries, drugs, poems, family feelings, sports, personal experiences, and most anything else should be discussed.

They think the role of the facilitator should be to direct the conversation, give them the freedom to talk about anything, help them feel comfortable with one another, help the group out of the silences, answer questions, be a good listener, share thoughts and feelings with them, help them to see the good and bad, and be their friend.

Many questions from the siblings to the facilitator deal with feelings, responses, pain, and awareness of the dying child. Questions frequently arise of a medical nature, on mortuary practices, body care, and transport, all of which would be difficult to answer were the facilitator not to have a strong medical knowledge base.

SUMMARY

Most children have a great capacity for dealing with death. Successful resolution of grief can help them confront the relationship between life and death. Many facts of life can be learned from death. Death is the end of life, but not the end of relationships.

The goals of assisting a child through grief should include the following:

1. To help the child grow in inner resourcefulness
2. To assist the child toward a sense of accomplishment
3. To help the child grow in moral courage; when they have the courage to say "I did it," then they have experienced growth
4. To help the child grow in trust
5. To help the child grow toward an awareness of self and help him or her to gain the ability to mediate between the conscious and unconscious
6. To help the child move to the future with strengthened concepts of family living

Significant help can be gained for children and their parents by their association with others who have experienced a similar loss, either on a one-to-one basis or as a group experience. Sharing another's pain is not easy, but this sharing can assist family unity and help all of the family members to heal. Families who are able to cope with the impact of the circumstances and to mourn appropriately are better able to resume and continue their emotional life in harmony.

ACKNOWLEDGMENT

The case examples included in this text were gleaned from the ~~ own and children's experiences in the setting of a sibling grief group. The author wishes to gratefully acknowledge the insights provided by the children in the group, many of whom are quoted in this chapter.

REFERENCES

Anthony, E.J. A working model for family studies. In E.J. Anthony, & C. Koupernick (Eds.), *The child in his family: The impact of disease and death* (Vol. 2: *[International Yearbook for Child Psychiatry and Allied Disciplines* Vol. 2]. New York: Wiley, 1973, 3–20.

Barnes, M. Crisis and adaptation in the families of fatally ill children. In E.J. Anthony, & C. Koupernick (Eds.), *The reactions of children and adolescents to the death of a parent or sibling: The child in his family.* Vol. 2. *The impact of disease and death.* *[International Yearbook for Child Psychiatry and Allied Disciplines* Vol. 2]. New York: Wiley, 1973.

Binger, C.M. Childhood leukemia—emotional impact on siblings. In E.J. Anthony & C. Koupernick C. (Eds.) *The child in his family: The impact of disease and death.* Vol. 2. *[International Yearbook for Child Psychiatry and Allied Disciplines* Vol. 2]* New York: Wiley, 1973, 2, 127–143.

Cain, A.C., Fast, I., & Erickson, M.E. Children's disturbed reactions to the death of a sibling. *American Journal of Orthopsychiatry,* 1964, *20,* 481–494.

Futterman, E.H., & Hoffman, I. Crisis and adaptation in families of fatally ill children. In E.J. Anthony, and C. Koupernick (Eds.). *The child in his family; The impact of disease and death.* Vol. 2. [International Yearbook for Child Psychiatry and Allied Disciplines]. New York: Wiley, 1973, 2, 127–143.

Gauthier, Y. The mourning reaction of a ten and a half year old boy. *Psychoanalytic Study of the Child,* 1965, *20,* 481–494.

Gourevitch, M. A survey of family reactions to disease and death in a family member. In E.J. Anthony, & C. Koupernik, (Eds.) *The child in his family: The impact of disease and death.* Vol. 2. [International Yearbook for Child Psychiatry and Allied Disciplines.] New York: Wiley, 1973, 2, 21–28.

Jackson, E. Helping children cope with death. *Archives of Foundation of Thanatology,* 1969, *1,* 1.

Jackson, E. Understanding the teenager's response to death. *Archives of Foundation of Thanatology,* 1968, *1,* 1.

Levitt, C., Linder, M., Sauer, S., & Pierce, S. Parent support groups for the grieving parent. In I.M. Martinson, (Ed.) *Home care for the dying child.* New York: Appleton Century Crofts, 1976.

Nagera, H. Children's reactions to the death of important objects: A developmental approach. *The Psychoanalytic Study of the Child.* 1970, *25,* 360–400.

Sugar, M. Normal adolescent mourning. *American Journal of Psychotherapy,* 1968, *22,* 258–269.

Woolsey, S., Thornton, D., & Friedman, S. Sudden Death. In E.J. Anthony, & C. Doupernik (Eds.). *The child in his family: The impact of disease and death.* Vol. 2. [International Yearbook for Child Psychiatry and Allied Disciplines]. New York: Wiley, 1973, 2, 3–20.

Yudkin, S. Children and death, *Lancet,* 1967, *1:*7480, 37–41.

Carolyn L. Williams,
Marvin L. Logel,

12

Chronic Pain in Adolescents: Psychological Considerations

During the past 15 years, chronic pain has been the subject of numerous monographs and review articles. During this same period, more than 100 multidisciplinary pain clinics and pain treatment programs have been established in the United States. For the most part, publication interest has focused on the clinical manifestations of chronic or recurrent pain in adult populations. Chronic pain in adolescents has not been embraced with the same enthusiasm. Nevertheless, in the health care setting, a significant number of adolescents present with complaints of pain. Consequently, the management of chronic pain in adolescents represents an important challenge to the health care provider.

This chapter will consider chronic or recurrent pain that occurs with some frequency in adolescents. The discussion will focus on adolescent pain problems in which psychological factors are thought to play a significant role. The term "psychogenic pain" is often applied to this type of problem. However, for several reasons the phrase *chronic or recurrent pain* is preferable to *psychogenic pain*. One advantage of this alternative designation is that it encompasses a wider range of clinical phenomena than does psychogenic pain. A second advantage is that it carries no etiological implications, an important consideration in light of the multiple manifestations of adolescent pain.

CHRONIC ILLNESS AND DISABILITIES IN CHILDHOOD AND ADOLESCENCE ISBN 0-8089-1635-1

DEFINITIONS AND TYPES OF PAIN

Pain is an extraordinarily complex phenomenon. Accordingly, the task of arriving at a satisfactory definition of pain is fraught with conceptual and philosophical difficulties. A detailed discussion of these difficulties would probably contribute little to the understanding of the clinical manifestations of pain and is not within the purview of the present chapter. For the sake of this discussion, however, and by way of introduction, the problems in defining pain may be succinctly summarized as follows: First, pain is a private experience that is not accessible to public observation (Sternbach, 1974). Second, the term "pain" is sometimes used to designate a specific sensory modality and is at other times used to refer to an aversive motivational–affective state (Weisenberg, 1977). Finally, pain is not invariably the result of tissue injury, nor is it always proportional to the degree of tissue injury. As documented by Melzack and Wall (1983), it is possible for injury to occur without pain, and pain, without injury.

It is generally accepted that pain is subject to the influence of a variety of psychological and social factors. Cultural background or ethnicity, personality, and emotional state of the individual have all been viewed as prominent among these factors. Weisenberg (1982) reviewed evidence suggesting wide variation among culturally defined groups in pain tolerance and mode of pain expression but not in sensory threshold for pain. Beecher's (1959) classic study of battlefield injury has been taken as unequivocal evidence of the influence of psychological factors, such as expectancy and anxiety, on pain. In that study, wounded soldiers were found to request fewer pain medications than did civilian hospital patients (25 percent versus 80 percent).

The Subcommittee on Taxonomy of the International Association for the Study of Pain (IASP) (Merskey, 1979) has arrived at the following definition of pain: "An unpleasant sensory and emotional experience associated with actual or potential tissue damage, or described in terms of such damage" (p. 250). Although not immune from criticism (e.g., Melzack & Wall, 1983), the foregoing definition is the most comprehensive and useful definition of pain proposed to date.

The expressions *emotional pain* and *painful experience* are commonly used to refer to unpleasant feelings (roughly, *mental suffering)* associated with stressful events or traumatic life situations. Strictly speaking, the type of pain denoted by these expressions is different from that constituting the major focus of this chapter, in which pain will be used strictly to refer to the type subsumed under the IASP definition.

Psychogenic and Organic Pain

Organic pain is usually associated with identifiable tissue damage or a known pathophysiological process. On the other hand, organic pain is frequently differentiated from functional or psychogenic pain. Fordyce (1976) noted that psychogenic pain has been used in two different ways. In its first use, the term is applied to pain for which there is no medical explanation, or for which overt pain responses (verbal complaints of pain and pain behavior) are judged by the clinician to be disproportionate to the degree of physical impairment. In this sense, psychogenic pain implies a discrepancy between pain behavior and nociceptive stimulation. The second use of psychogenic pain refers to situations in which psychological or emotional factors are believed to play a primary role in the etiology of pain. The implication of this definition is that psychological factors have been identified that are significant to the onset, exacerbation, or persistence of pain.

Fordyce (1976) presented cogent criticisms of the concept of psychogenic pain. He noted that it is often difficult to ascertain which of the two aforementioned uses of the term is intended by its users. He further noted that the concept of psychogenic pain tends to raise philosophical issues related to mind–body dualism that add little except confusion to the management of pain in the clinical setting. Clinically, the term frequently is used as a pseudoexplanation to denote pain not readily accounted for by findings from the physical examination or medical diagnostic procedures. In this application, psychogenic pain is a diagnosis arrived at by exclusion of somatic disease and not by inclusion of psychological factors.

Barr and Feuerstein (in press), in a recent discussion of recurrent abdominal pain in children and adolescents, questioned the basic clinical assumption that recurrent abdominal pain indicates the presence of either organic or psychogenic disease. To support their position, the authors note that a sizable number of patients with nonorganic abdominal pain displayed neither the emotional nor the behavioral problems necessary for a psychogenic explanation of their pain. For example, 51 percent of Apley's (1975) school children with abdominal pain were labeled *normal, average, good.* After reviewing the pain literature, Barr and Feuerstein (in press) concluded that psychogenic factors may play a role in an important subgroup of patients with nonorganic recurrent abdominal pain but by no means could account for all cases of nonorganic pain.

Recent studies of lactose intolerance in patients with recurrent abdominal pain (Barr, Levine, & Watkins, 1979; Liebman, 1979) suggest that the pain is not necessarily indicative of either psychogenic or organic disease but could be the "result of the interaction between a normal constitutional factor (low levels of small intestinal lactose activity during school-age) and a normal environmental factor (ingestion of lactose)" (Barr & Feuerstein, in press). Instead of assuming that all patients with recurrent abdominal pain fit into either an organic disease category or a psychogenic disease category, Barr and Feuerstein propose the use of a revised clinical model that allows "a category in which neither organic nor psychogenic etiology is presumed, nor is the symptom presumed to imply disease."

Although Szasz (1957) advocated use of psychogenic pain to describe pain for which psychological or emotional factors are of greater relative importance than organic factors, no completely satisfactory method has been devised by which psychological or organic factors can be weighted objectively in proportion to their relative importance to pain (see Brena, Chapman, Stegall, & Chyatte, 1979, for an attempt to do so).

An additional criticism of particular significance to pain in the clinical setting is that the diagnosis of psychogenic pain is often viewed as a pejorative epithet or term of opprobrium. Initially, the patient with chronic or recurrent pain may request medical or surgical evaluations or treatment procedures aimed at relief of symptoms from the health care system. With the passage of time, the behavioral manifestations of the pain problem may become more pronounced, with little or no change in the patient's medical status. At best, the response to noninvasive treatments or advice and reassurance is marginal. Eventually, the patient may feel blamed for the pain. The patient may believe that his or her pain is seen as imaginary. A power struggle transpires thereafter, with the frustrated patient (or family) trying to prove to the medical establishment that the patient's pain is real. The interaction and miscommunication between the patient and clinician may culminate in mutual rejection and hostility.

PAIN AND PSYCHIATRIC DISORDER

Conversion Disorders

The primary feature of conversion disorders is loss of, or alteration in, physical functioning that is suggestive of a physical disorder. The physical symptom is not under voluntary control, is without medical explanation, and is assumed to be related to psychological or emotional factors. The symptoms diagnosed as conversion disorders typically mimic neurological disorders such as paralysis, anesthesia, seizures, aphonia, and blindness.

According to diagnostic criteria, conversion symptoms involving the complaint of pain are not diagnosed as conversion disorders but instead are classified as psychogenic pain disorders. While some have argued that such differentiation is therapeutically or diagnostically important (Guze, 1967; Goodwin & Guze, 1979), there is no convincing evidence to support the segregation of conversion symptoms involving pain from those not involving pain (Bishop & Torch, 1979). Except for the nature of the predominant symptom, psychogenic pain disorders and conversion disorders are diagnosed according to identical criteria. The degree of conviction that a conversion symptom requires medical attention may be more important with respect to a number of variables related to clinical management (e.g., doctor shopping, overuse of medications, unnecessary medical procedures, response to medical advice and reassurance) than the nature of the symptom per se.

A significant proportion of conversion symptoms in children and adolescents involve the complaint of pain. Herman and Simonds (1975) reported that in a small sample of pediatric patients, 60 percent of conversion symptoms included the complaint of pain. Maloney (1980) reported similar data for 105 pediatric inpatients. Taken together, conversion symptoms that involved the complaint of abdominal pain, headache, or general pain were found in 47 percent of the patients. The most frequent conversion symptom was abdominal pain, which was diagnosed in 26 percent of the patients. Interestingly, a major family crisis occurred prior to the onset of exacerbation of the conversion symptom in 97 percent of the patients. In addition, a majority of patients were shown to have a problem with family communication (88 percent), a clinically depressed parent (85 percent), or unresolved grief reaction (58 percent)—usually related to loss of a parent or grandparent. These results were consistent with those of other studies (McKegney, 1967; Rock, 1971).

Maloney (1980) observed that few patients with conversion symptoms showed the classic *la belle indifference*—the outward disregard for their physical symptoms. In fact, the majority of patients demonstrated intense preoccupation with their symptoms.

It should be noted that there is not always an association between conversion symptoms and the so-called hysterical (histrionic) personality. In adults, conversion symptoms have been found to be associated with a wide variety of personality types. The occurrence of histrionic personality types has been found to range from approximately 10 to 55 percent in patients with conversion symptoms (Chodoff & Lyons 1958; Lewis &

Berman, 1965; McKegney, 1967; Ziegler & Imboden, 1960). Comparable findings would be expected for children and adolescents.

Hysteria

In the current diagnostic nomenclature, conversion disorder is differentiated from somatization disorder or hysteria. Goodwin and Guze (1979) proposed the following definition of hysteria:

A polysymptomatic disorder that begins early in life (usually in the teens, rarely after the 20s), chiefly affects women, and is characterized by recurrent, multiple, somatic complaints often described dramatically.

The syndrome of hysteria usually includes conversion symptoms, but the presence of conversion symptoms does not imply hysteria.

The relevance of the diagnosis of hysteria to the present discussion is twofold: the disorder typically has its onset in late adolescence or early adulthood, and a high percentage of patients with hysteria report pain. In fact, the presenting complaint of pain or a history of multiple pain complaints is in some respects an indispensable feature of the disorder (Perley & Guze, 1962; Purtell, Robins, & Cohen, 1951).

The course of hysteria is characterized by temporary remission of symptoms followed by subsequent reemergence of the same or similar complaints.

Hypochondriasis

A disorder that has much in common with hysteria is hypochondriasis. The essential feature of hypochondriasis is "an unrealistic interpretation of physical signs or sensations as abnormal, leading to preoccupation with fear or belief of having a serious disease" (DSM-III, 1982). In a recent review, Barskey and Klerman (1983) described hypochondriasis as characterized by disease conviction, somatic preoccuapation, disease phobia, and persistent overuse of the health care system, with failure to respond to medical advice and reassurance. Pain, usually judged by the clinician to be disproportionate to the degree of organic pathology, is the most frequent complaint in hypochondriasis (Kenyon, 1964, 1965, 1976). The disorder generally is thought to follow a chronic but irregular course similar to that of hysteria. Unlike hysteria, however, the age at onset is typically in adulthood (Kenyon, 1964). In addition, multiple physical complaints, if present in hypochondriasis, are presented by the patient as evidence of a specific somatic disease.

It is not uncommon for children and adolescents to employ physical complaints to avoid life situations they find unpleasant (e.g., school, domestic responsibilities, or certain family activities). These so-called hypochondriacal complaints usually are not associated with organic disorders and are interpreted by others as largely manipulative. These factors probably account for the view held by many parents and physicians that hypochondriacal complaints are fabricated or imaginary, and for the association of hypochondriasis with malingering.

The difficulty with the concept of hypochondriacal complaints described in this way is that the symptom of hypochondriasis (physical complaints) is confused with the syndrome of hypochondriasis (disease phobia, disease conviction, somatic preoccupation, and nonresponse to advice or reassurance). Physical complaints as a form of manipulative behavior are relatively frequent in children and adolescents. The syndrome of hypochondriasis is, in all likelihood, rare in the same population.

Hypochondriasis has been conceptualized by some authors (Dorfman, 1968, 1975; Kral, 1958; Lesse, 1968, 1974) as a defense against or mask of depression in adulthood. Recently, Lesse (1981) has extended this notion to hypochondriacal complaints in adolescents. The concept of masked depression is, to say the least, controversial. The evidence in support of the hypothesis with respect to hypochondriasis in adolescents has been in large part anecdotal, primarily consisting of unsystematic observation and clinical case reports. In addition, the manifestations of covert depression have yet to be specified in a manner that would permit the development of reliable and valid methods of measurement. Carlson and Cantwell (1980) presented data indicating that the majority of so-called masked depressions in children and adolescents meet research criteria for adult depressive disorders. These authors also reported that covert depression can be readily identified by the skilled clinician conducting a thorough interview.

These comments should not be interpreted as rejection of the notion that pain may be a symptom of adolescent depression. In fact, various physical complaints, including complaints of pain, may be prominent features of depression in children and adolescents. For example, Frommer (1968) subclassified a sample of depressed children and adolescents into three groups: enuretic depressives, depressives, and phobic depressives. Of significance to the present discussion was the finding that the incidence of abdominal pain in the three groups was 46 percent, 47 percent, and 68 percent, respectively. Headaches were also common, occurring in 24 to 31 percent of the depressed patients. However, the reader should be aware that the occurrence of clinical depression in childhood and adolescence is infrequent and there is controversy over whether some behaviors should be considered symptoms of depression (see Lefkowitz & Burton, 1978 for a discussion).

DEVELOPMENTAL CONSIDERATIONS

As with any other symptom or behavior occurring during adolescence, pain should be viewed from a developmental perspective. Despite the blurring of age distinctions in some studies and the lack of longitudinal research on the development of pain, there is information that allows comparison of pain experienced by adolescents with that experienced by older or younger people.

Adolescent Versus Adult Pain

A major source of differences between adolescents and adults is the localization of pain symptoms. The two most common types of chronic pain in adults are headaches and back pain (Bonica, 1980). Headaches are also common in adolescents but rank second in frequency to abdominal pain, which is a relatively infrequent complaint in adult chronic pain patients. The prevalence of chronic back pain is low in adolescents. However, a recent study (Fritz, Bleck, & Dahl, 1981) of knee pain in adolescents suggests that the incidence of mulculoskeletal pain may be higher than is generally assumed.

On a number of potentially important variables, comparison of adolescent with adult chronic pain problems is not possible because of lack of empirical data. Clinical experience suggests, however, that the incidence of dependence on prescription medications and of any type of pain-related surgery, necessary or unnecessary, is higher in adults than in adolescents. Furthermore, psychological precipitants to the onset of pain are more readily identified in adolescents than in adults, and financial compensation is less often a complicating factor for youth. Although there are always exceptions, the psychological treatment of choice for adolescents who suffer chronic or recurrent pain is often individual or family psychotherapy. Behavioral treatment methods, alone or in combination with individual or group psychotherapy, are considered by many to be most appropriate for the management of chronic pain in adults.

Another important difference between adolescents and adults is in the temporal characteristics of their chronic pain problems. The majority of adolescent pain patients report pain that occurs in discrete but repeated episodes. Although recurrent pain is not infrequent in adults (e.g., chronic recurrent headache), they tend to report pain that is continuous but variable in intensity more often than do adolescents. In addition, adults are more frequently disabled by chronic pain and tend to show greater functional impairment when they are disabled than do adolescents.

Adolescent Versus Child Pain

There is still debate in the literature about the age at which an individual is first capable of experiencing pain (Beales, 1982; Gross & Gardner, 1980; Swafford & Allan, 1968). Beales (1982) indicates that some surgeons' practice of performing certain procedures on their youngest patients without anesthetics is based on an unsubstantiated belief that the neural connections necessary for pain perception are still undeveloped at very young ages. On the other hand, Swafford and Allan (1968) suggested that pediatric patients seldom require medication for pain, even after general surgery. These results were not obtained in another experimental study of children's pain, however, in which a pressure algometer was used to measure pain thresholds in 150 children between 5 and 18 years of age. Haslam (1969) found that younger children had lower pain thresholds than older children. Weisenberg (1977) cited several studies indicating that pain threshold increased with age. Clearly, the results from experimental studies are equivocal.

The results from a recent study by Lollar, Smits, and Patterson (1982) showed a difference in children's ratings of their pain intensity and their parents' ratings of the children's pain. The adults underestimated the intensity of their children's reactions. Lollar et al. (1982) found that six-year-old children judged pain to last a significantly shorter time than did older children. They suggest that this could be due to younger children's immature concepts of time rather than to a difference in their perception of pain.

It is widely recognized that adolescents are more likely to complain of pain than are younger children. Swafford and Allan (1968) reported that the adolescents in their sample of 180 pediatric intensive care patients were given most of the analgesics for pain on that unit. Beales (1982) describes several reports of younger children experiencing less pain than adolescents or adults. However, given the current state of knowledge about children's and adolescents' experience of pain, it is uncertain whether these reports describe the young person's pain experience or relative lack of commmunication skills and level of cognitive development. A further complicating factor in understanding young people's pain behavior is the role of anxiety (Lollar, et al., 1982). Swafford and Allan's (1968) suggestion that tranquilizers may have a beneficial effect with pediatric pain patients is an example of the blurred distinction between pain and anxiety. Poznanski (1976) also has noted the close association of anxiety and pain.

The work of Beales et al. with young people with juvenile rheumatoid arthritis highlights some of the differences in the experience of pain in adolescents and younger children (Beales, Keen & Holt, personal communication). Younger children (ages 6–11 years) and adolescents (ages 12–17 years) reported similar sensations from their affected joints, but the adolescents attributed a more unpleasant meaning to their sensations. The adolescents had a greater understanding of the internal pathology of their joints and indicated more joint pain than did the younger children. The younger patients tended to be more disturbed by minor (visible) cutaneous injuries than by the presence of serious (but not visible to them) internal pathology.

Beales* et al. report that the differences in children's and adolescents' concerns about pain are easily understood when the increased cognitive capabilities of the adolescent are considered. According to Piaget's theory of cognitive development, it is only at adolescence that the individual becomes capable of thinking abstractly and considering possibilities not immediately present. Thus the adolescent is less tied to concrete reality than is the younger child.

COMMON PEDIATRIC PAIN COMPLAINTS

Much of what is known about pain in adolescence is from clinical studies of patients with chronic or recurrent complaints of pain. In some cases these complaints are associated with an underlying chronic disease, although in most cases no organic basis for the complaint has been found. Three complaints occur with such frequency in the pediatric population that they warrant special consideration: abdominal pain, headaches, and limb pain ("growing pains").

The Periodic Syndrome

Wyllie and Schlesinger (1933) are frequently credited with first naming attacks of headache, vomiting, fever, and abdominal pain the "periodic syndrome." They also noted that severe limb pains are common in the periodic syndrome. Apley (1975) discovered two earlier descriptions of the syndrome, one from 1802 and the other from 1882. These recurrent pain episodes have probably been enigmatic to physicians since the beginning of the treatment of disorders of childhood.

Like researchers who followed them, Wyllie and Schlesinger (1933) noted that children with the periodic syndrome were "for the most part

---

* Beales, J.G., Keen, J.H. & Holt, P.J.L. The child's perception of the disease and the experience of pain in juvenile chronic arthritis. Personal communication.

of a nervous type of disposition'' (p.6). The children's families had a positive history of similar complaints in childhood or as adults still suffered from similar complaints (i.e., biliousness or migraine). Unlike later researchers who indicate that the first occurrence of symptoms is usually after 2–3 years of age (e.g., Apley, 1975; Green, 1967; Stickler & Murphy, 1979), Wyllie and Schlesinger (1933) believed that the periodic syndrome could make its first appearance almost immediately after birth; although like others, they believed it was more common at 3–4 years of age.

   Estimates of the prevalence of recurrent abdominal pain, headaches, and limb pain vary among studies. Oster (1972), investigating a school population of 2178 children from 6–15 years of age, found that headaches occurred most frequently (20.6 percent), followed by limb pains (15.5 percent), and abdominal pain (12.3 percent). In a longitudinal study of healthy adolescents, Rauste-von Wright and von Wright (1981) found that limb pains were the second most common symptoms (following dry mouth and cough) for all age groups and both sexes. Headache and feelings of pain were also common in their female group. Of these three common symptoms, the psychological aspects of recurrent abdominal pain have been the most studied.

Recurrent Abdominal Pain

   Children and adolescents with recurrent complaints of abdominal pain, like those with frequent headaches and limb pains, present a particularly difficult diagnostic dilemma for the clinician; the pain may be a symptom of organic disease, but it may occur even more frequently in the absence of organic disease (Apley, 1975; Lebenthal, 1980). The British pediatrician John Apley contributed significantly to the current understanding of the symptom through both clinical descriptions and epidemiological work in schools (see Apley, 1975).

   Apley and Naish's (1958) field study of 1000 British school children indicated that 10.8 percent of those in primary and secondary school experience recurrent abdominal pains, defined as "at least three bouts of pain, severe enough to affect his activities, over a period of not less than three months, with attacks continuing in the year preceding the examination" (Apley & Naish, 1958, p. 165). This definition has limitations because it does not include a consideration of the quality of pain, its duration, any alleviating factors, or the child's physical condition between attacks (Lebenthal, 1980).

   The Apley and Naish (1958) field study used more stringent diagnostic criteria and found that recurrent abdominal pain was more frequent among girls (12.3 percent) compared with boys (9.5 percent). However, other studies of clinical cases have not found a higher incidence in girls (e.g.,

Apley, 1975; Liebman, 1978). Apley (1975) suggests that this inconsistency may exist because the symptom is seen as more trivial in girls, and thus, it is less likely to be brought to the attention of clinicians. The peak occurrence of the symptom in girls appears to be between 12 and 13 years of age (Apley, 1975; Apley & Naish, 1958). Boys show a different pattern, with peak occurrence at age 6 and smaller peaks between 9 and 10 years and then again at 14 years (Apley, 1975; Apley & Naish, 1958). These distributions indicate that reports of abdominal pain in both sexes increase around the time of entry into school; it appears to be a problem primarily of childhood and early adolescence.

Recurrent abdominal pain often occurs concurrently with other symptoms. Stone and Barbero's (1970) group of 102 patients (ages 2½–14 years) reported additional symptoms of headache, pallor, nausea, vomiting, obstipation, dizziness, poor appetite, transient weight loss, low-grade fever, pellet stools, and diarrhea. Others report similar lists (e.g., Apley, 1975; Apley & Naish, 1958; Liebman, 1978; Stickler & Murphy, 1979).

The initial obligation is to rule out organic disease, which typically accounts for less than one case in ten of those hospitalized for the complaint (Apley, 1975). In an outpatient sample of 119 children and adolescents from 3½ to 17 years of age, Liebman found no evidence of organic illness. After reviewing the records of 161 children and adolescents from under 5 years to 14 years of age seen at the Mayo Clinic for recurrent abdominal pain, Stickler and Murphy (1979) concluded that the more experienced physicians ordered fewer tests and the less-anxious parents were satisfied with fewer tests and fewer procedures.

Blendis, Hill, and Merskey (1978) reported that "there is substantial evidence that too many normal appendices are removed in patients with psychological illness." They reported the results of a study (Harding, 1962) in which histological examinations of 1300 appendices revealed that the removed appendix was completely normal in 515 cases (39.6 percent). It is particularly noteworthy that the appendices of two thirds of the females in the sample between 11 and 20 years of age were normal. Lebenthal (1980) notes that the pediatrician "has the main responsibility of assuring the family of the benign course of the entity and preventing deplorable practices, such as exploratory laparotomy," and that otherwise, endless diagnostic tests and doctor shopping may needlessly occur.

Both Liebman (1978) and Stone and Barbero (1970) presented information on the early medical history of children and adolescents with recurrent abdominal pain suggestive of a greater than expected number of problems. Forty-one percent or a sample of 102 children between 2½ and 14 years had mothers who experienced increased physiological symptoms during their pregnancies, which included nausea and vomiting of greater than five months' duration and excessive tiredness requiring protracted bed rest (Stone & Barbero, 1970). In addition, 31 percent of the mothers had a complicated labor or delivery. Liebman (1978) reported similar findings: 34 percent of the mothers of a sample of 119 patients (ages 3½–17 years) had pregnancies characterized by excessive nausea, vomiting, tiredness, headaches, or medical illnesses of greater than ten days' duration. The neonatal history of their samples was also indicative of problems. For example, 31 percent of the children in the Stone and Barbero (1970) and 29 percent in the Liebman (1978) studies had colic lasting more than three months. Unfortunately, these reports were unclear as to whether the studies were retrospectively based on parental recollections or medical records.

Although Apley (1975) reported no difference in intelligence in children with recurrent abdominal pain compared with a control group, problems with school attendance have been noted. In one sample of 119 children ages 3½–17 years, only 9 percent attended school regularly (Liebman, 1978). The "back to school tummy ache" has been suggested as masking school phobia or school refusal (Berger, 1974). Mauroner (1978) presented a psychodynamic explanation of the child's or adolescent's pain complaint, whereby the pain allows the child or adolescent to return home to a parent who is anxious about separation.

Emotional or personality problems have long been recognized as associated with recurrent abdominal pain. Wyllie and Schlesinger (1933) indicated that "they are for the most part a nervous type of disposition." More recently, Apley (1975) presented information comparing school children with and without recurrent abdominal pain and found that the children with the pain were more likely to be high strung, fussy, excitable, anxious, timid, or apprehensive. Furthermore, children with recurrent abdominal pain were more likely to show signs of emotional disturbance, such as undue fears, sleep disorders, and appetite difficulties. Liebman (1978) classified 30 percent of the children he studied as being perfectionistic or "superachievers."

Apley (1975) also indicated that parents of these children tended toward overprotection, likely due to excessive parental anxiety. One or both parents of children in both Apley's school and hospital series often showed intensive or obsessional preoccupation with the child's health. Marital discord, separation, or divorce were temporally related to a child's abdominal pain in 39 percent of Liebman's (1978) families.

There have been a few reports of follow-up studies of children and adolescents with recurrent abdominal pain (Apley & Hale, 1973; Christensen & Mortensen, 1975; Stickler & Murphy, 1979). Two studies offer reassurance that organic disease is only rarely missed. In Stickler and Murphy's (1979) sample of 161 children, only three instances of organic disease were later discovered. Apley and Hale (1973) similarly found only two instances of late diagnoses of organic cause in 60 cases.

The long-term prognosis of these children with nonorganic abdominal pain is guarded at best. Approximately one third of them, regardless of whether they were treated with reassurance, continued to have abdominal symptoms as adults (Apley & Hale, 1973). Another follow-up study found a similar pattern: one fourth of the patients in Stickler and Murphy's (1979) sample continued to have symptoms after five years. Christensen and Mortensen (1975), perhaps because they followed their subjects for a longer period of time (up to 29–30 years after the patients' hospitalization in childhood), found that one half of the children with recurrent abdominal pain also suffered from abdominal symptoms as adults, compared with one fourth to one third of the control sample. Some of the patients with symptoms in adulthood had been symptom free during adolescence. The patients in the Christensen and Mortensen (1975) study had also been treated with reassurance and explanation.

Stickler and Murphy (1979) were particularly concerned with the sizable percentage of their sample who continued to have symptoms and to seek medical intervention. They joined Christensen and Mortensen (1975) in wondering whether further psychosomatic or hypochondriacal illnesses could have been avoided with more intensive psychological or psychiatric intervention.

Apley and Hale (1973) suggested indications of good and bag prognoses for children with recurrent abdominal pain. Children were more likely to grow up and have pain if they came from "painful families" (i.e., one or both parents having recurrent pains or serious disturbances). Christensen and Mortensen (1975) reported a similar finding: children with parents who had current abdominal symptoms were more likely to have abdominal pain than children of adults with no current abdominal complaints. Interestingly, children of parents who had a history of abdominal pain in childhood were not more likely to suffer from abdominal pain than children whose parents did not have such a history (Christensen & Mortensen, 1975). The parents' current behavior, apparently, was more significant than their past medical history.

Age of onset, sex, and the duration of the symptoms before treatment were also found to be related to prognosis (Apley & Hale, 1973). A poorer prognosis was associated with being male, onset of symptoms before age six years, and pain of more than six months' duration before onset of treatment.

Headaches

As is the case with recurrent abdominal pain, organic abnormalities are very infrequently found in pediatric patients with headaches (Jay & Tomasi, 1981; Krupp & Friedman, 1953; Oster, 1972; Rigg, 1979; Rothner,

1979). However, there is limited information on the psychosocial characteristics of adolescents with recurrent headaches, perhaps because there has not been an investigator with the interests and talent of John Apley studying this condition. Many authors do not include psychosocial information in their reports on children and adolescents with headaches (e.g., Congdon & Forsythe, 1979; Hockaday, 1979; Jay & Tomasi, 1981; Rigg, 1980a, 1979). Hockaday (1979), in fact, eliminated children from her sample if their headaches appeared to be psychogenic.

An even more basic problem in considering the psychological aspects of headaches in adolescents is the problem of definition. For example, there is no widely accepted definition of migraine headaches in children (Congdon & Forsythe, 1979; Hockaday, 1979). Some investigators (e.g., Oster, 1972) do not elaborate about the different types of headaches. On the other hand, Rigg (1979) presents a rather exhaustive classification system. Conflicting reports about incidence, sex prevalence, and age at onset may arise simply because of classification.

Prensky and Sommer (1979) helped with some of the definition problems of migraine headaches in children and adolescents by enumerating criteria for that diagnosis. They suggested the following diagnostic criteria:

1. Recurrent headaches, separated by symptom-free intervals.
2. Any three of the following six symptoms: (a) abdominal pain, nausea, or vomiting with the headaches, (b) hemicrania, (c) a throbbing, pulsatile quality of pain, (d) complete relief after a brief period of rest, (e) an aura, either visual, sensory, or motor, and (f) a history of migraine headaches in one or more members of the immediate family (Prensky & Sommer, 1979, p. 506).

Others (e.g., Jay & Tomasi, 1981) accepted this definition and used it in further research.

Although Prensky and Sommer (1979) did not routinely use psychometric tests with their 84 migraine patients, they collected psychosocial information during clinical interviews. They reported a high incidence of depressive symptoms in their sample, and they suggested that this was the reason these patients were referred to a specialist. One group of the patients was treated with antidepressant medication in hopes of preventing headache attacks. In over 50 percent of this group the medication "did not substantially reduce the frequency of headaches within the first six months of treatment" (Prensky & Sommer, 1979, p. 504).

Other symptoms of psychological disturbance were also found in this same Prensky and Sommer (1979) sample. Several children were labeled overactive with a short attention span. Compulsive behavior and recurrent symptoms of severe anxiety were also noted. Below average performance in school was a problem with several of the children.

An earlier study by Krupp and Friedman (1953) described some of the psychosocial characteristics of 100 children from 3 to 14 years of age who were seen at the Montefiore Hospital Headache Clinic for chronic recurring headaches. They divided their sample into 75 patients with migraine defined as "headache which is characteristically unilateral, occurs in bouts usually associated with gastrointestinal or ocular symptoms, is often preceded by visual or psychologic disturbances, and is followed by sleep," and 17 patients with tension headaches, defined as "that type which is limited to head pain occurring in relation to constant or periodic emotional conflicts which may be conscious or unconscious" (p. 43).

Krupp and Friedman (1953) described the children with migraines as having superior intelligence and being good students. This is in contrast to Rigg's (1980b) report that there is no correlation between migraines and intelligence. According to Krupp and Friedman (1953), approximately one-fourth of migraine sufferers in their sample could have been diagnosed as psychoneurotic, although there were not diagnoses of primary behavior disorder or psychoses. Feelings of inadequacy and guilt were also common. A sizable portion of the migraine patients exhibited aggressive thoughts and actions; their headaches were thought to be related frequently to unexpressed hostility toward authority figures. Although only a few of the tension-headache patients underwent psychiatric evaluation, Krupp and Friedman (1953) believed that the psychopathology was similar to that of the migraine patients.

While Rigg (1980b) suggests that there is no specific personality type associated with migraine in general, stress is believed to be the most important trigger factor in children and adolescents. In some patients stress is ongoing and is related to the patients' life situation rather than to situational problems. Most investigators report a positive family history of headaches or other pain complaints.

There is conflicting information about the prognosis of migraine headaches that begin in childhood and adolescence. Krupp and Friedman (1953) indicated a poor prognosis. Blanchard and Andrasik (1982, p. 875) would concur and suggest that "more attention needs to be given to treatment of headache in children, which may also prevent these children from becoming troubled adult headache sufferers." The opposite opinion is presented by Congdon and Forsythe (1979) who state that childhood migraine is thought to have a good prognosis. Prensky and Sommer (1979) found that after several years two thirds of their sample were either completely free of headaches or had them only rarely. However, Congdon and Forsythe (1979), among others, point to the need for long term follow-up of these patients, since there have been reports of remissions lasting up to a decade. Furthermore, Oster (1972) suggests that headache–abdominal pain–limb pain patients may experience the different forms of pain as the years go by, leading him to conclude that "the total prognosis appears to be dubious."

Limb Pains

Like the other two common pediatric pain complaints, recurrent limb pains can be associated with organic illnesses, but more often, an organic basis for the complaint cannot be found (Passo, 1982). With this syndrome as well as the other two, definitional problems abound, leading to difficulties in estimating its prevalence. For instance, Calabro, Wachel, Holgerson, & Repice (1976) report frequencies of the complaint ranging from 4 percent to 50 percent due to the differences in diagnostic criteria. Passo (1982, p. 209) suggests that persistent or recurrent limb pain in children could be "a symptom of 1) an underlying systemic disease; 2) a serious primary musculoskeletal disease; or 3) a benign syndrome with no obvious organic etiology." He also contends that psychological factors could contribute to any of these three types of pain.

One type of limb pain has been called *growing pain* from time immemorial, as Oster and Nielsen (1972) note. The term is typically limited to pain complaints without organic origins. Naish and Apley (1951) defined it as limb pain of at least three months' duration that is not specifically located in the joints and is severe enough to limit normal activities. A more precise definition was offered by Oster and Nielsen (1972):

The symptoms consist of intermittent and frequently quite incapacitating pain localized deeply in the arms and/or legs in children and young people. The pain is not articular. Occasionally, it is accompanied by sensations of restlessness but never by tenderness, redness, or local swelling. Similarly, pain in the legs is not provoked by walking and the gait is always normal. The pain disappears in the morning (p. 329).

Growing pain is really a misnomer because growth, as characterized by height, weight, and weight/height ratio, does not influence the occurrence of growing pains (Oster & Nielsen, 1972; Passo, 1982).

Calabro et al. (1976) presented a clinical description of growing pains based on a review of earlier studies. They reported that it was more common among girls than boys and that it occurs during childhood and early adolescence. There is usually a positive family history of similar pain complaints. The pains usually occur at night and are most often felt in the thigh, calf, and posterior of the knee. The attacks of pain may occur for months or even years, but they eventually subside. It is, however, important to remember Oster's (1972) suggestion that growing pains, like headaches and abdominal pain, may converge. Calabro et al. (1976) point out that if the pain is generalized, differential diagnosis is more difficult, and juvenile rheumatoid arthritis, rheumatic fever, polymyositis or dermatomyositis, and leukemia must be ruled out.

Passo (1982) suggested that there is a group of children who do not quite fit the classic benign picture of growing pains but rather suffer from what he has labeled "psychogenic rheumatism." He indicates that these complaints do not fit established organic diagnoses but may be a manifestation of hysteria in childhood. The patients that he has seen complain of fleeting joint pain, occasional stiffness, transient swelling, and low-grade fevers. In some cases there is a history of an antecedent organic insult, such as trauma or a viral-like syndrome. The symptoms tend to linger rather than subside as with growing pains. However, on physical examination, these children appear normal.

While Passo (1982) did not present data from a systematic evaluation of children with psychogenic rheumatism, he described them psychologically as overachievers who often have a history of prolonged school absenteeism because of fatigue and recurrent pain. Other children are underachievers or learning disabled. Depressive symptoms and low-self-esteem may be common.

Fritz et al. (1981) reported on a group of 28 adolescents referred to an orthopedic clinic for knee pain. Of the 28, 5 were identified as having functional knee pain, 17 had clear organic pain, and 6 had signs that were ambiguous or insufficient for a definitive diagnosis. Unfortunately, the questionnaire they used (the Junior–Senior High School Personality Questionnaire) was not helpful in differentiating between the functional and organic groups.

ASSESSMENT OF THE PSYCHOLOGICAL COMPONENTS OF ADOLESCENTS' PAIN

Screening

The first health professional to see an adolescent with a pain complaint is most likely to be a medical provider. An alert school nurse may notice frequent school absences because of recurrent pain complaints and refer the adolescent to a physician for an evaluation, or, concerned parents may initiate a referral to their family practitioner or pediatrician. The physician usually begins the assessment with a complete history, physical examination, and routine laboratory tests. Given the nature of the pain that occurred in the adolescents described earlier, it is clear that this assessment must also include an initial evaluation of the psychological functioning of the adolescent and his or her parents. During this screening process, it is recommended that the physician avoid classifying the pain as either organic or functional (psychogenic), but rather recognize that psychological factors may be operating regardless of whether the pain has an organic etiology. Furthermore, Barr and Feuerstein's (in press) suggestion that there may be a category of patients with recurrent abdominal pain for whom no organic or psychogenic etiology is assumed should be kept in mind.

In screening for psychological problems, the physician can play an important role in the education of the adolescent and his or her parents. School nurses also have ample opportunity to provide this information to the adolescent. Both the parents and the adolescent can become aware of the role of stress and other psychological factors in disease by the types of questions the clinician asks. Green (1967) suggests that psychological issues be explored from the beginning of the assessment instead of after an organic etiology has been eliminated.

The words used by physicians during their screening may facilitate or hinder the evaluation. Adolescents with chronic pain complaints are quite sensitive to being told that the pain is not real, all in their heads, or due to emotional problems, or that they are crazy. Parents and adolescents may not listen to a physician if they believe he or she is saying that the pain is psychological. Therefore, language is important. Berger et al. (1977) suggest that words such as stress and tension are much less threatening than are words such as emotional and psychological problems.

The screening process is facilitated by seeing the adolescent and parent together first, then separately. Green (1967) provides a thorough list of psychological factors to explore including school problems, marital discord, deaths or separations of significant others in the adolescent's life, illness or handicaps in parents or siblings, mental illness in parents, parent–adolescent relationship problems, parents' preoccupation with adolescents' illness, inappropriate sleeping arrangements, and difficulties in expressing feelings (aggressive, hostile, or sexual). Green (1967) also provided a list of questions to ask including

1. What prompted the referral at this time?
2. Who suggested they seek the evaluation?
3. What do they think is wrong?
4. What do the parents expect from the evaluation?
5. What gains does the pain provide for the adolescent?

Passo (1982) suggested that the review of systems might be helpful to the physician in providing evidence for psychological problems, in that polysystemic pain may be indicative of a psychosomatic process. In some cases the adolescent or parent may not cooperate with the screening for psychological problems. "I know that the pain is physical" is frequently heard from an adolescent or a parent; therefore, there will be reluctance to share information about stress or turmoil in the family. The pain symptoms may be a cover for other concerns or problems. The sensitive physician is aware of this and continues the probe into problem areas. Of course, there are cases in which psychological factors are noncontributory to the pain complaint, but loud and vehement denials may be a signal of problems.

An adolescent's primary responsibility is school attendance and performance. Difficulties in meeting that responsibility can indicate the necessity of a thorough psychological evaluation. Berger (1974) describes how somatic complaints are often associated with the problem of school phobia or school refusal. Further exploration is suggested when an adolescent is able to continue with his or her highly valued activities (e.g., dance lessons, swim meets) but is in too much pain to meet the obligations of school.

The parent's attitude toward school is also important to assess. Who makes the decision that an adolescent should stay home because of illness or pain? In some cases it is the adolescent, but in others it is the parent who keeps an adolescent, otherwise willing to attend school, at home. Some parents actively work to keep their "sick" child out of school by arranging homebound tutors and instruction. Even if the adolescent's educational needs are met in that fashion, social development may be hindered with home instruction, and he or she often assumes the identity of a sick person.

The reasons for poor school attendance or performance are numerous. It may be the result of separation anxiety or an actual fear of school. Poor peer relationships may be contributory. The academic demands on the adolescent may be too stringent or too lenient. Adolescents whose pain complaints began with an illness resulting in an absence from school may feel overwhelmed by the amount of work they have to make up. They may also be hesitant about reentering their peer group. Because of this complexity, a psychological evaluation may be necessary to explore the various aspects of the adolescent's functioning.

MANAGEMENT OF THE PSYCHOLOGICAL COMPONENTS OF ADOLESCENTS' PAIN

The adolescent with a chronic pain complaint traditionally is treated by a pediatrician or other physician. The first step in the process is to rule out an organic basis for the complaint. Apley (1975) suggested that there are then three aspects of the treatment of a child with recurrent abdominal pain:

1. Convincing the parents that there is no organic cause for the pain.
2. Allowing the patient and parents to release emotional tension (achieved by attentive listening by the physician).
3. Friendly guidance about how to modify harmful aspects of the child's environment.

Hospitalization for the more intractable cases is often used as a means of facilitating the diagnosis and assuring the patient and parents that the evaluation is complete (e.g., Hughes & Zimin, 1978; Lebenthal, 1980; Liebman, 1978; Stone & Barbero, 1970). The hospitalization also allows for an extended period of observation of the patient's behavior and interaction with parents.

The hospital staff members may serve as models for the parents on how to deal with their adolescent's pain (Hughes & Zimin, 1978). Educating patients and parents about the benign nature of the pain complaints is frequently used (e.g., Calabro et al., 1976). The adolescent is instructed to resume his or her responsibilities, particularly at school. Reassurance by the physician that the adolescent is physically capable of meeting these responsibilities may be all that is needed (Lebenthal, 1980).

Along with assuring the patient and parents of the benign nature of the pain, it is useful to point out that the pain is real, and not imagined. Lebenthal (1980, p. 347) suggests describing the pain as a normal psychosomatic reaction to stress. The physician is then able to discuss with the parents the need to teach the adolescent to deal with tension or stress in a different way (Berger et al., 1977). Stickler and Murphy (1979) make the important suggestion of providing the adolescent with a face-saving device (i.e., an excuse for the symptoms that can be given to inquisitive peers or family about prolonged absences from school).

Some physicians then focus on family dynamics and direct suggestions to the parents about their own behavior. Krupp et al. (1953), for example, suggest that parents be instructed to minimize their own headaches in the presence of their children. Parental attitudes about the adolescent (e.g., seeing him or her as sick and unable to meet age-appropriate responsibilities) can have an effect on the adolescent's pain behavior. Encouraging the parents to accept the attitude that the adolescent can control or live with the symptoms can be an effective intervention (Berger et al., 1977).

Even with reassurance from the pediatrician, some adolescents and their parents continue to seek a medical explanation for the pain (Apley, 1976; Stickler & Murphy, 1979). This is of particular concern in those who continue to go through more and more invasive medical procedures or surgery without relief. Many of these adolescents continue to have pain into adulthood. It has been suggested that this group may benefit from more intensive psychological treatment, although there currently are no well-controlled studies to support this approach (Miller & Kratochwill, 1979; Wasserman, 1978).

Psychological treatment for the adolescent with recurrent pain and significant psychological or family dysfunction is clearly indicated. The types of treatment for these ..dolescents are quite varied, depending upon the individual's needs, and range from behavioral techniques such as relaxation training and biofeedback to more traditional insight-oriented psychotherapy. For some, simple reassurance is all that is needed, while others may require intense psychotherapy for depression or a change in school placement. Treatment programs for adolescents must be individualized, based on the results of the psychological and medical evaluation.

CONCLUSIONS

Recurrent pain complaints in adolescence range from being a mere nuisance for some to having more drastic effects on other adolescents who are seriously debilitated by the pain and on their families. Organic etiologies are rarely found for these recurrent complaints. The search for an organic basis for the complaint can become quite expensive and invasive to the patient. Because of frequently missed school, adolescents with recurrent pain may lag behind their peers both socially and academically.

Given the pervasiveness of the problem, a team approach is likely to be the most effective. The adolescent and parents should work with a health care team that includes a physician, a psychologist, and school personnel (e.g., school nurse, teachers, and counselors). All aspects of the adolescent's life should be explored. Further research and health care models should go beyond the old organic versus psychogenic model and allow for a more substantial understanding of the adolescent and his or her pain complaint.

REFERENCES

Apley, J. *The child with abdominal pains* (2nd ed.). Oxford: Blackwell, 1975.

Apley, J., & Hale, B. Children with recurrent abdominal pain: How do they grow up? *British Medical Journal,*1973, *3,* 7–9.

Apley, J., Naish, L. Recurrent abdominal pains: A field survey of 1000 school children. *Archives of Diseases of Children, 1958, 33,* 165–170.

Barr, R.G., & Feurerstein, M. Recurrent abdominal pain syndrome: How appropriate are our basic clinical assumptions? In P. Firestone, & P. McGrath (Eds.), *Pediatric and adolescent behavioral medicine.* New York: Springer, in press.

Barr, R.G., Levine, M.D., & Watkins, J.W. Recurrent abdominal pain in childhood due to lactose intolerance, a prospective study. *New England Journal of Medicine* 1979, *300,* 1449–1452.

Barsky, A.J., & Klerman, G.L. Overview: Hypochondriasis, bodily complaints, and somatic styles. *American Journal of Psychiatry, 1983, 140,* 273–283.

Beales, J.G. The assessment and management of pain in children. In P. Karoly, J.J. Steffen & D.J. O'Grady (Eds.), *Child health psychology: Concepts and issues.* New York: Pergamon Press, 1982.

Beecher, H.K. *Measurement of subjective responses.* New York: Oxford University Press, 1959.

Berger, H.G. Somatic pain and school avoidance. *Clinical Pediatrics,* 1974, *13,* 819–826.

Berger, H.G., Honig, P.J., & Liebman, R. Recurrent abdominal pain. Gaining control of the symptom. *American Journal of Diseases of Children,* 1977, *131,* 1340–1344.

Bishop, E.R., & Torch, E.M. Dividing "hysteria": A preliminary investigation of conversion disorder and psychalgia. *Journal of Nervous and Mental Disease,* 1979, *167,* 348–356.

Blanchard, E.B., & Andrasik, F. Psychological assessment and treatment of headache: Recent developments and emerging issues. *Journal of Consulting and Clinical Psychology,* 1982, *50,* 859–879.

Blendis, L.M., Hill, O.W., & Merskey, H. Abdominal pain and the emotions. *Pain,* 1978, *5,* 179–191.

Bonica, J.J. Pain research and therapy: Past and current status and future needs. In L., Ng, & J.J. Bonica (Eds.), *Pain, discomfort and Humanitarian Care.* New York: Elsevier, 1980, 1–46.

Brena, S.F., Chapman, S.L., Stegall, P.G., & Chyatte, S.B. Chronic pain states: Their relationship to impairment and disability. *Archives of Physical Medicine and Rehabilitation,* 1979, *60,* 387–389.

Calabro, J.J., Wachtel, A.E., Holgerson, W.B., & Repice, M.M. Growing pains: Fact or fiction? *Postgraduate Medicine,* 1976, *59,* 66–72.

Carlson, G.A., & Cantwell, D.A. Unmasking masked depression in children and adolescents. *American Journal of Psychiatry,* 1980, *137,* 445–449.

Christensen, M.F., & Mortensen, O. Long-term prognosis in children with recurrent abdominal pain. *Archives of Diseases of Children,* 1975, *50,* 110–114.

Chodoff, P., & Lyons, H. Hysteria: the hysterical personality and hysterical conversion. *American Journal of Psychiatry,* 1958, *114,* 734–740.

Congdon, P.J., & Forsythe, W.I. Migraine in childhood: A study of 300 children. *Developmental Medicine and Child Neurology,* 1979, *21,* 209–216.

Dorfman, W. Hypochondriasis as a defense against depression. *Psychosomatics,* 1968, *9,* 248–251.

Dorfman, W. Hypochondriasis-revisited: A dilemma and challenge to medicine and psychiatry. *Psychosomatics,* 1975, *16,* 14–16.

Fordyce, W.E. *Behavioral methods for chronic pain and illness.* St. Louis: Mosby, 1976.

Fritz, G.K., Bleck, E.E., & Dahl, I.S. Functional versus organic knee pain in adolescents. *American Journal Sports Medicine,* 1981, *9,* 247–249.

Frommer, E.A. Depressive illness in childhood. *British Journal of Psychiatry,* 1968, (Special Publication No. 2), *118,* 117–123.

Goodwin, D.W., & Guze, S.B. *Psychiatric diagnosis* (2nd ed.) New York: Oxford University Press, 1979.

Green, M. Diagnosis and treatment: Psychogenic recurrent, abdominal pain. *Pediatrics,* 1967, *40,* 84–89.

Gross, S.C., & Gardner, G.G. Child Pain: Treatment approaches. In W.L. Smith, H. Merskey, & S.C. Gross (Eds.), *Pain: Meaning and management.* Lancaster: MTP Press, 1980.

Guze, S.B. The diagnosis of hysteria: What are we trying to do? *American Journal of Psychiatry, 1967, 124,* 491–498.

Harding, H.E. A notable source of error in the diagnosis of appendicitis. *British Medical Journal,* 1962, *2,* 1028–1029.

Haslam, D.R. Age and perception of pain. *Psychosomic Science,* 1969, *15,* 86.

Herman, R.M., & Siminds, J.G. Incidence of conversion symptoms in children evaluated psychiatrically. *Missouri Medicine*, 1975, *72*, 597–604.

Hockaday, J.M. Basilar migraine in childhood. *Developmental Medicine and Child Neurology*, 1979, *21*, 455–463.

Jay, G.W., & Tomasi, L.G. Pediatric headaches: A one year retrospective analysis. *Headache*, 1981, *21*, 5–9.

Keating, D.P. Thinking processes in adolescence. In J. Adelson (Ed.), *Handbook of adolescent psychology*. New York: John Wiley, 1980.

Kenyon, F.E. Hypochondriasis: A clinical study. *British Journal of Psychiatry*, 1964, *110*, 478–488.

Kenyon, F.E. Hypochondriasis: A survey of some historical, clinical and social aspects. *British Journal of medical Psychology*, 1965, *38*, 117–133.

Kenyon, F.E. Hypochondrical states. *British Journal of Psychiatry*, 1976, *129*, 1–14.

Kral, V.A. Masked depression in middle aged men. *Canadial Medical Association Journal*, 1958, *79*, 1–5.

Krupp, G.R., & Friedman, A.P. Recurrent headache in children: A study of 100 clinical cases. *New York State Journal of Medicine*, 1953, *53*, 430–446.

Lebenthal, E. Recurrent abdominal pain in childhood. *American Journal of Diseases of Children*, 1980, *134*, 347–348.

Lefkowitz, M.M., & Burton, N. Childhood depression: A critique of the concept. *Psychological Bulletin*, 1978, *85*, 716–726.

Lesse, S. The multivariate masks of depression. *American Journal of Psychiatry*, 1968, *124*, 35–40.

Lesse, S. Hypochondriasis and psychosomatic disorders masking depression. In S. Lesse (Ed.), *Masked depression*. New York: Aronson, 1974, 53–74.

Lesse, S. Hypochondriacal and psychosomatic disorders masking depression n adolescents. *American Journal of Psychotherapy*, 1981, *35*, 356–367.

Lewis, A. 'Psychogenic': A word and its mutations. *Psychological Medicine*, 1972, *2*, 209–215.

Liebman, W. Recurrent abdominal pain in children. *Clinical Pediatrics*, 1978, *17*, 149–153.

Liebman, W.M. Recurrent abdominal pain in children: Lactose and sucrose intolerance, a prospective study. Pediatrics, 1979, *64*, 43–45.

Lollar, D.J., Smiths, S.J., & Patterson, D.L. Assessment of pediatric pain: An empirical perspective. *Journal of Pediatric Psychology*, 1982, *7*, 267–278.

Maloney, M.J. Diagnosing hysterical conversion reactions in children. *Pediatrics*, 1980, *97*, 1016–1020.

Mauroner, N.L. The family and GI problems. *Psychosomatics*, 1978, *19*, 137–139.

McKegney, F.P. The incidence and characteristics of patients with conversion reaction: A general hospital consultation service sample. *American Journal of Psychiatry*, 1967, *124*, 542–551.

Melzack, R., & Dennis, S.G. Neurophysiological foundations of pain. In R.A. Sternback (Ed.), *The psychology of pain*. New York: Raven Press, 1978, 1–26.

Melzack, R., & Wall, P.D. *The challenge of pain*. New York: Basic Books, 1983.

Merskey, H., & IASP Subcommittee on Taxonomy. Pain terms: A list of definitions and notes on usage. *Pain*, 1979, *6*, 249–252.

Miller, A.J., & Kratochwill, T.R. Reduction of frequent stomachache complaints by time out. *Behavior Therapy*, 1979, *10*, 211–218.

Naish, J.M., & Apley, J. Growing pains: Clinical study of non-arthritic limb pains in children. *Archives of Diseases of Children*, 1951, *26*, 134–140.

Osborne, D. Use of MMPI with medical patients. In J.N. Butcher (Ed.), *New developments in the use of the MMPI*. Minneapolis: University of Minnesota Press, 1979.

Oster, J. Recurrent abdominal pain, headache, and limb pains in children and adolescents. *Pediatrics*, 1972, *50*, 429–436.

Oster, J., & Nielsen, A. Growing pains: A clinical investigation of a school population. *Acta Paediatrica Scandinavica* 1972, *61*, 329–334.

Passo, M.H. Aches and limb pain. *Pediatric Clinics of North America*, 1982, *29*, 209–219.

Perley, M.J., & Guze, S.B. Hysteria—The stability and usefulness of clinical criteria. *New England Journal of Medicine*, 1962, *266*, 421–426.

Poznanski, E.A. Children's reactions to pain: A psychiatrist's perspective. *Clinical Pediatrics*, 1976, *15*, 1114–1119.

Prensky, A.L., & Sommer, D. Diagnosis and treatment of migraine in children. *Neurology*, 1979, *29*, 506–510.

Purtell, J.J., Robins, E., & Cohen, M.E. Observations on clinical aspects of hysteria. *Journal of the American Medical Association*, 1951, *146*, 902–909.

Rauste-von Wright, M., & von Wright, J. A longitudinal study of psychosomatic symptoms in healthy 11–18 year old girls and boys. *Journal of Psychosomatic Research*, 1981, *25*, 525–534.

Rigg, C.A. Cluster and intracranial headaches. *Journal of Current Adolescent Medicine*, 1980a, *2*, 29–30.

Rigg, C.A. Episodic vascular headaches–migraine. *Journal of Current Adolescent Medicine*, 1980b, *2*, 25–30.

Rigg, C.A. Introduction, extracranial headache, and referred pain. *Journal of Current Adolescent Medicine*, 1979, *1*, 44–46.

Rock, N.L. Conversion reactions in childhood: A clinical study on childhood neuroses. *Journal of American Academy of Child Psychiatry*, 1971, *10*, 65–77.

Rothner, A.D. Headaches in children: A review. *Headache*, 1979, *19*, 156–162.

Sternbach, R.A. *Pain patients: Traits and treatment.* New York: Academic Press, 1974.

Stickler, G., & Murphy, D.B. Recurrent abdominal pain. *American Journal of Diseases of Children*, 1979, *133*, 486–484.

Stone, R.T., & Barbero, G.J. Recurrent abdominal pain in childhood. *Pediatrics*, 1970, *45*, 732–738.

Swafford, L.I., & Allen, D. Pain relief in the pediatric patient. *Medical Clinics of North America*, 1968, *52*, 131–136.

Szasz, T.S. *Pain and pleasure: A study of bodily feelings* London: Tavistock Publications, 1957.

Wasserman, T.H. The elimination of complaints of stomach cramps in a 12-year-old child by covert positive reinforcement. *The Behavior Therapist*, 1978, *1*, 13–14.

Weisenberg, M. Pain and pain control. *Psychological Bulletin*, 1977, *84*, 1008–1044.

Weisenberg, M. Cultural and ethnic factors in reaction to pain. In I. Al-Issa (Ed.), *Culture and Psychopathology*. Baltimore: University Park Press, 1982.

Wyllie, W.G., & Schlesinger, B. The periodic group of disorders in childhood. *British Journal of Children's Diseases*, 1933, *30*, 1–21.

Ziegler, F.J., Imboden, J.B., & Meyer, E. Contemporary conversion reactions: A clinical study. *American Journal of Psychiatry*, 1960, *116*, 901–909.

Melissa Hamp

13
The Diabetic Teenager

Optimal care of the adolescent with chronic disease includes attention not only to medical needs but to the life situation and developmental tasks of the teenager as well. Nowhere is this requirement more apparent than in the management of the adolescent with diabetes.* Diabetes, more than most other medical conditions, requires active participation on the part of the patient in the daily assessment and treatment of the condition. The need for daily monitoring, injections, and attention to diet, when combined with the striving for autonomy and experimentation associated with the adolescent years, may create conflicts and frustration for the patient, the patient's family, and the professionals who are providing health care.

While many adolescents successfully manage both their diabetes and their transition to adulthood, others do not. For some, the teenage years are fraught with poor diabetic control, recurrent hospitalization for diabetic ketoacidosis, and the resulting labels of brittle, out of control, and difficult to manage. The potential for adverse psychological sequelae and premature onset of diabetic complications is indeed real in these young people. During adolescence, emotional factors play a significant role in the development and maintenance of brittle diabetes (Greydanus & Hoffmann, 1979). Additionally, much of the diabetic teenager's behavior, which is regarded by family and health professionals as problematic, might be considered normal in a healthy teenager (Tattersall & Lowe, 1981).

Thus, comprehensive medical management of the adolescent diabetic

---

*Unless otherwise specified, the term diabetes used in this chapter refers to insulin-dependent mellitus (IDDM).

CHRONIC ILLNESS AND DISABILITIES IN CHILDHOOD AND ADOLESCENCE   ISBN 0-8089-1635-1

must incorporate an understanding of both the developmental contexts of adolescence and the emotional and psychosocial aspects of chronic disease.

ADOLESCENCE AND DIABETES

Developmental Tasks of Adolescence

The developmental tasks of adolescence are essentially those of emancipation and identity formation. More than a transition from childhood to adulthood, adolescence is a segment in the continuum of human development. Adolescents can be viewed as persons with specific qualities, roles to perform, and skills to develop (Konopka, 1973). Physically, the young person attains an adult form during puberty, and with it, the capacity for reproduction. Socially, the adolescent moves from the childhood dependence on parents and family to the interdependence of adulthood. Peers become an important reference group in this transition period, providing support for separation and a forum for the testing of psychosocial and sexual identity. Coincident with physical and social change, the adolescent becomes a keen self-observer with reflective consciousness of self in interaction with others. With an increased capacity for abstract thought, previously accepted values and standards of behavior (often parental) may be rejected by the adolescent and alternative possibilities discovered and explored. Inherent in all of these changes is the adolescent's awareness of the potential for change, growth, and mastery. The experimentation and risk-taking behavior that are characteristic of adolescence may be viewed as natural responses of testing this new potential. Such developmental changes are, of course, generalizations and do not apply to all adolescents to the same degree. Neither do these changes occur in a discrete, irrevocable manner. The adolescent may vacillate between the desire for autonomy and mastery and the relative security of childhood behavior. Such ambivalence in part explains much of what Konopka (1973) regards as the healthy and normal characteristics of adolescence: audacity and insecurity, loneliness and psychological vulnerability, mood swings, peer-group need, and the tendency to be argumentative and emotional.

Influence of Diabetes on Developmental Tasks

The diagnosis of a chronic disease such as diabetes necessarily influences or threatens the teenager's accomplishment of the developmental tasks of adolescence. As reviewed by Hoffmann (1975), the impact of chronic illness is felt throughout the chronological stages of adolescence.

The early adolescent, in the midst of puberty, is preoccupied with bodily changes, normalcy, and body image. Poorly controlled IDDM may lead to stunted growth or delayed pubertal maturation (Laron, Volovitz, & Karp, 1977). Frequent medical exams or hospitalizations subject the body-conscious young teenager to embarrassment and invasion of privacy (Tattersall & Lowe, 1981).

In mid-adolescence, teenagers are increasingly and often ambivalently involved in struggles with their parents for autonomy and control. In certain families parental overconcern may result in the focusing of all conflict on the diabetic condition and its therapy to the exclusion of other, more traditional issues, such as the teenager's appearance or peer activities (Tattersall & Lowe, 1981). In such cases, the adolescent's efforts to exert control and independence may similarly focus on the disease and its treatment through rebellion against the daily therapy schedule, resulting in poor control of the diabetes. The mid-adolescent has great allegiance to the peer group, and is primarily concerned with conforming. Much of adolescent peer-group socializing centers around eating. The erratic eating patterns and consumption of ready made foods, both of which are typical of this stage of development, are disallowed in the traditional dietary regimen of IDDM. The diabetic teenager's sense of being different is further heightened by the potential occurrence of insulin-induced hypoglycemia and the social stigma associated with the attendant loss of consciousness. Finally, the mid-adolescent's concern with attracting the opposite sex, if combined with actual or perceived deficits of physical integrity due to the chronic illness, may adversely affect the developing psychosexual identity (Hoffmann, 1975).

The late adolescent is concerned with intimacy, education, career, marriage, procreation, and other future-oriented issues. The very real possibility of morbidity or mortality from diabetic complications in young adulthood may blunt this future orientation, interrupting or destroying personal or vocational plans. Awareness of progressive disability in the adolescent with IDDM can be a source of great pressure and conflict for the youth and his or her family (Frish, Galatzer, & Laron, 1977; Gil, Frish, Amir, & Galatzer, 1977). Even the otherwise healthy young adult with diabetes may suffer from discrimination by employers and loading of insurance premiums as a result of the disease (Tattersall & Lowe, 1981).

PSYCHOSOCIAL ASPECTS OF DIABETES

The Adolescent

As discussed, the diagnosis of diabetes in childhood or adolescence poses potential problems for normal psychosocial development. The literature on the psychosocial aspects of diabetes is voluminous and has been recently reviewed (Greydanus & Hoffmann, 1979). Two main themes of this literature are the impact of diabetes on the healthy development of the adolescent and factors in the adolescent's family and emotional environment that influence control of the disease.

Many researchers have sought to determine the psychosocial attributes of diabetic teenagers compared with their normal peers. General intelligence of diabetic youths has not been found to be significantly different from that of nondiabetic controls (Etzwiler & Sines, 1962; Steinhauser, Borner, & Koepp, 1977). In spite of this, a higher incidence of teacher-rated academic difficulties, ranging from motivational problems to specific learning skill deficiencies, has been reported (Etzwiler & Sines, 1962; Gath, Smith, & Baum, 1980). Additionally, many investigators have found personal and social adjustment to illness to be a potential problem for diabetic teenagers. In this context, adjustment is a broad descriptor of self-esteem, body image, and psychological health in the face of chronic illness. Kaufmann and Hersher (1971) reported significant alterations in body image in a small sample of hospitalized diabetic teenagers. These patients described incomplete, distorted, or "diseased" images of their internal anatomy, although they were all healthy in appearance. Sullivan (1979) also found body-image concerns and lower than average self-esteem among a portion of adolescent girls at a diabetes camp. Although the majority of the girls appeared to be well adjusted with a positive attitude toward their diabetes, Sullivan noted a significant minority with low self-esteem and depression as assessed by difficulties with peers and families, dependence–independence conflicts, school adjustment, and body-image concerns. Hauser, Pollets, and Turner (1979), in contrast, found slightly higher degrees of self-esteem, but lower levels of ego development, among diabetic adolescents when compared with controls.

In a much quoted study, Swift and Seidman (1967) found evidence of a high percentage of psychopathology and poor adjustment to their illness in 37.5 percent of 40 diabetic youths. Social and emotional adjustment and acceptance of diabetes were significantly related to control of diabetes. Psychosocial problems occurred more frequently among diabetics who were in poor metabolic control. Simonds (1977) found that diabetic teens in good control showed psychosocial adjustment equal to or better than nondiabetic controls, but poorly controlled diabetics displayed more anxiety, depression, behavior problems, and dependency conflicts. Additionally, Koski (1969) noted better differentiated ego boundaries and more imaginative and sensitive personalities in adolescent diabetics who were in good control. In contrast, poorly controlled diabetics showed less personality integration, more pathological ego boundaries, and greater aggressiveness. In a study of self-concept and acceptance of diabetes among a group of adolescents surveyed once in 1966 and again in 1975, Galatzer, Fritz, and Laron (1977) noted improved self-concept and better acceptance of diabetes over the interval. They noted, however, that over time the study subjects also had developed an increased (and realistic) anxiety over the possibility of diabetic complications.

Finally, a 1980 study by Kellerman, Zeltzer, and Ellenberg, found no significant differences in anxiety, self-esteem, and health locus of control between healthy controls and chronically ill adolescents, including those with IDDM. The authors speculated that high levels of control over health evidenced by diabetic teenagers are an accurate assessment of the role of the diabetic in his or her own disease management.

As can be noted in this small sampling of studies, the literature on psychosocial development of diabetic adolescents fails to delineate a discrete profile of developmental problems. While some adolescents cope well with their disease, others have problems, particularly in the areas of self-concept, anxiety, and depression. One common finding, however, is that adjustment to disease and self-concept seems to be correlated with relatively successful management of diabetes.

Finally, mention must be made of the relationship of emotional stress to diabetic control. Anecdotal reports of diabetic ketoacidosis precipitated by emotional upset, particularly in adolescent females, are common in the literature. Hinkle and Wolf (1952) demonstrated that life events perceived as stressful produced changes in urine, plasma glucose, and plasma ketones, and this response was accentuated in diabetics relative to controls. Chase and Jackson (1981) administered a stress checklist to diabetic children and adolescents and found a correlation between elevated stress scores and lower levels of biochemical diabetic control, particularly in older adolescents. Other empirical studies of life stress in diabetics seem to support the view that emotional stress plays a role in fluctuation of disease control (Hauser & Pollets, 1979). Though supportive research is necessary, a psychophysiological model of stress incorporating hormonal response, metabolic changes, and learned behavioral responses leading to diabetic decompensation, has been proposed (Tarnow & Silverman, 1981). If proved valid, such a model would at least partially explain the labile nature of IDDM in even the well-adjusted and previously well-controlled teenager who is experiencing the normal emotional vicissitudes of adolescence. Furthermore, such a construct might provide some clues to better understanding the relationship between family functioning and diabetic control.

The Family

Since treatment of diabetes in childhood and adolescence occurs primarily within the family context, it is important to understand family characteristics that influence good or poor control of diabetes. The diagnosis of any chronic and progressive illness in a child obviously has effects on that child's family. Paramount among the reactions experienced by the diabetic's family are fear of death of the affected child (Tietz & Vidmar, 1972), guilt related to the inheritable nature of the disease (Koski, 1969), and problems surrounding the changes in family routines necessitated by the regulated schedule of monitoring and treating diabetes. How the family copes with these issues is critical to success or failure in managing the child's disease. Family adjustment to diabetes has been shown to reflect previously established family behavior patterns and coping styles (Bruch, 1949).

Traditionally, the diabetic child's mother assumes a primary role in the management of the treatment regimen (Etzwiler & Sines, 1962). Thus, maternal attitudes and coping styles may influence both the control of the diabetes and the child's acceptance of the diabetes and its therapy. Using a questionnaire given to 76 mothers of insulin-dependent diabetic children and adolescents, Jochmus (1977) found that the majority (71 percent) displayed a child-rearing style that was either domineering and constricting or overprotective and indulgent. Twenty percent showed indifference, anxiety, or resentment, and only the remaining 9 percent displayed the optimal pattern of consistency and tolerance. Anderson and Auslander (1980) related the overcontrolling and perfectionistic maternal style to good disease control but disturbed personality development in the diabetic child. One might speculate that both the domineering and the overprotective parenting styles lay the groundwork for resentment and rebellion when the child reaches adolescence, with poor control of diabetes as the probable result. The indifferent and rejecting maternal styles are associated with poor control of diabetes as well as disturbed psychological functioning in the child and adolescent; conversely, the consistent yet flexible mothers would tend to have children with fair to good diabetic control and healthy personalities (Anderson and Auslander, 1980).

Diabetics in good metabolic control generally come from families with the following attributes:

1. Incorporation of the diabetic regimen into the family routine (Quint, 1970)
2. High family cohesion and less conflict (particularly marital) (Anderson, Miller, & Auslander, 1981)
3. Equal treatment of the diabetic child and his or her siblings (Anderson, et al., 1981)
4. Self-sufficiency and self-management encouraged and supported in the diabetic child (Anderson, et al. 1981)
5. Familial and financial stability over time (Koski, Ahlas, & Kumento 1976)

Children and parents from such families seem to accept the demands of diabetes; they generally attain successful management such that the disease becomes predictable (Simonds, 1977). Thus, the diabetic youth is usually more accepting of the disease, better adjusted, and better prepared to face the developmental tasks of adolescence.

In contrast, diabetics in poor control are more frequently from families with the following characteristics:

1. Coping styles based on recurring crises (Quint, 1970)
2. Lack of parental acceptance of the disease (Bruhn, 1974) and parental view of diabetes mellitus as having a pervasively negative impact on the child (Anderson, et al., 1981)
3. Family disintegration through death and divorce (Koski, et al., 1976)
4. More rigidity, enmeshment and intergenerational conflicts (Koski, et al., 1976; Minuchin, Baker, Rossman, Liekman, Milman, & Todd, 1975)
5. Poverty (Bruhn, 1974)
6. Attitudes of distrust, indifference, and differential treatment of the diabetic member (Anderson, et al., 1981)

The diabetic child in such a family has a much lower tendency to attain mastery over his or her condition. Diabetes may be seen as a source of conflict in an often chaotic family with poorly established patterns of conflict resolution. The illness is "bad" and its treatment may become a means to manipulate other family members, particularly during the adolescent's struggle for independence. Such an adolescent is much more likely to go on sprees of dietary indiscretion, to falsify urine tests, and "forget" to administer insulin. Alternatively, poor acceptance of the illness may contribute to social isolation in adolescence and withdrawal into the role of invalidism (Bruhn, 1974).

ISSUES IN THERAPY OF TEENAGE DIABETICS

Therapy for management of diabetes in adolescence should incorporate the goal of optimal metabolic control along with maximal healthy adolescent development.

As outlined by Bennett and Ward (1977), minimal goals for disease management include:

1. Freedom from symptoms, acidosis, and insulin-induced hypoglycemia
2. Normal serum lipids
3. Normal growth and pubertal development

The higher-order goal of prevention of microvascular complications through tighter control of blood glucose, (approaching normoglycemia), although not practical for all youths is applicable to selected highly motivated adolescents.

Also guiding any treatment plan are the following developmental goals appropriate to the adolescent patient:

1. Ongoing education of the adolescent and family regarding IDDM and its management
2. Responsibility for self-management of diabetes, closely tied to:
   Normal separation and individuation
   Normal school attendance and activity level, and appropriate vocational planning
3. Fostering of normal psychosocial and sexual identity in the emerging young adult with diabetes (Bennett & Ward, 1977)

Self-Care

Ideally, by the time a child reaches adolescence he or she will have assumed the primary responsibility for daily insulin injections and monitoring of control. Self-care can usually be accomplished in late childhood; intelligence, emotional maturity, ocular or other handicaps, motivation, and family dynamics are all factors to be considered in the timing of the transition from parental care.

The focus of the diabetic care team should shift from the adult care giver to the diabetic teenager. The adolescent should be encouraged to take over the jobs of appointment making, record keeping, and communication of progress or problems to the physician. Because of the documented evidence of widespread misinformation about diabetes and its treatment, even in patients with long duration of disease (Etzwiler & Sines, 1962; Johnson, Pollak, & Silverstein, 1982), it is essential that education regarding the nature of diabetes, complications, symptoms, injection and testing techniques, diet, and exercise is reviewed for the adolescent and family at this time and repeated as often as necessary.

Responsibility for self-care and successful management of diabetes can be a positive contribution to the adolescent's sense of mastery and control over his or her life. The family is encouraged to gradually relinquish responsibility for daily diabetic management while remaining supportive of the adolescent's efforts toward self-care. Anticipatory counseling by the health team is essential so that issues surrounding diabetic care do not become the focus of the normal parent–teen conflicts that occur in adolescence. Finally, as the adolescent nears adulthood, the transition from pediatrician to internist should be facilitated by the health care team to ensure continuity of care.

Insulin

Insulin requirements for prepubertal children are usually between 0.5 and 1.0 U/kg/day. Insulin requirements increase with puberty (often to approximately 1.5 U/kg/day) and then begin to decline and level off in adulthood. Total insulin doses of greater than 1.5 U/kg/day in an adolescent with poorly controlled symptoms or frequent ketoacidosis should prompt investigation to rule out either insulin-resistant states or the Somogyi phenomenon (over-insulinization leading to hypoglycemia followed by rebound hyperglycemia).

For acceptable control of blood glucose, most adolescents require two insulin shots every day, each consisting of a mixture of regular and intermediate-acting insulin, (*split-mixed* regimen). Split-mixed insulin therapy consists of one injection 30 minutes before breakfast, usually consisting of two thirds of the total daily insulin dose, in a ratio of NPH (or lente) to regular insulin of 2:1 or 3:1. The second injection, one half hour before the evening meal, consumes the remainder of the day's dose in a similar mix of intermediate-acting and regular insulin.

Adjustment of dose is made according to urine or blood test results and knowledge of peak action times of each type of insulin in order to maintain as normal a diurnal serum glucose pattern as possible, while avoiding hypoglycemia. Daily requirements will vary according to diet, activity, and illness. Highly motivated adolescents, with the supervision and support of the diabetic care team, may use self-monitoring of serum glucose and a multicomponent insulin regimen to obtain control approaching euglycemia (Skyler, Lasky, & Skyler, 1978).

With the adolescent growth spurt, changing insulin requirements should be anticipated. Poor control resulting from underinsulinization or the Somogyi phenomenon can significantly affect the rate and magnitude of pubertal growth. Jackson, Holland, Chatman, Guthrie, and Hewett (1978) demonstrated accelerated growth associated with improved diabetic control in youths previously in fair or poor control. These authors also stress the need to similarly anticipate decreased calorie and insulin requirements after maturation is complete, so as to avoid obesity, particularly in adolescent girls.

One of the few obvious physical stigmata of insulin therapy, potentially problematic for body-conscious adolescents, is lipodystrophy, or atrophy of subcutaneous fatty tissue at insulin injection sites. This problem can be avoided by regular rotation of the injection sites (anterior thighs, lateral upper arms, abdomen, and buttocks), and the use of purified pork insulin (Bacon et al., 1982).

Monitoring of Diabetic Control

Traditionally, outpatient self-assessment of diabetic control has consisted of urine testing for glucose and ketones. Minimal glucosuria is the goal and may be defined as an average glucose spill of 1 percent, obtained over the day's urine testing (before breakfast, lunch, dinner, and bedtime). Episodic elevations over 1–2 percent may result from erratic eating or activity patterns, infection, and emotional excitement or stress. These transient elevations are acceptable in the adolescent, for whom attempts at rigid control using urine testing result in frequent hypoglycemic episodes. Chronic elevations in urine glucose spill indicate inadequate disease control or impending ketoacidosis and mandate adjustment of insulin dose.

Difficulties for patients using urine testing include inconvenience, embarrassment, and the practical difficulty of repeatedly performing double-voided urine collections. More important, the renal threshold for glucose spill into the urine (approximately 160 mg/dl) is significantly higher than euglycemic diurnal variations in blood glucose. Thus, even consistently negative urine tests, which expose the patient to potential hypoglycemia, may not reflect adequate blood sugar control.

Recent advances in techniques for home self-monitoring of blood glucose helped to make optimal control of blood glucose an attainable goal (Skyler et al., 1978). Increasing numbers of insulin-dependent diabetics are being taught home glucose monitoring using finger pricks for capillary blood sampling, glucose-sensitive reagent strips, and reflectance meters for assessment of blood glucose concentration.*

Home glucose monitoring enables the diabetic to directly measure current control; assess the effects of diet, insulin, and exercise on blood sugar levels; and objectively evaluate symptoms of hypoglycemia. Because blood testing facilitates prevention of hyperglycemia and hypoglycemia to a degree unobtainable with urine testing, the American Diabetes Association (ADA) recently issued a policy statement in support of home glucose monitoring as the preferential means of assessing control for any insulin-dependent patient (ADA, 1982). Specifically, the ADA strongly encourages use of home glucose monitoring in certain groups of diabetic patients, including those with severe hypoglycemic reactions, those who

---

*Glucometer: Manufactured by Ames (Division of Miles Laboratories), P.O. Box 70, Elkhart, Indianapolis 46515

Accu-Chek-b.G.: Manufactured by Bio-Dynamics, 9115 Hague Road, Indianapolis 46250

are pregnant, those with unusually high or low renal glucose thresholds, and those with insulin-resistant states that make control difficult.

As outlined by Skyler and associates (1978), blood glucose monitoring may be used for continual, intermittent, or problem assessment of control. Continual assessment utilizes glucose testing before meals and at bedtime. Additional information for patients utilizing continual assessment can be obtained with the addition of postprandial blood tests to provide intermittent diurnal profiles. Alternatively, patients who prefer to utilize urine testing as their basic means of daily assessment can periodically obtain diurnal blood glucose profiles to compare and correlate urine test results with blood sugar control. Blood glucose tests for problem assessment can include nocturnal testing if hypoglycemia is suspected during sleep, or spot checks can be performed any time problem symptoms occur.

The use of home glucose monitoring requires a motivated patient who understands and accepts the goals of rigid diabetic control. Ongoing support and patient education regarding testing patterns and insulin adjustment are essential. The benefits of this intensive effort on the part of both patient and health provider, as measured by patient acceptance of home glucose monitoring, are better insight into daily patterns of blood sugar and facilitation of better diabetic control (Skyler et al., 1978).

In addition to increasing the accuracy of diabetic management, home glucose monitoring can provide several psychological benefits to the adolescent with IDDM. As better control is attained, a sense of predictability and mastery over the diabetic condition contributes positively to the teenager's realization of autonomy, self-esteem, and acceptance of a chronic illness. Dupuis (1980) noted increased self-reliance, reduced anxiety, and improvement in depression scores concomitant with improved diabetic control in a group of adolescents and young adults participating in a self-monitored blood glucose program. Better monitoring allows more flexibility in the treatment regimen to accommodate daily therapy to the often erratic life-style of the teenager. A large majority of adolescents studied by Sonksen, Judd, and Lowy (1980) felt that the advantages of home glucose monitoring (speed, accuracy, simplicity, and social acceptability) were well worth the disadvantage of daily finger pricks.

For chronic assessment of control, hemoglobin A_{Ic} (HbA_{Ic}) has proved to be a useful indicator for outpatient monitoring by the physician. The HbA_{Ic} results from glycosylation of normal hemoglobin and is elevated in diabetics (Koenig, Peterson, & Kylo, 1976). With prolonged hyperglycemia, the percentage of glycosylated hemoglobin rises and remains elevated for the life of the red cell. HbA_{Ic} can be measured, and thus provides an index of control over the preceding several months. HbA_{Ic} levels in nondiabetic persons average between 3 and 6 percent; elevations significantly above this level suggest inadequate diabetic control.

Medical follow-up of diabetic control should include routine surveillance for complications. Serum lipids should be monitored and the appropriate dietary modifications made for abnormal lipid elevations. Insulin injection sites need routine inspection for evidence of lipodystrophy. Regular dental care should be encouraged because of the higher than normal prevalence of periodontal disease in young people with IDDM (Cianciola, Park, & Brock, 1982).

Diabetic retinopathy is a leading cause of blindness in the United States. Although rarely noted before puberty, microaneurysms or proliferative changes develop in postpubertal insulin-dependent diabetics within 15 years unless a relatively high degree of disease control is maintained (Jackson, Ide, Guthrie, & James, 1982). Baseline ophthalmologic examination should be obtained at diagnosis, and adolescents should receive periodic follow-up evaluations.

The earliest signs of diabetic neuropathy are usually sensory abnormalities and decreased reflexes in the lower extremities. Routine screening should include specific questions about pain or numbness localization and symptoms of autonomic dysfunction. Adolescent males should be questioned about erectile function. Serial neurological exams are essential for detecting subtle deficits, particularly in vibration sense and ankle jerks.

While renal transplants are possible in individuals with end-stage diabetic nephropathy, kidney disease remains the most significant cause of mortality in diabetics with long-standing illness. Microvascular diabetic renal disease generally presents first with proteinuria, followed by hypertension and decreased renal function. Urinalysis and blood pressure measurement are thus routinely indicated during follow-up visits for the diabetic adolescent.

NUTRITION AND DIABETES MELLITUS

Although the importance of diet in the management of insulin-dependent diabetes mellitus is widely recognized, the composition of the diet as well as the type of dietary regimen (an uncontrolled or *free* diet versus a highly calculated or weighed diet) remains controversial. Dietary management plays a primary role in control of the blood glucose concentration and the prevention of hypoglycemia; however, whether dietary changes can significantly delay or prevent the long-term complications of diabetes is unconfirmed. Over the years, nutritional recommendations for individuals with diabetes mellitus have undergone several modifications. The current dietary recommendations from the Committee on Food and Nutrition of the American Diabetes Association for Insulin-Dependent

Diabetic Persons emphasize a decrease in the total fat and an increase in the complex carbohydrate content of the diet. Specifically, the recommendations include a protein intake of 12–20 percent of total energy intake, with carbohydrates accounting for 50–60 percent of total energy intake and fats comprising the difference. It was recommended that the level of saturated fats in the diet be decreased to less than ten percent of total calories; polyunsaturated fats should supply up to ten percent of the total calories and monosaturated fat should make up the rest of the fat intake (American Diabetes Association, 1979).

Since atherosclerotic disease has become the most common complication of diabetes, the recommended changes for fat were based on the premise that the atherosclerotic process is enhanced by a high saturated-fat diet. It is uncertain whether a reduction or restriction of dietary saturated fat and cholesterol will slow progression of atherosclerosis. The dietary fat recommendations are consistent with the recommendations of the American Heart Association for a prudent diet and should be incorporated into the diet of the entire family. In fact, the basic recommended dietary plan for insulin-dependent individuals, which is high in complex carbohydrates, low in sucrose and fat, and moderate in the use of salt, is one that is nutritionally adequate and health promoting for the entire family.

For insulin-dependent adolescent diabetics, the dietary recommendations and meal plans should be as flexible as possible. The life-style, preferences, and eating habits of the individual all need to be taken into consideration. A flexible meal plan may result in better patient acceptance and increased dietary compliance. The factors to be considered when planning diets for insulin-dependent individuals include (1) the timing of meals, (2) diet composition, (3) energy content of the diet, and (4) level of physical activity (American Diabetes Association, 1979). The timing of meals and daily consistency in amount and distribution of carbohydrates, protein, and fat are of vital importance in maintaining good metabolic management and should be a major goal in the dietary management plan. However, there can be flexibility in determining the distribution pattern of the diet.

Generally, both an afternoon and an evening snack are recommended for insulin-dependent teenagers. Snacks should be high in protein and complex carbohydrates. Both meals and snacks should be eaten on a regular schedule. Adolescents in general are notorious meal skippers, and they often have a penchant for snacking on foods that are high in sugar; therefore, special dietary counseling is needed when working with insulin-dependent youths. Because of occasional unavoidable delays in meals and snacks, teenagers need education and information so they can make wise decisions when in these situations. When meals are delayed for an hour, approximately 10–12 grams of carbohydrates are needed in the interim (Franz, 1981). Likewise, adolescent diabetics need counseling and education as to the effects of alcohol on blood sugar levels.

As was mentioned, current dietary recommendations for insulin-dependent diabetics advocate increased consumption of carbohydrates. High carbohydrate diets have been repeatedly found to improve oral glucose tolerance in insulin-dependent diabetics (Arky, Wylie- Rossett, & El-Beheri, 1982). Recently, there has also been emphasis on increasing the fiber content of the diet, as it has been reported to lower postprandial plasma glucose levels (American Diabetes Association, 1979). The American Diabetes Association recommends incorporating high-fiber foods into diabetic meal plans whenever acceptable to the patient. Adolescents should be encouraged to eat whole grain cereals and breads as well as to increase consumption of fibrous fruits, vegetables, and legumes. Admittedly, this is a difficult request to make of almost any teenager.

Most authorities advise restriction of refined sugar, as ingestion of concentrated simple carbohydrates aggravates hyperglycemia and causes wide fluctuations in the blood glucose (Arky et al., 1982; El-Beheri Burgess, 1982). Sucrose or table sugar is of primary concern. Some authorities recommend that children and teenagers with diabetes consume at least 60 percent of their carbohydrates in the form of breads, cereals, and potatoes, and 40 percent or less from the mixture of monosaccharides and disaccharides (lactose from dairy products and fructose from fruit) and severely limit the extent of consumption from sucrose sources (Drash, Becker, Henian, & Sterenchak, 1981).

Most insulin-dependent diabetic individuals are thin when first diagnosed; therefore, a diet high in energy to allow for catch-up weight is needed. A diet sufficient in energy for normal growth and development to occur should be a major goal when working with adolescent diabetics. If obesity occurs, appropriate caloric restriction is warranted.

One reason for failure to comply with dietary recommendations is an inadequate individualized educational and follow-up program. For adolescents, the follow-up and reevaluation of the diet are recommended every six months. The nutritionist needs to work closely with the diabetic adolescent to adequately teach the skills for managing his or her own nutritional care. Adolescents will need to learn the relationships between meals, activities, and insulin so as to adjust all three appropriately. Furthermore, the need to understand what foods are needed for normal weight and growth development, how to choose foods for activity and exercise, how to use snacks to prevent hypoglycemia, how to minimize the effects of alcohol when consumed, and how to use it appropriately (Franz, 1981).

Exercise

The interrelationships between diabetes and exercise have been recently reviewed (Skyler, 1979). Optimal physical fitness should be encouraged for all teenagers with IDDM. For cardiovascular health and diabetic control, regular daily exercise is recommended. Teenagers should be encouraged to participate in sports and other physical activities appropriate to their physical fitness and desire. Communication among the diabetic athelete, the coach, and the health care team will best facilitate this.

The adolescent should be familiar with the effects of exercise on reducing blood sugar and the consequent necessity of consuming extra food prior to physical exercise and carrying quickly utilized carbohydrates at all times to avoid hypoglycemia during activities. Exercise accelerates insulin mobilization when injections are made in the body part to be exercised; therefore, sites should be avoided when the limb is to be involved in physical activity (i.e., a leg should not be injected before running).

Additionally, it should be stressed to the adolescent that exercise alone is not sufficient to control hyperglycemia; in fact, insulin-antagonistic, counter-regulatory hormones induced by exercise in an insulin-deficient state will worsen impending ketoacidosis (Skyler, 1979).

Sexuality, Contraception, and Pregnancy

Sexuality and sexual activity among adolescents is a fact of life, regardless of diabetes. It has been estimated that in the United States nearly half of adolescent males and one third of adolescent females are sexually active by the age of 15–17 (Alan Guttmacher Institute, 1981). Thus, anticipatory counseling regarding the relationship between diabetes and sexuality—including sexual function, contraception, and pregnancy—is part of the total care of the adolescent with diabetes. These issues should be discussed openly and objectively with the adolescent, with due consideration given to the patient's level of cognitive development and sense of modesty. Teenaged males may harbor a fear of impotency related to their condition. It should be emphasized that in most instances, diabetes in good control does not alter sexual libido or function; however, the relationship between long-term poorly controlled IDDM and impotence should be discussed.

Routine aspects of self-management of IDDM should be incorporated into dating activities, as required. Teenagers of both sexes should be encouraged not to conceal their diabetes from friends or dating partners; rather, it should be stressed that open communication is essential for developing mature relationships. Group discussions among diabetic adolescents or the use of peer counselors may ease anxiety and help the adolescent to solve problems related to dating and being diabetic. The more open the diabetic can be with others about the condition, the less likely it is that he or she will use the illness manipulatively.

Prepregnancy counseling should be offered to diabetic females before marriage or childbearing plans are established. The importance of good diabetic control in the early weeks of gestation, prior to the first missed period, and its effect on pregnancy outcome should be explained.

Contraception should be offered to the sexually active adolescent, but, because of the reported higher incidence of pill-related complications in women with IDDM (Steel & Duncan, 1978), oral contraceptives should be prescribed judiciously and monitored closely. The relation of estrogen-containing oral contraception to serum lipids and the risk of cardiovascular and thromboembolic disease in women with IDDM is still in question. A higher than average failure rate has been reported in diabetic women using IUDs (Steel & Duncan, 1980). This, combined with the increased risk of pelvic infections with this device, make the IUD inappropriate for most adolescents with IDDM. These authors recommend progesten-only minipills or barrier methods as the appropriate initial contraceptive for young diabetic women. Others advocate the more fool-proof low-dose combination pill because of the medical consequences were a diabetic teenager to unwittingly become pregnant. For women who have completed their families or have serious diabetic complications (e.g., renal failure) that make the risk of pregnancy unacceptable, voluntary sterilization should be considered.

A discussion of the management of pregnancy in women with IDDM is beyond the scope of this chapter. Mintz, Skyler, and Chez (1978) have noted, however, that improved monitoring and intensive insulin therapy have significantly improved pregnancy outcome and decreased the incidence of complications. The care of the pregnant diabetic should be a cooperative effort between diabetologist and obstetrician. Delivery should take place at a high-risk center with personnel who are experienced in perinatal management of mother and infant.

Alcohol, Smoking, and Drug Use

Experimentation and risk-taking behavior in adolescence often includes the use of potentially harmful substances. Cigarette smoking, a risk factor in cardiovascular disease, is of course to be discouraged in all teenagers but even more so in those with IDDM.

Large amounts of alcohol, particularly if unaccompanied by food, may precipitate hypoglycemia in IDDM. Additionally, impaired judgment secondary to excess alcohol consumption may complicate recognition and treatment of problems. Although excessive use of alcohol is contraindicated in IDDM, a rigid ban on alcohol usually is not realistic for diabetic adolescents and young adults. An open discussion on the impact of alcohol consumption should be incorporated into the nutritional instruction provided for diabetics (McDonald, 1980).

Abuse of alcohol or street drugs by teenagers should prompt investigation into other areas of functioning, especially those involving school, peers, and family. A search should be made for underlying depression; referral for chemical use counseling, family therapy, or individual psychotherapy may be indicated.

Employment

Adolescents and young adults with IDDM may face prejudice in the marketplace. Fear or ignorance of diabetes on the part of potential employers may cause them to regard even well-controlled diabetics as bad risks for performing and keeping a job. In a study of employment experience of young adults with IDDM (Kantrow, 1961), over 50 percent of those surveyed reported job rejection on the basis of their medical condition. Of these, nearly one half subsequently denied their illness in order to gain employment.

The adolescent who is looking for work should be encouraged to be truthful about his or her diabetes but may justifiably benefit from advocacy on the part of the physician or other health provider. Prospective employers can be informed of current advances in therapy and assured that the well-controlled diabetic can maintain normal job attendance and performance.

The Brittle Diabetic Teenager

The term "brittle diabetic" generally is used to refer to a patient whose disease is very difficult to control, with wide and rapid fluctuations in blood glucose between hyperglycemia and hypoglycemia and frequent episodes of ketoacidosis and hospitalization.

Although some adolescents have very labile blood sugar control due to physical causes (e.g., insulin antibodies or Somogyi phenomenon) or treatment errors (e.g., incorrect measuring of insulin or poor understanding of IDDM and its therapy), the majority of brittle teenaged diabetics can attribute their unstable control to emotional or psychosocial factors (Greydanus & Hoffmann, 1979). As noted earlier, family acceptance of a chronic disease, family economic and social resources, and family communication patterns may all affect the child's acceptance and subsequent management of diabetes. Maladaptive coping styles in youths with poor acceptance of their condition include such characteristics as extreme denial, frustration and rejection, rebellion, depression, and self-destructive behavior (Simonds, 1979). When combined with the dependence–independence conflict of normal adolescence, this lack of acceptance may be acted out via noncompliance with the therapeutic regimen, including dietary indiscretion, "forgetting" to take insulin, or falsifying urine or blood sugar tests.

Alternatively, the brittle adolescent diabetic may be deliberately manipulating his or her condition as a way out of an intolerable situation (Rosen & Lidz, 1949). The hospital ward may be viewed as preferable to school problems, family turmoil, or conflict with peers.

Treatment of the brittle diabetic should be directed at improving the adolescent's acceptance and sense of mastery over the condition. Diabetes education review and instruction in home glucose monitoring improve knowledge and acceptability of diabetes. Peer experiences, such as diabetic rap groups (Warren-Boulton, Anderson, Swartz, & Drexler, 1981) or summer camps for diabetics, can provide the opportunity for learning, socializing, and peer support. The teenager's knowledge of diabetic management should be incorporated into a flexible treatment plan, and goals for therapy should realistically reflect developmental stage and life situation.

If the hospital is viewed as a refuge from problems at home, hospitalization for diabetic control should be avoided whenever possible. When hospitalization is necessary, prompt discharge after problem resolution, restriction of hospital visitors and activities, and inpatient family counseling may help break the cycle of repeated hospitalization (Parker, Gunder-Hunt, & Spencer, 1980). Minuchin, Baker, and Rossman (1975) have demonstrated significant reduction in hospital admissions of brittle diabetics when dysfunctional family-relating styles are modified by family therapy.

Continuity of care, patience, a multidisciplinary approach, and attention to the adolescent as an individual often suffice to support the brittle teenaged diabetic and his or her family through the years of adolescence (Tattersall & Lowe, 1981). Occasionally, further psychiatric or social service measures are needed, and in such instances referral should be made promptly.

CONCLUSION

Since the discovery of insulin in 1922, significant strides have been made in the treatment of diabetes mellitus. Current knowledge and technology facilitate the goal of better glucose control and provide new approaches to achievement of that goal. Future studies involving diabetics with tight control are necessary to confirm the hypothesized role of rigid diabetic control in the prevention of complications. Unless such research refutes the hypothesis, the goal of optimal control of blood glucose will remain the cornerstone of prudent medical therapy (Kaplan, 1982). Current and future investigative approaches to achieving this goal include safe and practical techniques of continuous insulin infusion for outpatient use (Santiago, Clemens, Clarke, & Kipnis, 1979; Skyler, Seigler, & Reeves, 1982), and the synthesis of human insulin by recombinant DNA techniques (Hansen, Lernmark, Nielsen, Owerback, & Welinder, B., 1982; Henehan, 1983). Such efforts toward improving treatment of diabetes are essential until either prevention of diabetes or a definitive cure (e.g., islet-cell transplantation) becomes a reality.

For health professionals who care for adolescents with IDDM, the challenge is one of combining the best of modern clinical knowledge and technique with the developmental needs of the teenager. The result, when this challenge is successfully met, is an independent young adult with a healthy personality, who competently handles the day to day demands of a chronic disease.

ACKNOWLEDGMENT

The section on Nutrition and Diabetes Mellitus was written by Mary Story, R.D., Ph.D.

REFERENCES

Alan Guttmacher Institute. *Teenage pregnancy: The problem that hasn't gone away.* New York: Alan Guttmacher Institute, 1981.

American Diabetes Association. Principles of nutrition and dietary recommendations for individuals with diabetes mellitus. *Diabetes Care,* 1979, *2* (6), 520–523.

American Diabetes Association. Indications for use of continuous insulin delivery systems and self-measurement of blood glucose. *Diabetes Care,* 1982, *5* (2), 140–141.

Anderson, B.J., & Auslander, W. Research on diabetes management and the family: A critique. *Diabetes Care,* 1980, *3,* 696–702.

Anderson, B.J., Miller, J.P., Auslander, W.F., & Santiago, J.V. Family characteristics of diabetic adolescents: Relationship to metabolic control. *Diabetes Care,* 1981, *4* (6), 586–594.

Arky, R., Wylie-Rossett, L., & El-Beheri, B. Examination of current dietary recommendations for individuals with diabetes mellitus. *Diabetes Care,* 1982, *5* (1), 59.

Bennett, D.L., & Ward, M.S. Diabetes mellitus in adolescents: A comprehensive approach to outpatient care. *Southern Medical Journal,* 1977, *70* (6), 705–708.

Bruch, H. Physiological and psychological interrelationships in diabetes in children. *Psychosomatic Medicine,* 1949, *11,* 200–210.

Bruhn, J.G. Psychosocial influences in diabetes mellitus. *Postgraduate Medicine*, 1974, *56* (2), 113–118.

Chase, H.P., & Jackson, G.C. Stress and sugar control in children with insulin-dependent diabetes mellitus. *Journal of Pediatrics*, 1981, *98* (6), 1011–1013.

Cianciola, L.J., Park, B.H., Bruck, E., et al. Prevalence of periodontal disease in insulin-dependent diabetes mellitus. *Journal of the American Dental Association*, 1982, *104*, 653–660.

Drash, A. Diabetes mellitus in childhood: A review. *Journal of Pediatrics*, 1971, *78* (6), 919–941.

Drash, A.L., Becker, D.J., Henien, A.G., & Steranchak, J. Nutritional considerations in the treatment of the child with diabetes mellitus. In R.M. Suskind (Ed.), *Textbook of pediatric nutrition*. New York: Raven Press, 1981.

Dupuis, A. Assessment of the psychological factors and responses in self-managed patients. *Diabetes Care*, 1980, *3* (1), 117–120.

El-Beheri Burgess, B. Rationale for changes in the dietary management of diabetes. *Journal of the American Dietetic Association*, 1982, *81* (3), 258.

Etzwiler, D.D., & Sines, L.K. Juvenile diabetes and its management: Family social and academic implications. *Journal of the American Dental Association*, 1962, *181* (4), 304–309.

Franz, M. The dietitian: A key member of the diabetes team. *Journal of the American Dietetic Association*, 1981, *79* (3), 302.

Frish, M., Galatzer, A., & Laron, Z. Child–parent attitudes toward diabetes. In Z. Laron (Ed.), *Pediatric and adolescent endocrinology*, Vol. 3. Basil, Switzerland: S. Karger, 1977, 55–58.

Galat er, A., Frish, M., & Laron, Z. Changes in self-concept and feelings toward diabetes in a group of juvenile diabetic adolescents; Psychological aspects of balance of diabetes in juveniles. In Z. Laron (Ed.), *Pediatric and adolescent endocrinology*, Vol. 3. Basil, Switzerland: S. Karger, 1977, 17–21.

Gath, A., Smith, M.A., & Baum, J.D. Emotional, behavioral, and educational disorders in diabetic children. *Archives of Diseases in Childhood*, 1980, *55*, 371–75.

Gil, R., Frish, M., Amir, S., & Galatzer, A. Awareness of complications among juvenile diabetics and their parents. In Psychological aspects of balance of diabetes in juveniles. In Z. Laron (Ed.), *Pediatric and adolescent endocrinology*, Vol. 3. Basil, Switzerland: S. Karger, 1977, 59–63.

Greydanus, D.E., & Hoffmann, A.D. Psychological factors in diabetes mellitus—A review of the literature with emphasis on adolescence. *American Journal of Diseases in Children*, 1979, *133*, 1061–1066.

Hansen, B., Lernmark, A., Nielsen, J.H., Owerbach, D., & Welinder, B. New Approaches to therapy and diagnosis of diabetes. *Diabetologia*, 1982, *22*, 61–62.

Hauser, S.T., & Pollets, D. Psychological aspects of diabetes mellitus: A critical review. *Diabetes Care*, 1979, *2* (2), 227–232.

Hauser, S., Pollets, D., Turner, B., et al. Ego development and self-esteem in diabetic adolescents. *Diabetes Care*, 1979, *2*, 465–471.

Henehan, J. More studies show human insulin's benefit. *Journal of the American Dental Association*, 1983, *249* (3), 328.

Hinkle, L., & Wolf, S. Importance of life stress in the course and management of diabetes mellitus. *Journal of the American Dental Association*, 1952, *148*, 513–520.

Hoffmann, A.D. The impact of illness in adolescence and coping behavior. *Acta Paediatrica Scandinavica*, 1975, Suppl. 256, 29–33.

Jackson, R.L., Holland, E., Chatman, I.D., Guthrie, D., & Hewett, J.E. Growth and maturation of children with insulin-dependent diabetes mellitus. *Diabetes Care*, 1978, *1* (2), 96–107.

Jackson, R.L., Ide, C.H., Guthrie, R.A., & James, R.D. Retinopathy in adolescent and young adults with onset of insulin-dependent diabetes in childhood. *Ophthalmology,* 1982, *89* (1), 7–13.

Jochmus, I. The influence of maternal patterns of child-rearing upon diabetic children and adolescents; Psychological aspects of balance of diabetes in juveniles. In Z. Laron (Ed.), *Pediatric and adolescent endocrinology,* Vol. 3. Basil, Switzerland: S. Karger, 1977, 52–54.

Johnson, S.B., Pollak, T., Silverstein, J.H., et al. Cognitive and behavioral knowledge about insulin-dependent diabetes among children and parents. *Pediatrics,* 1982, *69* (6), 708–713.

Kantrow, A.H. Employment Experiences of juvenile diabetics. *Diabetes,* 1961, *10* (6), 476–481.

Kaplan, S.A. (Moderator). UCLA conference—Diabetes mellitus. *Annals of Internal Medicine,* 1982, *96,* 635–649.

Kaufman, R.V., & Hersher, B. Body image changes in teen-age diabetics. *Pediatrics,* 1971, *48* (1), 123–128.

Kellerman, J., Zeltzer, L., Ellenberg, L., et al. Psychological effects of illness in adolescence. I. Anxiety, self-esteem and perception of control. *Journal of Pediatrics,* 1980, *97* (1), 126–131.

Koenig, R.J., Peterson, C.M., Kilo, C., et al. HgA$_{1c}$ as an indicator of the degree of glucose tolerance in diabetes. *Diabetes,* 1976, *25,* 230–232.

Konopka, G. Requirements for healthy development of adolescent youth. *Adolescence,* 1973, *8* (31), 1–26.

Koski, M.L. The coping process in childhood diabetes. *Acta Paediatrica Scandinavica,* 1969, Suppl., 198, 1–56.

Koski, M.L., Ahlas, A., & Kumento, A. A psychosomatic follow-up study of childhood diabetics. *Acta Paedopsychiatrica* (Basel), 1976, *42,* 12–26.

Laron, A., Volovitz, B., & Karp, M. Linear growth and insulin dose as indices of control in children with diabetes mellitus; Medical aspects of blance of diabetes in juveniles. In Z. Laron (Ed.), *Pediatric and adolescent endocrinology,* Vol. 2. Basil, Switzerland: S. Karger, 1977, 60–69.

McDonald, J. Alcohol and diabetes. *Diabetes Care,* 1980, *3* (5), 629–637.

Mintz, D.H., Skyler, J.S., & Chez, R.A. Diabetes mellitus and pregnancy. *Diabetes Care,* 1978, *1* (1), 49–63.

Minuchin, S., Baker, L., Rossman, B., Liekman, R., Milman, L., & Todd, T. A conceptual model of psychosomatic illness in children. *Archives of General Psychiatry,* 1975, *32,* 1031–1038.

Parker, L., Gunter-Hunt, G., & Spencer, M. Reducing diabetic ketoacidosis hospitalization. *Diabetes,* 1980, *29,* Suppl. 2, (106), 27a.

Quint, J.C. The developing diabetic identity: A study of family influence. In M.V. Batey (Ed.), *Communicating nursing research,* Vol. 3. Boulder: Western Interstate Commission of Higher Education, 1970, 14–32.

Rosen, H., & Lidz, T. Emotional factors in the precipitation of recurrent diabetic acidosis. *Psychosomatic Medicine,* 1949, *11* (4), 211–15.

Santiago, J.V., Clemens, A.H., Clarke, W.L., & Kipnis, D.M. Closed-loop and open-loop devices for blood glucose control in normal and diabetic subjects. *Diabetes,* 1979, *28* (1), 71–81.

Simonds, J.F. Psychiatric status of diabetic youth matched with a control group. *Diabetes,* 1977, *26,* 921–925.

Simonds, J.F. Emotions and compliance in diabetic children. *Psychosomatics,* 1979, *20* (8), 544–551.

Skyler, J.S. Diabetes and exercise: Clinical implications. *Diabetes Care,* 1979, *2* (3), 307–311.

Skyler, J.S., Lasky, I.A., Skyler, D., et al. Home blood glucose monitoring as an aid in diabetes management. *Diabetes Care*, 1978, *1* (3), 150–151.

Skyler, J.S., Seigler, D.E., & Reeves, M.L. Optimizing pumped insulin delivery. *Diabetes Care*, 1982, *5* (2), 135–139.

Sonksen, P.H., Judd, S., & Lowy, C. Home monitoring of blood glucose: New approach to management of insulin-dependent diabetic patients in Great Britain. *Diabetes Care*, 1980, *3* (1), 100–107.

Steel, J.M., & Duncan, J.J.P. Serious complications of oral contraception in insulin-dependent diabetics. *Contraception*, 1978, *17* (4), 291–295.

Steel, J.M., & Duncan, L.J.P. Contraception for the insulin-dependent diabetic woman: The view from one clinic. *Diabetes Care*, 1980, *3* (4), 557–560.

Steinhauser, H.C., Borner, S., & Koepp, P. Personality of juvenile diabetics. In Psychological aspects of balance of diabetes in juveniles. In A. Laron (Ed.), *Pediatric and adolescent endocrinology*, Vol. 3. Basil, Switzerland: S. Karger, 1977, 1–7.

Sullivan, B.J. Adjustment in diabetic adolescent girls: I. Development of the diabetic adjustment scale. II. Adjustment, self-esteem, and depression in diabetic adolescent girls. *Psychosomatic Medicine*, 1979, *41* (2), 119–138.

Swift, C.R., & Seidman, F.L. Adjustment problems of juvenile diabetes. *Psychosomatic Medicine*, 1967, *29*, 555–571.

Tarnow, J.D., & Silverman, S.W. The psychophysiologic aspects of stress in juvenile diabetes mellitus. *International Journal of Psychiatry in Medicine*, 1981, *11* (1), 25–44.

Tattersall, R.B., & Lowe, J. Diabetes in adolescence. *Diabetologia*, 1981, *20*, 517–523.

Tietz, W., & Vidmar, J.T. The impact of coping styles on the control of juvenile diabetes. *Psychiatry in Medicine*, 1972, *3*, 67–74.

Warren-Boulton, E., Anderson, B.J., Swartz, N.L., & Drexler, A.J. A group approach to the management of diabetes in adolescents and young adults. *Diabetes Care*, 1981, *4*, 620–623.

Barbara J. Leonard

14

The Adolescent with Epilepsy

Epilepsy is a term that is applied to a group of central nervous system disorders that result from recurring abnormal electrical discharges of nerve cells in the brain. A seizure is the result of an abnormal discharge of electrical energy by the brain. This can be focal—limited to a small part of the brain—or generalized, involving larger segments or even the entire brain.

CHARACTERISTICS OF EPILEPSY

Epilepsy is a prevalent neurological disorder occurring in approximately 4 million Americans. It is estimated that from one to one and one half percent of the population is affected with a seizure disorder; the incidence is highest in the first year of life and after the age of 55 (Gumnit, 1981).

Onset and Causes

While epilepsy may begin at any age, etiology varies with age at which onset occurs. Perinatal hypoxia or trauma, congenital malformations, infections, and metabolic disorders account for the majority of the seizure disorders when epilepsy begins in infancy. If it begins in childhood or adolescence, it is the idiopathic type of seizure diathesis that is first observed. Fever and central nervous system infections can also be causative

CHRONIC ILLNESS AND DISABILITIES IN CHILDHOOD AND ADOLESCENCE ISBN 0-8089-1635-1

agents, as can head injury, lead toxicity, and drug use. Adult-onset epilepsy can be the result of head injury, brain tumors, and vascular diseases.

Epilepsy is a complex, multifaceted disorder that can result from numerous underlying causes. Generalized seizures may result from inborn errors of metabolism or from any disease that affects the entire brain, including electrolyte disturbances and infection or inflammation of the brain, its linings, or blood vessels; poisons or drug reactions must be ruled out as well, as should degenerative disorders of the nervous system, tumors, allergic and immune reactions following viral infections, and immunizations.

Focal seizures are usually the result of disease caused by irritation or scars of a specific part of the brain. Possible causes of focal seizures include blood vessel abnormalities, masses, malformations, and trauma. The idiopathic focal seizure is associated with a familial tendency; in families with one member with the disorder, there is about a three and one half percent chance of seizures occurring in another near relative (Chabria & Shope, 1982). Whether this increased familial incidence is due to an inheritable predisposition is not known. The concordance rate of epilepsy in monozygotic twins is 20 times higher than the rate of epilepsy in dizygotic twins (Scott, 1977).

Prognosis

Approximately 60 percent of epileptic individuals will become seizure free with treatment. An additional 25 percent can achieve sufficient control to live functional lives. In the remaining 15 percent, no consistent relief of symptoms can be achieved. For those individuals, larger doses of the anticonvulsant will be ineffective in controlling the seizures and will complicate their lives. They are less likely to be able to carry on normal activities because of the interference of attacks and side effects of the anticonvulsants (Gordon, 1982).

ISSUES FOR THE ADOLESCENT WITH EPILEPSY

Developmental Issues

The adolescent in our society is faced with four major developmental tasks. The consolidation of identity is foremost and forms the basis for achieving independence from parents. In addition to gaining emotional independence from parents, the adolescent must establish new love objects outside the family and achieve economic independence. While many factors affect the rate of accomplishing these tasks, the first three (all but economic independence) take roughly six years (Strax, 1976). Duvall stresses that the adolescent must come to an acceptance of his body and the changes of sexual development. A satisfying masculine or feminine social role is also necessary to develop. The adolescent must form mature relationships with peers and achieve emotional independence from parents. The need to select a career requires the adolescent to develop the necessary cognitive and social skills to be successful in the work place. When the adolescent is able to achieve the tasks of adolescence they become the foundation for adjustment as an adult.

The adolescent with epilepsy is, first of all, an adolescent, and has the same developmental task requirements as all youths. Epilepsy can add considerable stress to the already complicated issues faced by adolescents. The psychological and behavioral disturbances correlated with epilepsy are primarily the result of problems in the home, the school, or the peer group. That is, most adolescents with epilepsy will develop normally if given the chance (Hartlage, Green, & Offutt, 1972). Unfortunately, the adolescent with epilepsy often lacks a normal social milieu in which to make adaptations requisite to completing developmental tasks.

Psychological Issues

Rutter, Graham, and Yule (1970) found that the percentage of psychiatric disorders among the general population of children and adolescents was 6.6 percent. For individuals with nonneurological chronic disease, the rate was 11.6 percent. Blind children had a rate of 16.6 percent, and children and adolescents with epilepsy associated with organic brain disease had a rate of 58.3 percent. Those with organic brain diseases, uncomplicated by seizures, had a rate of 37.5 percent, and those with epilepsy and no other pathology had a rate of 28.6 percent. The authors concluded that children and adolescents with chronic physical disorders involving the brain show a marked increase in psychiatric disability. The presence of this disability could not be accounted for by age or sex differences, visibility of the handicap, or lower intelligence. Neither was any significant association found between the severity of the handicap imposed by the epilepsy and the likelihood of psychiatric disorder. The authors assert that the most important feature in relation to the much higher rate of psychiatric disorders in epileptic children is the presence of neurological dysfunction.

Learning Problems

The association between learning or school problems and the presence of epilepsy has been supported in carefully conducted studies over the past two decades (Rutter, Tizare, & Whitmore, 1970; Green & Hartlage,

1970; Holdsworth & Whitmore, 1974; Stores, 1978). These studies conclude that many adolescents have learning disabilities superimposed on their epilepsy, and this complicates their problems in academic achievement. For some individuals, the learning deficit is more responsible for school failure than is the epilepsy itself. Rutter, Tizard, and Whitmore (1970) state that 18 percent of epileptic children over eight years of age are retarded in reading by at least two years, irrespective of level of intelligence. Hartlage and Green (1972) reported similar findings. Holdsworth and Whitmore's findings (1974) suggest that only one third of the 85 children with epilepsy in their sample achieved satisfactory progress according to their teachers. These children were in regular classrooms. One in six was falling behind in work, and one in five presented a behavior problem in the classroom. The frequency of their seizures and their occurrence during the previous 12 months or in school had no bearing on educational outcome. In addition, the authors report that all of those with behavior problems were educationally delayed, while one quarter of the educationally retarded had behavior problems.

Stores (1978) found that there were striking differences in inattentiveness between epileptic and nonepileptic children and preadolescents. Epileptic boys were generally adversely affected, and were rated by teachers or parents as more inattentive, overactive, and having significantly poorer performance on tests of both sustained attention and accuracy of visual scanning than epileptic girls. Stores concluded that epileptic boys are behaviorally more vulnerable than epileptic girls; however, this finding may parallel the general population. Except for the association between the presence of a persistent left temporal lobe spike discharge and retardation or disturbed behavior, Stores found no explanation for the inattentiveness attributable to drug effects, type of epilepsy, or EEG abnormalities.

Although research on the subject of school performance is relatively sparse, it is quite convincing that children and adolescents with epilepsy have academic and behavioral problems in the school setting. They are a group with significant learning disabilities. A multifaceted explanation for their problems is only reasonable.

Factors Associated With Poor School Progress

Stores (1976) views drug therapy, the disease itself, seizure control, and attitudinal factors as more relevant explanations for both behavioral and academic school problems than poor attendance. Two general factors are important in drug therapy: overdosage with antiepileptic drugs can result in an increase in seizure frequency as well as a range of psychiatric disorders; and phenobarbital and related drugs at or above therapeutic levels can be responsible for restlessness, irritability, mental slowing, and depression in many children.

The locus of epileptic activity in the brain can result in specific learning problems. For example, if electrical discharges are in the speech area of the brain, the individual will have difficulty with expressive language and verbal ability. However, more common than these specific limitations are defects of attention that appear to be associated with bursts of generalized abnormal activity recorded on the EEG, rather than from one particular area. The clinical or behavioral effects of this activity can be subtle, and the altered consciousness is not infrequently misinterpreted as daydreaming or mannerisms. Though there may be no perceptible change in behavior, the individual's consciousness is impaired; thus he or she may register incoming information imperfectly or not at all. The term "subclinical seizure discharge" describes these more insidious behavioral effects of seizure activity.

In addition to the subtle form of seizure, generalized activity may continue without interruption for extended periods of time, producing the condition known as *minor epileptic status*. Stores (1976) describes the clinical picture of this condition as one of perplexity, subnormality, even psychosis. Both focal and generalized epileptic activity can be very sensitive to emotional and attentional factors; seizures of all kinds can be precipitated by boredom or stress in the classroom or even by particular subjects at school.

While psychological explanations are critical components of the cause and treatment of learning disabilities associated with epilepsy in children and adolescents, attitudinal issues also contribute to this complex picture. Responsible adults, such as parents and teachers, can be overly concerned and protective toward the individual. The effect of their behavior on adolescents with epilepsy may well dampen developing initiative and independence. In addition, peer problems can play a significant role in adjustment and academic progress (Strax, 1976). Acceptance by peers, so essential to the development of self-esteem in the normal adolescent, is no less important to the individual with epilepsy.

Family Issues

Just as adolescents must resolve individual developmental tasks, so do families with adolescents have developmental tasks that require resolution. The family is expected to accommodate its patterns of interaction and behavior to permit healthy adjustment of all family members (Minuchin, 1975). The tasks specific to the family with adolescents include provision of suitable housing to accommodate widely different needs within the family, provision for ever-changing financial demands, division of responsibilities for family living, preservation of the marital relationship, communication between the generations, expansion of the teenager's as well as the parents' horizons, and maintenance of ethical and moral perspectives meaningful to the family members (Duvall, 1977). Parents must provide a secure home for individuals who are in the process of emancipating themselves from the family both emotionally and financially.

These difficult tasks may be even more complex and challenging for families with adolescents with special needs. No matter how functional, families confront barriers in the larger society that complicate the task of emancipation. Limitations in educational and vocational opportunities pose significant barriers for adolescents with epilepsy and, thus, for their families. Negative social attitudes further compound the problems of normal living.

The family is a matrix within which the adolescent forms an identity and acquires self-confidence and basic values. This foundation is tested in the peer group during adolescence. While a successful childhood does not guarantee a successful adolescence, the converse makes adolescence extremely difficult, especially if the diagnosis of seizures has been made in childhood. Pless (1975) emphasizes the relationship between early onset of disease and the presence of secondary psychological and academic problems.

Families initially react to the diagnosis of chronic illness with shock and disbelief (Hill, 1965). For most families, the acceptance of the child's problems will result in quality parent–child relationships. However, for some, the disappointment and grief associated with the diagnosis will psychologically cripple the child. Healthy parental behavior will greatly aid the adolescent in coming to terms with the illness and its developmental implications (Strax, 1976). Two examples highlight the difference:

> An adolescent girl with psychomotor seizures of early onset achieved competitive status as a diver. As an early adolescent, she regularly traveled with her team. Responsible for her anticonvulsant therapy, she was never known to be noncompliant. Her parents treated her as a capable, normal adolescent with a controllable problem. In contrast, another girl with the same diagnosis was alternately overprotected and treated permissively by her mother. She rebelled by using street drugs, which compounded her seizure disorder and subsequently resulted in school failure and addiction.

As Gliedman and Roth (1980) point out, every parent comes to the experience of raising a child or adolescent with the disability of being a novice. Unless the family has had prior experience with handicapped people, they are unprepared to parent the individual with special needs. In addition to acquisition of knowledge about the disease, its etiology, and treatment, parents of adolescents with epilepsy must develop positive, accepting attitudes toward their children. For some, the latter is a most difficult task (Bryant, 1971). Parental styles have been categorized by some as overprotective, overpermissive, and salutary.

PARENTING STYLES

Overprotection

Overprotection of the adolescent by parents tends to be the result of parental fear that the adolescent will come to harm if allowed to pursue the activities that are developmentally appropriate. This protective stance is manifested by prohibiting the teenager from managing his or her own anticonvulsant therapy or by not allowing socialization with peers. Even with good seizure control, such families will not allow the adolescent to obtain a driver's license. The list is endless. The parents' anxiety or fear for the adolescent's safety interferes directly with his or her ability to achieve emancipation. An overprotected adolescent tends to become angry and resentful at not being allowed the freedom and opportunity afforded peers. This may result in rebellion against parents for the restrictions, in turn creating new problems. Richardson and Friedman (1974) found the presence of significant psychosocial problems in 13 of 17 families they interviewed. Parents were overprotective, and the adolescents were resistant and rebellious in their response to it. Hostility, alienation, and depression are all too common adolescent emotional responses to such an environment.

An adolescent who has been overprotected because of epilepsy since childhood will have missed many opportunities to develop normal peer relationships and self-confidence as a child. In other words, the tasks required of the child during latency may be poorly accomplished, thus increasing the stresses of adolescence. The isolated individual is at high risk for withdrawal and depression resulting in both self-hatred and greater dependency on parents and family. Feelings of personal and social inadequacy and a sense of estrangement may predominate. Probably the most insidious response to overprotectiveness is that the individual will identify with the parents' overprotectiveness and become obsessed with personal vulnerability. This, in turn, engenders chronic anxiety and insecurity and ensures limited aspirations or goals for self-development.

Overpermissiveness

An equally problematic parental style is that of overpermissiveness. The parents may feel responsible for "causing" the child's seizures, and as means of compensation, they place few demands or boundaries on behavior. The impact of overpermissiveness fosters both short- and long-range problems. When adolescents prematurely assume responsibility for themselves and perhaps for their parents as well, they tend to be overwhelmed with a sense of insecurity. Such individuals are often manipulative and demanding and are not infrequently in conflict with authority figures. An adolescent's response to parental anger and embarrassment may take the form of guilt for causing their grief. Because of dependence on the parent, the adolescent directs the resultant anger toward himself or herself, peers, siblings, or other adults such as teachers. A common reaction to this parent–child conflict is the adolescent's denial of the disease and noncompliance with therapy.

Parental Expectations

In addition to parental overprotectiveness and permissiveness, parents of children with epilepsy often expect less of those children than they do of their normal offspring. Long and Moore (1979) found significant differences between epileptic children and their siblings. The children with seizures were expected to have more emotional problems and to be more unpredictable and high-strung. Siblings were expected to do better at school, to play more sports, to have greater powers of concentration, and to have a wider choice of occupation. On a behavioral checklist, parents rated their children with epilepsy as more neurotic than their siblings. When looking at the children themselves, the researchers found that the children with epilepsy had lower self-esteem than their siblings and that they tested below average for their chronological age in reading. The difference with their siblings was statistically significant in the predicted direction; that is, the siblings were doing better academically than was the child with epilepsy. Long and Moore conclude that given the presence of parental doubts and worries about their child's condition, in the absence of appropriate guidelines, many parents may adopt controlling and restrictive practices to ensure against the possible effects of the unknown.

Styles of Interaction

Hauck (1972) found that children of autocratic parents had seizures despite three years of adequate medication, while children of nonautocratic parents were seizure-free. Tensions, such as fear and aggression, can lead to seizures and lack of response to adequate therapy. Ritchie (1981) found that families with children with epilepsy were more matriarchal and autocratic in their decision-making style than were families whose children were seizure-free. While the autocratic style appears to be efficient in problem solving and meeting the family crisis and dependency needs of a chronically ill child, such an autocratic style may also lead to disturbed behavior in the long-term, if not modified.

Healthy Parental Behavior

Healthy parental behavior begins with the parents' successful resolution of the diagnosis of epilepsy. It exists when the parents come to accept the adolescent, along with the unique problems, and can reframe the situation into a challenge rather than an issue to be avoided. They do not deny presence of the disease or reject the child because of his or her problems. They are able to handle their own anxiety about the dangers involved in permitting age-appropriate activities and can recognize their fears while allowing the adolescent to have appropriate experiences with friends. They set limits when necessary without being arbitrary. Such parents tend to guide rather than control their adolescent's life and tend to negotiate and discuss potentially dangerous situations.

The parents of an 18-year-old girl with infrequent generalized tonic–clonic seizures had discussed with their daughter the risk of swimming unattended. Unfortunately, this young woman drowned at a pool party even though there were many people present. She had a generalized seizure and was not noticed until it was too late to save her. While this was a great tragedy to her parents, they were able to resolve their feelings about it, knowing that their daughter knew the risks involved and that her death was not due to carelessness.

Healthy parent behavior includes insistence on age-appropriate behavior on the part of the adolescent. These parents know their adolescent's capabilities and expect him or her to measure up to that standard. They recognize the stigma epilepsy has in the minds of many, and they prepare the adolescent to cope with it. They are also likely to be involved in their own individual pursuits, thus effectively balancing their parent role with their own personal interests. In short, healthy parents help their child by accepting his or her problem and expecting the child to perform up to age and ability standards.

In summary, the prevalence of negative parental behavior toward adolescents with epilepsy is not really known. The higher prevalence of psychological and academic problems in adolescents with the disease is, at best, an indicator of troubled parent–adolescent interaction, but it is not the whole story. The adolescent's problems result from a complex interaction of factors including negative parental interactions, the type of disease and response to treatment, the individual's personality and response to the disease, and responses from the larger society, including the school staff and peers.

SIBLING INTERACTIONS

Siblings as well as parents are affected when an adolescent has special needs. Most of the literature on the subject of siblings with an ill brother or sister focuses on the impact of the sick child on the healthy sibling. Reciprocal impact has not been addressed. In those families with dysfunctional parental style, such as overprotectiveness or overpermissiveness, the sibling subsystem will be equally vulnerable to dysfunction (Minuchin, 1975). Intense parental concern and overprotection of one child or adolescent will put stress on the other children. Spinetta and Deasy-Spinetta (1981) reported that siblings of children with cancer were the least well provided for emotionally of all family members. This finding held over the three years of their study. In fact, even when the child with cancer was in remission, the siblings were emotionally neglected. Healthy siblings described their family as significantly lower in cohesion and higher in conflict that did the ill child. The healthy siblings related that they were continually reminded that the disease's effects were part of their day to day lives. Their concerns were broader than the concerns of the child with cancer.

Leonard (1983) compared healthy siblings with a brother or sister with newly diagnosed cancer, diabetes, cystic fibrosis, or epilepsy. These siblings viewed the disease of the ill children or adolescents as more serious than did the patients themselves. The healthy children described themselves as moderately to highly anxious and admitted to being angry with their parents for time they spent with the ill sibling. Even though most of the healthy subjects reported having good communication with their parents, their relationships with their ill sibling had changed. It was not as open, especially with regard to the disease. The siblings were hesitant to talk with their ill brother or sister about the condition. A 15-year-old sibling, who had witnessed his older sister's first seizure and had accompanied her to the emergency room with his mother, had not talked to his sister about her problems until one month after the incident. Even then he did not know how she really felt about her diagnosis and its treatment. While he expressed concern for her, he was reluctant to talk with her for fear of touching on sensitive issues. Most of the siblings in the study had never talked with each other about their feelings concerning the disease. Most said that they wanted to but were afraid of hurting their ill sibling. The ill children and adolescents, on the other hand, did not think that their brother or sister really was that interested in their problems. One young adolescent said of his sister, "I never talk with her; she's got her own life . . . why should I, anyway? It's a long, boring story" (Leonard, 1983). The long-term implications of the lack of sibling communication are not known.

Certainly, critical benefits of the sibling relationship may be diminished or lost if the disease presents a barrier to sibling interaction. Such benefits typically include companionship as well as identification and introduction and inclusion in friendship groups—especially if siblings are close in age and of the same sex. In addition, the sibling subsystem may be used to soften or interpret parental behavior. Disruption in the siblings' relationship may have significant effects in both the healthy sibling and the adolescent with epilepsy. The scarcity of literature makes it virtually impossible to determine whether the lack of communication between siblings on critical issues is potentially harmful. The health care team is usually unaware of sibling concerns, but these relationships should be considered important and assessed periodically by health care providers.

THE SCHOOL AND THE ADOLESCENT WITH EPILEPSY

While it has been noted that children with epilepsy have learning problems disproportionate to their intelligence, the reasons for this discrepancy are not well understood. The school is probably the second most important environment for the adolescent. Here, in addition to the acquisition of critical academic and vocational skills, the adolescent develops significant social skills. It is through peer relationships that the individual satisfies the developmental tasks of emancipation. The milieu of the school can either support or hinder the acceptance of handicapped individuals. The school administration and teachers' attitudes toward the adolescent with epilepsy appear to be important variables in the success or failure of social and academic development. Unfortunately, many adults are ignorant of the nature of the disease and its consequences for the adolescent, so, rather than normalize the school environment, they tend to overprotect the individual with epilepsy. They set their expectations lower and are satisfied with less productivity from the adolescent with epilepsy than from his or her peers (Holdsworth, 1974).

The milieu of the school not only sets the stage for academic success or failure for the adolescent with epilepsy, but to an extent, it also structures the quality of peer interactions. Overly restrictive schools will prevent the adolescent from participation with peers in activities that help to establish friendships. Being excluded from sports and field trips can have devastating effects. Strax (see Chapter 4) points out that the adolescent with a handicap—in this case, physical mobility—is left behind by the peer group. This has a profound effect on the individual's self-esteem and confidence, the result of which, Strax notes, is that adolescents with chronic illness need a longer time to work out the critical developmental issues of adolescence. He says that in the majority of such cases, adolescent development must come from the nuclear and extended family because experience with peers is limited. Peer groups will not admit individuals who are different; without friends, life for the adolescent is extremely lonely. The rejected individual may tend toward inappropriate behavior, which leads to further rejection.

The school environment can contribute to greater understanding of the individual with epilepsy, and classroom situations can be structured to integrate the individual with epilepsy, thereby breaking down barriers with classmates. Teacher expectations should coincide with the individual's potential, not his diagnosis. Appropriate expectations build self-esteem. While the school cannot make friends for the adolescent with epilepsy, it can structure the atmosphere of the environment so as to allow friendships to occur. It should not contribute further barriers for adolescents with epilepsy.

PEERS

Adolescents with epilepsy may well come to the teenage years socially deprived and immature. If the individual has not made strong friendships during the elementary school years, he or she will be at a serious disadvantage during adolescence. By this time subconscious self-rejection may have taken place. Worry about acceptability to others, particularly those of the opposite sex, is common among normal adolescents; such worry is heightened in the individual with epilepsy who does not have a healthy self-concept. Even if the individual has the emotional maturity, self-esteem, and confidence needed to make friends, he or she must learn to deal with the problem of not being acceptable to some people. Depression in adolescents with chronic illness is not uncommon. It is an understandable result of feeling different and being rejected by others. Families and schools need to support these individuals as they develop the skills and confidence to deal with peer relationships. These institutions must encourage and support appropriate developmental tasks rather than structuring situations so as to avoid conflict, failure, and pain, and consequently denying the possibility of healthy development.

HEALTH CARE OF THE ADOLESCENT WITH EPILEPSY

This section describes the health care needs of adolescents with epilepsy and those of their family. The following issues are discussed: the physical aspects of care, including medical diagnosis and therapy with anticonvulsants; the psychosocial component of care; and coordination of care with other relevant institutions. Since epilepsy is a chronic condition by definition, it must be treated within the context of chronic illness (see Table 14-1). Chronically ill adolescents require comprehensive, continuous, and coordinated care. The following discussion assumes the presence of these three essential components of health care for the adolescent with epilepsy.

Table 14-1
Differences Between Acute Illness and Chronic Diseases in Childhood

Factor	Acute	Chronic
Causative agent	Single	Multicausal
Diagnosis	Usually easily made	Often complicated, time-consuming
Treatment	Specific, not pervasive, short	Difficult, trial and error, pervasive, ongoing
Child Involvement		
Organ systems	One or two	Many
Psychological/social	Minimal	Extensive
Participation in care	Minimal, short-term	Highly involved, long term
Long-Term Outcome		
	Highly predictable, no residual losses	Ambiguous, often poor, many residual losses
Parental Involvement		
	Minimal	Extensive, every aspect of life affected
Health Care System Involvement		
	Minimal	Extensive
Other Social Systems		
	Usually none	Extensive, education vocational–rehabilitation

Medical Care

Initial Evaluation

The first task the physician must undertake is classification of the seizure disorder. This is done according to the clinical description, etiology, and EEG. Specific studies will vary according to the age of the patient, past history, seizure type, and local facilities. A detailed history and complete physical and neurological examination of the patient (and family members if indicated) are the most important parts of the initial evaluation and subsequent follow-up. The detailed history of the seizures should include information pertaining to frequency, precipitating causes and events, presence or absence of an aura, ictus, and postictal periods, and the pattern of seizure recurrence. For example, is the ictus a true seizure? Syncope, benign paroxysmal vertigo, hypoglycemia, tics and movement disorders, migraine, psychosis, and hysterical seizures must all be considered in the diagnosis. Laboratory studies must include complete blood count, urinalysis, fasting blood glucose, serum calcium and phosphorus, and more extensive studies depending on the findings of the aforementioned. All patients with suspected seizures should have an EEG for diagnosis and classification. This should be done within three or four days of the seizure. The tracing is made while the patient is awake and during light sleep. Lumbar puncture, skull x-rays, and computed tomography are frequently useful, especially in cases of head trauma, suspicion of tumor, determination of congenital brain abnormalities, pathological eleification, demyelinization, intracranial hemorrhages, and vascular abnormalities. Once epilepsy is confirmed, the appropriate therapy—usually an anticonvulsant—is begun.

Anticonvulsant Therapy

Seizure management in adolescents with epilepsy is a complex task involving more than just the central nervous system. Anticonvulsant therapy is a critical component of that management; the aim is to control seizures while minimizing side effects. Ideally, this is done by avoiding barbiturates whenever possible and minimizing the use of phenytoins in females. The principles of anticonvulsant therapy can be summarized as follows:

1. The EEG is the basis for determining the type of seizure disorder and consequently the type of drug therapy necessary.
2. Therapy is initiated with the smallest dose possible and gradually increased at weekly intervals until the therapeutic dose is reached. It is increased at monthly intervals until the seizures are controlled and the appropriate serum level is reached or toxic signs appear.

3. The drug's half-life determines the timing of dosage. If its half-life is less than 12 hours, three doses daily are given, and if greater than 12 hours, dosage is once daily.
4. Serum levels provide optimal or therapeutic levels in most anticonvulsants with the exception of valproic acid and carbamazepine.
5. Drug interactions should be avoided, especially those of drugs with similar side effects.
6. Anticonvulsants may decrease the effects of steroids, anticoagulants, antipyretics, antidepressants, and antirheumatics.
7. Teratogenicity is a known risk with phenytoin, phenobarbital, primidone, and tridione. Few abnormalities have been reported with carbamazepine, and none are known with valproic acid.

The decision to treat—and how to treat—an adolescent with anticonvulsants requires a delicate balance between risks and benefits. The first criterion is the age of the individual. The adolescent is set apart from his or her peers if seizures are uncontrolled. However, the rare seizure, while interfering with the individual's ability to drive, may be preferred to continuous drug therapy with its concomitant problems. This is a very delicate matter that must be decided by the adolescent and the physician together. Second, the severity of the seizures and their frequency are important aspects and should be considered in the decision-making process. Certainly, the "kindling" effect of untreated seizures is well recognized and cannot be ignored (Gordon, 1982). Third, family history and type of seizure disorder must be considered. Less is known about the long-term side effects of anticonvulsant therapy than the short-term problems. Side effects include interference with red and white blood cells and calcium metabolism, and behavioral and learning problems. The effects of phenobarbital are found to be a contributing factor in both memory and comprehension problems, although not in overall IQ. During growth the individual may be particularly vulnerable to the effect of drugs with respect to growth and learning. Research must establish the etiology of learning problems, whether it be drugs, seizures, or the underlying cerebral disorder. If the decision is made to begin therapy, the type of seizure disorder should guide the choice of the initial drug (see Table 14-2).

Monitoring the Drug

Monitoring drug therapy is an important part of epilepsy treatment. Monitoring includes careful history taking, physical examination, and neurological examination, as well as laboratory studies of blood, liver function, and therapeutic serum levels of the anticonvulsant. The frequency of monitoring is partly determined by the level of seizure control achieved and partly by the toxicity of the agent being used. When control

Table 14-2
The Primary Anticonvulsants, Seizure Type, and Side Effects

Trade name	Generic	Dosage (mg/kg)	Therapeutic range (mg/ml)	Indications	Principal side effects
Phenobarbital ® (Comatic, Purepac, Rexall)	Phenobarbital	4–6	10–20	Tonic–clonic psychomotor	Nausea, vomiting, drowsiness, hyperactivity, rash, learning problems
Dilantin '® (Parke-Davis)	Phenytoin	1–5	20–40	Tonic–clonic psychomotor	Gingivitis, hypertrophy, anemia, nausea, vomiting, ataxia, nystagmus, rash, malaise
Mysoline ® (Ayerst)	Primidone	10–20	5–10	Tonic–clonic	Nausea, vomiting, drowsiness, hyperactivity, rash, learning problems, ataxia, earache, gum pain, acne, psychological problems
Tegretol ® (Geigy)	Carbamazepine	7–15	—	Psychomotor	Nausea, vomiting, rash, vertigo, fever, aplastic anemia, liver damage, urinary frequency or retention
Zarontin ® (Parke-Davis)	Ethosuximide	20–30	40–80	Petit mal	Nausea, vomiting, anorexia, dizziness, hiccups, blood dyscrasias, liver damage, lupus
Depakene ® (Abbott)	Valproic acid	10–40	50–100	Petit mal, absence with automatisms	Drowsiness, weight loss or gain, hair loss, nausea and vomiting, liver damage, leukopenia

is well established, the adolescent should be seen no less frequently than every six months. Adolescents on sodium valproate should be seen at four-month intervals to monitor liver function.

Monitoring the level of the drug is a critical component of health care for the adolescent with epilepsy; however, drawing blood is often traumatic. For those individuals who have difficulty with venipuncture, reliable micromethods for use with blood, saliva, and other body fluids can be used to monitor some drugs (Brett, 1977; Zysset, Rudeberg, Vassella, Kupfer, & Birchner, 1981). Particularly in adolescents who are on phenytoin therapy, saliva samples appear to be as reliable as plasma.

For adolescents who require more than one anticonvulsant for seizure, the aforementioned authors caution practitioners to be aware of the nonlinear relationship between plasma and dose of certain anticonvulsants. For phenytoin, especially, a small increment in the drug can produce relatively large rises in plasma level, resulting in the sudden attainment of toxic levels. The measurement of blood (or saliva) levels allows the dose to be accurately tailored to the individual patient. Three aspects must be reviewed in order to determine the basis of toxicity in adolescents who are simultaneously on more than one anticonvulsant:

1. The offending drug must be identified.
2. A decision as to cause of failure must be determined—is it the multiple treatment, or is it due to drug interaction?
3. The intoxication must be distinguished from the effects of underlying disease. This is especially important in cases of degenerative brain disorder (Brett, 1977).

Richens (1981) has cautioned of the need to monitor the level of one drug both before and after adding another to the adolescent's treatment regimen. In doing so, the risk of drug interaction can be greatly minimized.

Many adolescents will want to withdraw from anticonvulsant therapy even when the odds of remaining seizure free are minimal. For those who have not had a seizure episode over a prolonged period of time, it is not uncommon to develop a notion of having been cured. Even at times when medically uncertain, it may be important for the physician to allow a trial without medication. If seizures return, however, the results may be devastating and may result in depression, anger and hostility, or acting-out behavior. Not all individuals are able to accept the implications of lifelong therapy with anticonvulsants. The return of seizures shatters any fantasies the adolescent may have developed about the absence of disease. The physician or another member of the health care team must be on hand to help the adolescent deal with the recurrence of seizures. Even though devastating, it may provide a means of communication about the significance of epilepsy in the patient's life and lead to a resolution of his or her feelings about it.

Psychosocial Component of Care

The development of secondary psychological and learning problems appears to be much higher in individuals with epilepsy than in those with other chronic diseases or in the general population (Rutter, Graham, & Yule, 1970). Because of these findings, every effort must be made to prevent psychological and learning problems in this population. The development of secondary sequelae is multicausal; therefore, prevention must be multifaceted. The approach to prevention includes patient and family education as well as psychological assessment and treatment of both adolescents and families.

Provider–Patient Relationship

The key ingredient in treatment of adolescents with epilepsy is the care provider–patient relationship. This relationship must be based on trust and mutual respect. The adolescent must get a clear sense of understanding from the health care provider. In turn, the care provider must always view the youth first as a person and an adolescent and second as a person with a seizure disorder. To build trust, the provider works directly with the adolescent and indirectly with the youth's parents. Conversations must be held in confidence unless to do so would be harmful to the patient or to others. An authoritarian approach will not be effective with most adolescents, while a democratic mode is more likely to increase compliance. The provider holds the teenager accountable for behavior and helps the adolescent with epilepsy to "own" his or her illness. The adolescent must become responsible for management of the disorder; this includes administration of anticonvulsants as well as monitoring of general health behavior. The road to ownership may be difficult for both the adolescent and the provider. A firm but patient approach appears to work best. The provider may need to set limits if care is flagrantly violated by the adolescent. This may mean directing the parents to structure their adolescent's life until he or she proves able to handle responsibility more effectively. This action generally can be avoided if a trusting relationship can be successfully fostered between provider and patient and if the provider works with the family and is supportive of their relationship with the adolescent. Through the use of contracts the teenager can come to understand and accept his or her role in disease management. Unlike those of acute illness, the goal of epilepsy treatment is control, not cure. Since control is a lifelong process, the patient must become an active participant if treatment is to be successful.

The relationship with the family is based on an understanding that the adolescent–provider relationship is central. This, however, does not preclude working with the family. The effective provider conveys a sense of respect for and support of the parents by seeking to know and understand their concerns and needs. He or she also can serve as a bridge between parent and teenager when needed.

Psychological Intervention

Prevention of psychological problems in adolescents and parents is a major goal of the provider. For most, the diagnosis of epilepsy is upsetting. For some, it will disrupt usual coping patterns; thus, providers must first communicate their understanding of the disruptions that a chronic illness such as epilepsy may cause. Clinicians need to allow for, and encourage, open expression of feelings. Many irrational fears and concerns can be put to rest if they are allowed to be voiced. Appolone (1978) identifies four areas of concern for families of children with epilepsy:

1. Resolving of fantasies and fears regarding epilepsy; parents are often afraid their child will die or come to physical harm during a seizure. They also fear brain damage, subsequent mental retardation, and increased emotional problems.
2. Interpreting facts about the disease; Appolone found that cognitive confrontation by the parents at the time of the diagnosis was a critical variable correlated with later good adjustment and high self-esteem in the children. It is thus essential to explore the parents' feelings about the disorder.
3. Assisting parents to establish realistic behavioral expectations and limits for the adolescent child; overprotection appears to be the main factor in maladjustment of epileptic individuals. Therefore, Appolone advocates helping parents work out reasonable expectations for the adolescents with epilepsy.
4. Disclosing information about the adolescent's condition in such a way as to benefit the individual; Appolone believes that parents who are able to interpret information about the adolescent's condition feel a sense of increased adequacy and power over the disease. When parents can enlighten others about the condition, they have a means of building their own sense of competence and control.

Psychological intervention remains a constant component in the health care of adolescents with epilepsy and their family. While the time of initial diagnosis provides a unique opportunity for counseling and education, both of family members and of the adolescent, ongoing involvement is necessary for assessing the adjustment of family members and the adolescent and for continuing education. Because adolescence is a time of rapid psychological growth and increased stress, the needs of parents and their teenagers will also change rapidly. What was appropriate parental behavior for the early adolescent will need revision for the mid-adolescent.

Continuing to let go emotionally may be very difficult when the parent witnesses the adolescent violating some aspects of the health care behavior they had tried to establish. For example, an adolescent whose parents no longer take responsibility for administration of anticonvulsants may provoke parental anger by not getting up in time to take the medication. The parents feel frustrated and attacked by the adolescent who is throwing away their earlier investment. Thus, the issue of parent–adolescent relationships is a constant concern of the provider. Hopefully, thorough initial education of the parents and the adolescent and resolution of their concerns about the disease will help to establish a healthy foundation with open communication, and only periodic time-limited interventions will be necessary.

Education

Education of the epileptic adolescent and his or her family regarding the disease and its treatment is a fundamental component of care. Long and Moore (1979) found that 50 percent of the families in their study were virtually uninformed about their child's epilepsy and its treatment. This disquieting finding alerts those who care for families and adolescents with seizures to provide appropriate and ongoing education. This same study also revealed that very few of the parents ever discussed the diagnosis with their child. Ziegler (1981) found that parental and adolescent attitudes about seizures significantly influenced the therapeutic course of the disease. He makes the following recommendations for the care provider:

1. Clarify what the patients and the parents believe about epilepsy, convulsions, and seizures and what their emotional responses are to seizures.
2. Determine the family's and patient's underlying fears about the disease so that the process of reeducation can address their concerns.
3. Discuss how to handle a seizure when and if one occurs.
4. Review their knowledge of anticonvulsant therapy and how it controls seizures, as well as its potential side and toxic effects.
5. Explain the seizure triggering mechanisms.
6. Help them to understand the process by which the patient can develop a healthy self-concept and continue to meet age-appropriate developmental tasks.

Coordination of Health Care

Coordination of epileptic care with other health care providers may occur; however, coordination of care with other institutions is often neglected. It is not always necessary to communicate with school personnel about an individual child, especially if the seizure disorder is well controlled and is not interfering with the child's learning process. If communication is warranted, however, the health care provider should make every effort to explain the exact nature of the individual's problem, its educational and functional impact, and how it should be handled by school personnel. Holdsworth and Whitmore (1974) found communication between teachers and doctors to be the exception rather than the rule. Few of the teachers were adequately informed about epilepsy and, as a result, they tended to set inappropriate expectations for the individual children. Most of the teachers in the study were unaware of absence seizures, and even more were unaware of the serious educational disability the seizures can create.

In some instances, school is the only place in which an adolescent with epilepsy can be adequately observed. Properly instructed teachers can be of primary importance in observing an adolescent for the presence of seizures. The importance of such observations for the individual's care must be stressed. Teachers need to feel that they can contact the health care team if they have concerns about the adolescent's condition. Teachers may, in fact, be the first to notice subtle changes in learning and behavior that may indicate need for medical attention.

CONCLUSION

This chapter has dealt with epilepsy in the adolescent. Monitoring and managing this condition is challenging for teenagers and for those who must guide and assist them. Epilepsy is unique in that it has at least as many secondary disabilities as it has primary effects. It appears that secondary sequelae have less to do with the seizure disorder than with maladaptation to a social environment that is generally ignorant about and prejudiced against the disease. Therein lies the challenge for the clinician who is caring for the adolescent with epilepsy. Health care for adolescents with seizures must be comprehensive, continuous, and coordinated if it is to be effective. Control of the seizures is the unique responsibility of the health care provider, but it must not eclipse the equally important responsibility of psychological support and education of the adolescent as an individual. For healthy development, the adolescent with epilepsy must be prepared to deal with an unfriendly environment in a way that does not kindle further rejection.

REFERENCES

Appolone, C. Preventive social work intervention with families of children with epilepsy. *Social Work in Health Care*, 1978, *4*(2), 139–148.

Brett, E. Implications of measuring anticonvulsant blood levels in epilepsy. *Developmental Medicine and Child Neurology*, 1977, *19*, 245–251.

Bryant, M.E. Parent–child relationships: Their effect on rehabilitation. *Journal of Learning Disabilities,* 1971, *4*(6), 325–329.

Chaabria, S., & Shope, J.T. Medical aspects of epilepsy: An overview. In R.B. Black, B.P. Hermann, & J.T. Shope (Eds.), *Nursing management of epilepsy.* Rockville, MD: Aspen Systems Corp. 1982, pp. 1–21.

Duvall, E. *Marriage and family development* (5th ed.). Philadelphia: J.B. Lippincott & Co., 1977.

Gliedman, J., & Roth, W. *The unexpected minority: Handicapped children in America.* New York: Harcourt Brace Jovanovich, 1980.

Gordon, N. Duration of treatment for childhood epilepsy. *Developmental Medicine and Child Neurology,* 1982, *24,* 84–88.

Green, J.B., & Hartlage, L.C. Comparative performance of epileptic and nonepileptic children and adolescents. *Diseases of the Nervous System,* 1971, *32,* 418.

Gumnit, R. (Ed.). Epilepsy: A handbook for physicians (4th ed.). Minneapolis: Comprehensive Epilepsy Program, 1981.

Hartlage, L.C., & Green, J.B. The relation of parental attitudes to academic and social achievement in epileptic children. *Epilepsia* (Amsterdam), 1972, *13,* 21–26.

Hartlage, L.C., Green, J.B., & Offutt, L. Dependency in epileptic children. *Epilepsia* (Amsterdam), 1972, *13,* 27–30.

Hill, R. Generic features of families under stress. *Crisis intervention.* New York: Family Service Assoc. of America, 1965.

Holdsworth, L., & Whitmore, K. A study of children with epilepsy attending ordinary schools. I. Their seizure patterns, progress and behavior in school. *Developmental Medicine and Child Neurology,* 1974, *16,* 746–758.

Holdsworth, L., & Whitmore, K. A study of children with epilepsy attending ordinary schools. II. Information and attitudes held by their teachers. *Developmental Medicine and Child Neurology,* 1974, *16,* 759–765.

Leonard, B. (1983) *The impact of chronic illness on the siblings of an affected child.* Unpublished doctoral dissertation, University of Minnesota, Minneapolis, Minnesota, 1983.

Lindsay, J., Ounsted, C., & Richards, P. Long-term outcome in children with temporal lobe seizures. I. Social outcome and childhood factors. *Developmental Medicine and Child Neurology,* 1979, *21,* 285–298.

Long, C.G., & Moore, J.R. Parental expectations for their epileptic children. *Journal of Child Psychology and Psychiatry,* 1979, *20,* 299–312.

Minuchin, S., Baker, L., Rosman, B., Liebman, R., Milman, L., & Todd, T. A conceptual model of psychosomatic illness in children. *Archives of General Psychiatry,* August 1975, *32,* 1031–1038.

Pless, I.B., & Roghmann, K.J. Chronic illness and its consequences, observations based on three epidemiological surveys. *Journal of Pediatrics,* 1979, p. 351.

Pless, I.B. The care of children with chronic illness. T. Moore, (Ed.), *Report of the 67th Ross Conference on Pediatric Research.* Ross Laboratories, 1975.

Richardson, D.W., & Friedman, S.B. Psychosocial problems of the adolescent patient with epilepsy: The epileptic's need for comprehensive care. *Clinical Pediatrics,* 1974, *13*(2), 121–126.

Richens, A., Dunlop, A. Serum-phenytoin levels in management of epilepsy. *Lancet,* 1981, *2,* 247–248.

Ritchie, K. Research note: interaction in the families of epileptic children. *Journal of Child Psychology and Psychiatry,* 1981, *22,* 65–71.

Rutter, M., Graham, P., & Yule, W. The prevalence of psychiatric disorder in neuroepileptic children. A neuropsychiatric study of childhood. *Clinics in developmental medicine,* 1970, Chap. 11, No. 35–36.

Scott, D. Psychiatric aspects of childhood and adolescent epilepsy. *The Practitioner,* 1977, *218,* 417–423.

Shukla, G.D., Strivastava, O.N., Katiyar, V., et al. Psychiatric manifestations in temporal lobe epilepsy: A controlled study. *British Journal of Psychiatry*, 1979, *135*, 411–417.

Spinetta, J., & Deasy-Spinetta, P. (Eds.). *Living with childhood cancer*. St. Louis: Mosby Company, 1981.

Stores, G. School-children with epilepsy at risk for learning and behavior problems. *Developmental Medicine and Child Neurology*, 1978, *20*, 502–508.

Stores, G. The investigation and management of school children with epilepsy. *Public Health* (London), 1976, *90*, 171–177.

Strax, T. Adolescence: A period of stress, the search for an identity. In D. Bergsma & A. Pulver, (Eds.), *Birth defects: Original article series*, 1976, 11, 63–70.

Ziegler, R.G. Impairments of control and competence in epileptic children and their families. *Epilepsia*, 1981, *22*, 339–346.

Zysset, T., Rudeberg, A., Vassella, F., Kupfer, A., & Bircher, J. Phenytoin therapy for epileptic children: Evaluation of salivary and plasma concentrations and methods of assessing compliance. *Developmental Medicine and Child Neurology*, 1981, *23*, 66–75.

BIBLIOGRAPHY

Allmond, B., Buckman, W., & Gofman, H. *The family is the patient*. St. Louis: Mosby, 1979.

Aminoff, M.D., & Simon, R.P. Status epilepticus: Causes, clinical features and consequences in 98 patients. *The American Journal of Medicine*, 1980, *69*, 657–666.

Anderson, S.V., & Bauwens, E.E. *Chronic health problems*. St. Louis: Mosby, 1981.

Andrulonis, P.A., Glueck, B.C., Stroebel, C.F., et al. Organic brain dysfunction and the borderline syndrome. *Psych. Clin. North America*, 1980, *4*(1), 47–66.

Bauer, E.W. Thoughts on parenting the child with epilepsy. *Comprehensive Epilepsy Program for the State of Minnesota*. Minneapolis, MN: [Paper originally prepared for presentation at the Epilepsy Conference for Nurses, Oct. 14, 1977, Lafayette Clinic, Detroit, Michigan].

Beniak, J. Patient education in epilepsy. *Journal Neurolsurgical Nursing*, 1982, *14*(1), 19–22.

Prognosis of temporal lobe epilepsy in childhood. *British Medical Journal*, March, 1980, 812–813.

Burr, W. Hill, R. Nue, F.I., et al. (Eds.). *Contemporary theories about the family*, Vol. I. New York: The Free Press, 1979.

Burt, M.R., & Rorabacher, J.A. The social world of young adults with epilepsy. [Paper read at the 85th Annual Meeting of the American Psychological Assn., San Francisco, CA, August 1977].

Burton, L. *Care of the child facing death*. London & Boston: Routledge & Kegan Paul, 1974.

Comprehensive Epilepsy Program. *Medical aspects of epilepsy*. Minneapolis: University of Minnesota, 1978.

Carozza, V.J. Understanding the patient with epilepsy. *Nursing Clinics of North America*, March, 1970, *5*(1), 13–22.

Ferguson, S.M., & Rayport, M. The adjustment to living without epilepsy. *The Journal of Nervous and Mental Disease*, 1965, *140*, (1), 26–37.

Fischbacher, E. Effect of reduction of anticonvulsants on wellbeing. *British Medical Journal*, August, 1982, *285*, 423–424.

Freeman, S. *The epileptic in home, school and society: Coping with the invisible handicap*. Springfield, Illinois: Charles C. Thomas Publisher, 1979.

French, A., & Berlin, I.N. *Depression in children and adolescents*. New York: Human Sciences Press, 1979.

Harvard Child Health Project, *Children's medical care, needs & treatments* (Vols. I, II, III). Cambridge, Mass.: Ballinger Press, 1977.

Hauser, S.T., & Shapiro, R.L. Differentiation of adolescent self-images. *Archives General Psychiatry,* July 1973, *29,* 63–68.

Ireton, H. Psychologic problems of children with seizures. *Postgraduate Medicine,* August 1969, 119–123.

Ireys, H. Health care for chronically disabled children and their families. In *Better health for our children: A national strategy.* U.S. Dept. of Health and Human Services/Public Health, 1981, 321.

Jeavons, P.M. Choice of drug therapy in epilepsy. *The Practitioner,* October 1977, *219,* 542–556.

Johnson, B.M. Nursing priorities in the management of epilepsy. In R.B. Black, B.P. Herman, & J.T. Shope (Eds.), *Nursing management of epilepsy.* Rockville, MD: Aspen Systems Corp. 1982.

Kempe, H. et al. *Pediatric diagnosis and treatment* (4th ed.). Los Altos, CA: Lange Medical Publications, 1976.

Koocher, G., & O'Malley, J.E. *The damocles syndrome: The psychosocial consequences of surviving childhood cancer.* New York: McGraw-Hill Book Co., 1981.

Landau, W.M. More on epilepsy and epileptic drivers. *Annals of Neurology,* August 1979, *6*(2), 140.

Lessman, S.E. *Accepting epilepsy: Social and emotional issues for patients and their families.* In R.B. Black, B.P. Herman, & J.T. Shope (Eds.), *Nursing management of epilepsy,* Rockville, MD: Aspen Systems Corp. 1982, 73–82.

Lewis, C., et al. *A right to health: The problem of access to primary medical care.* New York: John Wiley & Sons, 1976.

Lewis, D.O. Delinquency, psychomotor epileptic symptoms, and paranoid ideation: A triad. *American Journal of Psychiatry,* 1976, *133*(12), 1395–1398.

Lopez, K.A., & Seastrunk, J.W., II. Temporal lobe epilepsy: A new entity in psychiatry. *Journal of Psychiatric Nursing and Mental Health Services,* August 1980, 10–15.

Low, N.L. Seizure disorders in children. In J.A. Downey, & N. L. Low (Eds.), *The child with disabling illness: Principles of rehabilitation.* New York: Raven Press, 1982.

MacDougall, V. Teaching children and families about seizures. *The Canadian Nurse,* April 1982, 30–35.

Millspaugh, D., Kreminitzer, M., & Lending, M. Providing services for adolescents who live with seizures. *Children Today,* September–October, 1976, 7–9, 34–35.

Minuchin, S., et al. *Psychosomatic families,* Cambridge, MA & London: Harvard University Press, 1980.

Nielsen, H., & Kristensen, O. Personality correlates of sphenoidal eeg-foci in temporal lobe epilepsy. *Acta Neurol, Scandinav,* (Denmark), 1981, *64,* 289–300.

O'Leary, D.S., Seidenberg, M., Berent, S., & Boll, T.J. Effects of age on onset of tonic–clonic seizures on neuropsychological performance in children. *Epilepsia,* 1981, *22,* 197–204.

Palva, E.S., Linnoila, M., Routledge, P., & Seppala, T. Actions and interactions of diazepam and alcohol on psychomotor skills in young and middle-aged subjects. *Acta Pharmacol, et Toxicol,* 1982, *50,* 363–369.

Reiss, I. Family systems in America (3rd ed.). New York: Holt, Rinehart & Winston, 1980.

Romeis, J. The role of grandparents in adjustment to epilepsy. *Social Work in Health Care,* 1980, *6*(1), 37–43.

Ross, E.M., & Evans, D. Epilepsy in Bristol secondary school children. Epilepsia (Amst.), 1972, *13,* 7–12.

Rutter, M. Developmental neuropsychiatry: Concepts, issues and prospects. *Journal of Clinical Neuropsychology,* 1982, *4*(2), 91–115.

Rutter, M. *Changing youth in a changing society.* Cambridge, MA: Harvard University Press, 1980.

Rutter, M. *Helping troubled children.* New York & London: Plenum Press, 1975.

Schwartz, H., & Kart, C.S. *Dominant issues in medical sociology.* Reading, Mass: Addison-Wesley Publishing Co., 1978.

Shope, J.T. The clinical specialist in epilepsy. Nursing Clinics of North America, December 1974, 9(4), 761–772.

Spunt, A.L., & Black, R.B. Drug treatment of seizure disorders. In R.B. Black, B.P. Herman, & J.T. Shope (Eds.), *Nursing management of epilepsy.* Rockville, MD: Aspen Systems Corp. 1982, 25–41.

Stores, G., & Piran, N. Dependency of different types in school children with epilepsy. *Psychological Medicine,* 1978, *8,* 441–445.

Stores, G., Hart, J., & Piran, N. Inattentiveness in school children with epilepsy. *Epilepsia,* 1978, *19,* 169–175.

Talbot, N. *Raising children in modern America.* Boston: Little, Brown & Co., 1976.

Voeller, K.K.S., & Rothenberg, M.B. Psychosocial aspects of the management of seizures in children. *Pediatrics,* 1973, *51*(6), 1072–1081.

Wikler, L., & Stoycheff, J. Parental compliance with postdischarge: recommendations for retarded children. *Hospital and Community Psychiatry,* 1974, *25*(9), 595–598.

Williams, D.T., Gold, A.P., Shrout, P., et al. The impact of psychiatric intervention on patients with uncontrolled seizures. *The Journal of Nervous and Mental Disease,* 1979, *167*(10), 626–631.

Woodward, F.S. The total patient: Implications for nursing care of the epileptic. *Journal of Neurosurgical Nursing,* 1982, *14*(4), 166–169.

Stanley F. Battle

15
Chronically Ill Children with Sickle Cell Anemia

Sickle cell anemia is a unique physical disease. It is a painful, inherited blood disorder found predominantly in black children. It is one of the genetically inherited diseases with a specifically defined molecular derangement that results in physiochemical compromise (Phillips, 1973).

Because of its protean complications, the disease can be extremely disruptive of a family's structure, testing its capacity to cope and adjust. As a consequence of the sequelae of sickle cell anemia, youths often experience severe disability and social isolation. Frequently, parents must act as advocates for their children in both the medical and the school system. The most important role played by parents is assisting their child to cope with this physical condition.

In dealing with the family of a newly diagnosed individual with sickle cell anemia, helping professionals must assist family members in understanding the nature of the disease and the requirements of good home care. This knowledge must be assimilated in a relatively short period of time, with little previous scientific background, and under conditions of extreme emotional stress (Flanagan, 1980). Family members must also be assisted in adjusting to their initial shock, fear, and guilt. The process of adjustment and assimilation is often complicated by pressures from a misinformed public and misconceptions that cause unnecessary worry and alarm.

In the past, sickle cell anemia was referred to as "bad blood," and thought of as a condition similar to syphilis. It is, thus, important that parents receive information that is accurate and up to date. For instance, although parents often assume an early mortality for their children, this

CHRONIC ILLNESS AND DISABILITIES IN CHILDHOOD AND ADOLESCENCE ISBN 0-8089-1635-1

is no longer the rule. While a decade ago average life expectancy was 14.3 years (Wintrobe, 1974), the result of improved treatment is that many sickle cell patients live productive lives well into their 50s and 60s.

Sickle cell anemia is a major health problem of black people in Africa, South America, Latin America, and the West Indies, as well as in the United States. The incidence of sickle cell anemia among blacks is estimated at 1 in 400. Sickle cell trait occurs in about 1 of every 12 black Americans (Scott & Kessler, 1967).

Sickle cell anemia is a hereditary disorder characterized by painful crises, such as chronic anemia and chronic injury to the heart, spleen, and liver. The basic defect is a mutant autosomal gene effecting a substitution of valine for glutamic acid on the hemoglobin chain ($\alpha2_{\beta}6$ val). This can result in either sickle cell anemia or a healthy carrier with sickle cell trait. The individual who is a trait carrier is not ill, whereas the individual with sickle cell anemia actually has the disease, an important distinction to make to those who are screened for the trait. Complications from the disease tend to occur only under unusual conditions in individuals with the sickle cell trait, but those homozygous for sickle cell anemia bear the full brunt of the disease (White, 1974).

FEATURES OF SICKLE CELL ANEMIA

Characteristics During Adolescence

During adolescence a number of physical characteristics of the disease are extremely important to the affected individual and the parents. By this time there is a heightened awareness of the unpredictable occurrence of acute crises. Table 15-1 reports some of the physical complications that may occur during infancy, childhood, and adolescence. Clinically, crises attributable to vascular occlusions appear to be the most common. They are characterized by fever and severe pain in the extremities, chest, back, or abdomen. Pain in the extremities may be osseous or muscular, or it may be localized in a joint that becomes swollen and warm, closely simulating rheumatic arthritis (Diggs, 1965). Adolescents also frequently experience abdominal pain with associated ileus.

Painful crises may be precipitated by viral or bacterial infections; excessive cold, hot or damp weather; extreme emotional and physical conditions such as stress and overexertion; pregnancy; high altitude; excessive use of alcohol; immobility; and underwater swimming (Flanagan, 1980).

Because of the pain and physical limitations associated with a sickle cell anemia crisis, young people with the disease tend to miss a significant

Table 15-1
Features of Sickle Cell Anemia

Infancy (birth to age 2)	Childhood	Adolescence
Pain	Pain	Pain
Hand–foot syndrome (dactylitis)	Cerebral vascular accident	Cerebrovascular accident
Anemia	Hematuria	Pulmonary involvement
Jaundice	Anemia	Ocular hemorrhages
Fever	Impaired growth	Leg ulcers
Pneumonia	Increased heart size	Gallstones
Osteomyelitis *Salmonella*	Splenic sequestration	Impaired fertility
	Fever	Anemia
	Osteomyelitis *(Salmonella)*	Fever
		Pneumonia
		Priapism

amount of school. Diggs (1965) observed a group of children with the disorder over a two-year period and found that of the 18 who were in school, illness related to sickle cell anemia led to an average of 14 days of school missed per child per year. Such absence poses problems in educational programming as well in parental work and social schedules.

Adolescence is a demanding period for the parent and for the affected adolescent. For the healthy teenager, development can be viewed as progressive physical growth and social improvement, with advances built upon prior successes. For the adolescent with sickle cell anemia, however, adolescence may be marred by physical and emotional setbacks.

The onset of puberty is likely to be delayed in an adolescent with sickle cell anemia. These adolescents may consequently experience ridicule and humiliation from peers. Furthermore, the adolescent with sickle cell anemia may experience feelings of inferiority, resentment, and rejection; as a result, there may be a tendency to withdraw from the peer group and possibly from family relationships as well (Fischoff & Whitten, 1974).

Another important aspect of adolescent development is sexual maturation and the associated development of new sexual roles. Sickle cell anemia can cause difficulties in the development of normal role processes for young men and women due to depreciated body image and higher than average medical risks, such as for pregnancy. These problems take on even greater significance during adulthood.

ADAPTIVE TASKS IN SICKLE CELL PATIENTS AND
THEIR FAMILIES

The following case examples illustrate a number of issues faced by youths with sickle cell anemia and their families. While not all of the patients were teenagers at the time of interview, the problems and concerns raised are directly applicable to adolescents and need to be considered by those who work with affected young people and their families.

Case Studies

J.R. is a 32-year-old black male. An only child, he has never married and currently lives at home with his parents. He became aware of his illness approximately at the age of five and, since that time, his life has been complicated by the disease.

Currently, he walks only with great difficulty because of pain, swelling, and leg ulcers that, despite treatment, have persisted for 12 years. As a result, he is unable to work and cannot contribute financially to his family, who he sees as having sacrificed continually for him.

He reports that not only have his parents invested a large percentage of their limited financial resources, but their personal investment has been even greater. The last vacation he can recall their taking was 12 years ago. While Mr. R. reports feeling constant guilt about his condition and the impact it has had on his family, he believes that there is little he can do to alter the situation. He reports that at times he feels like giving up and asserts: "If I could make a pact with God to kill someone and in return receive good health, I would do so" (Battle, 1982).

Patients who have genetic conditions generally learn to adapt to their physical condition based on three factors: their environment (i.e., family and peers), ability to cope (personal intrinsic characteristic), and overall physical condition. Parents' and family members' tasks include providing a stable environment for the affected family member and assisting him or her in developing a positive self-identity. Family members attempt to provide hope, encourage development of a satisfactory self-image, preserve relationships, and prepare for the future in the face of uncertain day to day problems and long-term sequelae. Patients with long-term consequences, such as severe stroke, leg ulcers, liver damage, and visual impairment, can find that life planning becomes complicated, at best. There is no way that parents and family members can anticipate any of these problems. Parental support is frequently handicapped by their own feelings of guilt at "causing" the disease in their offspring. They blame themselves and generally carry this burden of guilt all their lives. In many instances, they shelter their affected child in an attempt to protect him or her from further physical and emotional injury; this, however, only increases developmental delays and social isolation.

L.B. is a 25-year-old male with sickle cell anemia and a healthy 3-year-old daughter. Mr. B. describes the feeling of a crisis: "Your entire body is in pain; you hurt all over. The arms, legs, and back may be the first areas you experience pain; but generally your mobility is affected because of pain—the joints of your body. Imagine lying in bed and somebody putting nails and knives into your body." Mr. B. has been hospitalized more than 100 times. While the frequency of his hospitalizations has decreased with age (which is characteristic of the condition), his concerns have not diminished. Sometimes he wonders how much he can take. Currently he has leg ulcers and lives in constant fear both of recurrent pain of and dying.

He laments the profound effect the disease has had on his parents and wife. He recalls how, as a child, his parents were considerate and caring, always trying to explain his medical problems and the need for hospitalization. However, he was always aware of the strain hospitalization placed on his parents, especially during his teenage years.

Peers were not always as kind. Mr. B. recalls being teased and ostracized: "It is very difficult for other children and adolescents to understand what you are going through!" Parental support helped overcome some of the social pain (Battle, 1982).

Parents who have a child with chronic conditions have different ways of perceiving their child's prognosis. Parents may adhere to defensive denial such that they may recognize the same physical and clinical clues that the doctor observes but may distort their conclusions so as to avoid facing certain realities. Such denial is a means of coping. Distortion of prognosis can be observed two ways: parents who themselves are physically impaired may perceive more serious symptoms in their child than parents who are unimpaired, or parents may be unable to make rational, objective observations with regard to their child's physical condition (Frydman, 1980).

For patients with sickle cell anemia, visits to the hosptial may be accompanied by depressive reactions resulting from loss of health and interpersonal relationships. It has been observed that patients in chronic pain may experience sleep loss, anhedonia, anorexia, weight loss, lowered energy levels, and heightened levels of anxiety. These conditions may have a profound effect on the family as well as on the patient. Family members are also vulnerable to depression and isolation (Morin & Waring, 1981).

S.J., a single mother with sickle cell anemia, is 20 years of age; her daughter is unaffected. Ms. J. indicates that for many years she would not accept her condition and went to the hospital only if she was in need of acute medical care. When eventually she admitted to herself that she had sickle cell anemia and physical limitations, she lapsed into a deep depression of two years' duration.

During her teenage years, Ms. J. used morphine and codeine to control her pain, and as a result she became chemically dependent—a dependency that was overcome with family and physician assistance. Ms. J. has been hospitalized on an average of six times annually, with medical complications including hepatitis, eight or nine episodes of pneumonia, gall bladder surgery, and hip replacement twice—once at the age of 15 and again three years later as the result of complications from a fall.

Ms. J. reports that because of the unpredictability of the condition, coupled with frequent hospitalizations, maintaining full-time employment and completing her education have been thwarted. She reports that she attempted to obtain degrees from a junior college and a business school; however, on both occasions, her education was interupted by hospitalizations, and school personnel were unsympathetic.

Because of Ms. J's physical condition, her employment situation, and the baby, she lives at home with her parents. Her child seems to give her emotional and moral drive, but she is concerned about her daughter's well-being when she is forced to go to the hospital as a result of a crisis.

Throughout her life, Ms. J.'s parents have been supportive. They assume full responsibility for Ms. J.'s daughter when she is hospitalized and have assured her of their willingness to rear her daughter were Ms. J. to die (Battle, 1982).

This case raises many difficult and complex issues. First, from a medical perspective, it is especially ill-advised for adolescents to bear children because of the additional risks attendant to their pregnancy. Second, because of the severe and chronic nature of the pain experienced, youths with sickle cell anemia are at especially high risk for drug addiction. The health care provider needs to walk a fine line between providing relief of pain and creating a second debilitating condition on top of an already complex problem.

Third, the case raises issues regarding parent-child relationships. While Ms. J.'s parents appear to be committed to both their daughter and their grandchild, one wonders about the outcome if this were not the case. What if they were not willing to put her interests and needs above their own? Certainly, the physical and psychological prognosis would be much worse.

Mr. F. was first hospitalized at age seven months as a result of developing pneumonia. It was then that physicians discovered that he had sickle cell anemia.

Five years ago, Mr. F.'s sister died as a result of sickle cell anemia. She was 20 years of age. Mr. F. is 30, and he lives at home with his parents. Over the years, Mr. F.'s parents have become experts on sickle cell anemia. They have faced numerous crises and death, yet remain very close-knit.

Like many others with sickle cell anemia in his age group, he is unemployed. He reports no vocational aspirations, neither does he want a family, for he feels he could not sustain the responsibility.

Mr. F talks only with difficulty about his physical condition, preferring to keep it a secret whenever possible. His parents, on the other hand, feel he should be more open; this has been the subject of family conflict in the past.

Mr. F. desires neither special treatment nor privileges because of having sickle cell anemia, nor does he use his condition as an excuse. Yet he still wonders why he has the disease. When he was younger, he believed that he was being punished.

Mr. F.'s parents recall his infancy as filled with constant medical problems and recurrent expenses. It was only their faith that sustained them. The school years were marked by numerous absences and, thus, for his parents, many days of work lost (Battle, 1982).

It is very difficult to isolate in concrete terms how parents cope with the emotional and physical demands of having a child with sickle cell anemia. Developmentally, from the time of onset, parents may be defensive. The actual birth of the child is a crisis. As a result of the child's physical condition, the parents will not only assume the role of caretaker, but hopefully, will also encourage the child to achieve his or her developmental goals. While children will benefit from these situations they may place severe pressure on the parent or parents. Children with sickle cell disease are likely to experience difficulty in attaining the developmental tasks of early infancy, especially the task of developing basic trust (Whitten, 1974). Sickle cell anemia precludes a successful, early stage of development between parent and baby. The parents are placed in a position of adjustment and readjustment at each stage of development (infancy, childhood, adolescence, and adulthood).

Sickle cell anemia can interfere with the development of healthy siblings as well. Parents may compare their unaffected child with the affected child, and as a result, the child who has the disease may be the recipient of more attention and direct care. Parents may worry less about the child who is physically normal.

Patients with sickle cell anemia are dependent on parents and siblings for emotional support. The family appears to be the primary source of emotional stability. Peer relationships do not assume the same level of significance as they do with healthy adolescents (Battle, 1980).

Parents of children with sickle cell anemia frequently assume the role of advocate for their child, consequently they may be viewed as hostile and defensive. These parents do not want pity for their child but appropriate care and treatment (Battle, 1982).

Perceptions, Adjustment, and Coping of Sickle Cell Patients

In a recent study the perceptions of adult sickle cell anemia patients were examined within an age range of 18–35 (Battle, 1982). The population consisted of 44 black men and women with sickle cell anemia. There were a total of 27 females and 17 males with a median age of 26 years. The study attempted to ascertain perceptions of sickle cell anemia patients

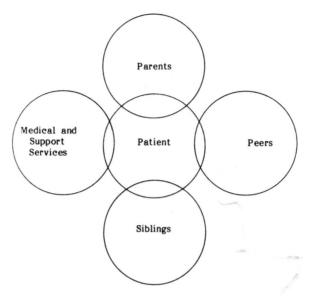

Figure 15-1.   Patient support network.

with regard to the nature and condition of their illness. The questions
focused on perceptions of physical condition, adjustment to crisis and
intercedent periods of illness, and coping mechanisms. Special interest
was directed toward use of sick role, use of denial, feelings of dependency,
future perceptions, role of patient within family, and self-identity.

The patient with sickle cell anemia depends on an immediate support
network (see Fig. 15-1). This network is essential to the emotional stability
of the patient; it can be viewed as a lifeline of support.

Physical characteristics of respondents varied depending on disease
complications. Several patients had strokes or leg ulcers, and several appeared healthy, which frequently is a characteristic of sickle cell anemia.

Employment

As a result of the various complications of the disease, some patients
suffered more physical pain, and others experienced greater emotional
stress. Patients expressed concern over the effect of sickle cell anemia
on their employment status, health, and financial well-being. Essentially,
all respondents who were employed were concerned that sickle cell anemia
could cause them to lose their jobs. Because of employment problems,
patients may be forced to rely on their family members for financial support. Only 15.9 percent of the respondents were employed. Of those who
were unemployed, 84.1 percent perceived sickle cell anemia as the cause
of their unemployment status. Based on data from the United States De-

partment of Labor's Commerce Bureau in 1978, unemployment for black males ranged from 10.6 percent between the ages of 25 and 34 to 37.0 percent between the ages of 16 and 19. For black females between the ages of 25 and 34, 12.9 percent were unemployed. The highest percentage was found in black women between 16 and 19 in which it was 39.9 percent. Clearly, the unemployment rates among black men and women were high. The question is whether the high rate of unemployment in this sample was attributed to race of the respondents, the disease, or both.

Family Coping

In the study population, family members generally shared the responsibility of caring for the family member with sickle cell anemia. This factor probably helped promote higher levels of adjustment in these patients and among family members. Family members and patients appeared to react to hardship with optimism, which appeared to be ingrained in their philosophy of life. Feelings of apprehension are often heightened or aroused during a sickle cell anemia crisis, but patients perceived their physical condition as good between crises. They felt they could function adequately with restrictions.

It became apparent that family members found strength in concentrating on more positive outcomes. For instance, patients and parents were strengthened in their ability to cope by the awareness of other patients who experienced greater pain or were disabled in some way as a result of the disorder. When patients and family members went to the hospital, they often reported being distracted from the negative aspects of their own situation by observing those who were worse off.

Patient Knowledge and Concerns

Respondents possessed good knowledge of their physical condition and a basic understanding of morphological principles associated with sickle cell anemia. Their primary concerns were with the effects of sickle cell anemia on their health. Generally, the areas in which they reported less concern included loss of friends, disruption of home life, disruption of self-respect, and shame regarding their physical appearance.

Respondents did not want pity or appear to demand excessive care either during or between crises. Overall, respondents rejected the notion of a sick role, despite the fact that many normal adult roles—breadwinner, parent, husband or wife—were seen to be unavailable to those with sickle cell disease. Despite these limitations, most respondents did not perceive their illness as serious. Parents and family generally tried to assist the affected family member in developing a reasonable outlook on the actual limitations of his or her condition.

The Role of Denial

The respondents' perceived primary method of coping appeared to be denial, which was viewed as defensive. Respondents wished to project an image of strength and to be viewed as normal, functioning individuals. They saw themselves as independent individuals and appeared proud when they could care for themselves. There was little acknowledgment of dependence on others, even during crises. Perhaps autonomy needs are met as much by the assertion of autonomy as by the reality.

Respondents felt they were a very important part of their family (84 percent) in areas of decision making and in providing the moral support they could. They felt it was important for them to participate in all aspects of family life. Only 18 percent of them indicated that they experienced unhappiness, rejection from peers, and a lack of self-reliance at any time.

Patients were extremely optimistic about the future. Whether employed or unemployed, respondents felt that their chances of continuing employment or securing employment were extremely high. They did not acknowledge concern about death; their concern was for a more complete and prosperous future. A degree of optimism, coupled with defensive denial, appeared to be the dynamic that allowed these adult sickle cell patients to persist in the face of overwhelmingly negative odds.

Adjustment Characteristics in Family Members and Patients

It is clear that the family plays a major role in assisting the family member who is affected with sickle cell anemia to adjust to his or her physical condition. Generally, families rely on extended family member relationships as well as deep religious ties as a means of coping with the stress of the disease.

It is difficult to present absolute adjustment characteristics utilized by family members and patients, primarily because of differences among and between people concerning values and generational differences. Family members are faced with uneven medical care, isolation, and uncertainty. Frequently, the mother takes the responsibility for supervising the care of the child with sickle cell anemia. The father has a greater tendency to avoid contributing to the child's direct care. It is not uncommon for the parent who is providing the majority of care to experience severe depression because of inadequate support and isolation from her spouse. The need to be sensitive to families' needs psychologically, socially, and emotionally is critical. Added to the emotional trauma and guilt of having a child with a hereditary disease is resentment over sickle cell anemia being a problem that primarily affects blacks (Anionwu & Beattie, 1981).

Undoubtedly, among family members, the mothers of sickle cell anemia patients have the greatest burden to bear; if support is provided by spouse, physician, and appropriate helping professionals, some of the stress may be reduced. With an adequate support system, the mother can confront her anxieties and more effectively handle the illness of the child. Real optimism, understanding of sickle cell anemia, and a support system are important factors in adjustment. According to Tropouer, Franz, and Dilgard (1970), the absence of obvious signs or complaints of emotional distress does not imply that the child or the parents are not experiencing emotional distress. Unexpressed feelings of anxiety, hostility, and despair can evolve into serious behavior patterns that can prevent the development of a normal treatment process and healthy supports between the patient and parents. When the presence of depression, guilt, rejection, denial or illness, or chronic behavioral disturbances in a patient or parent impairs therapeutic effectiveness, appropriate psychiatric consultation should be considered.

Parents and family members who are not emotionally supportive of one another will suffer greater difficulty in adjusting to the illness. In such an environment, family members affected by the strain may derive emotional support from sources outside the family, such as parent groups (through the Sickle Cell Society), religious, and counseling agencies.

Parents who are under stress may intensify their child's difficulties in coping. The parents' ability to adjust is closely linked to the child's ability to improve physically and develop normally.

Because sickle cell anemia is a chronic and progressive disorder with diverse manifestations, parents must be educated to deal with its effects. Children can suffer from subjective experiences of victimization and vulnerability, which may alter their attitude and hinder interpersonal relationships with their parents.

Parents who have children with sickle cell anemia seem to rely on interfamily relationships, and the disorder appears to generate a level of family privacy. The family responds to crises and hardships as a family unit. Comprehensive sickle cell programs and clincis are most helpful in providing educational and supportive counseling services. Parents seem to cope better with the responsibilities of caring for their child if they support one another emotionally. Overall, the ability of parents and family members to cope with the disease is linked to the severity of the affected child's condition.

CONCLUSION

Sickle cell disease is a complex hemoglobinopathy that stresses both individual and family resources. Frequent hospitalizations are a hallmark of the condition, as are exceedingly painful crises. Most children with the disease are diagnosed early and, because of their medical needs, are highly dependent upon the health care delivery system. As medical therapies for this condition improve, so does longevity. While there is evidence that those with sickle cell disease lag behind their healthy peers developmentally, this need not be the case. Through an integrated approach, in which the health care team works closely with the school personnel and the family, healthy adolescent development is a realistic goal.

REFERENCES

Anionwu, E., & Beattie, A. Learning to cope with sickle cell disease, a parent's experience. *Nursing Times*, 1981, *28*, 1214–1219.

Battle, S. *Psychosocial perspectives of sickle cell anemia patients*. Chicago: Eterna Press, 1982.

Diggs, L.W. Sickle cell crisis. *American Journal of Clinical Pathology*, 1965, *44*, 1–11.

Fischoff, J., & Whitten, C. Psychological effects of sickle cell disease. *Archives of Internal Medicine*, 1974, *133*, 681–689.

Flanagan, D. Home management of sickle cell anemia. *Pediatric Nursing*, 1980, *6*(2), A–D.

Frydman, M. Perception of illness severity and psychiatric symptoms in parents of chronically ill children. *Journal of Psychosomatic Research*, 1980, *24*, 361–369.

Morin, E., & Waring E. Depression and sickle cell anemia. *Southern Medical Journal*, 1981, *74*(6), 766–768.

Phillips, J. Mental health and sickle cell anemia—A psychosocial approach. *Urban Health*, 1973, *2*(6), 36–39.

Scott, R.B., & Kessler, A.D. A child with sickle cell anemia in your class(room). Washington, D.C.: Department of Pediatrics and child health, Howard University College of Medicine, 1967.

Tropouer, A., Franz, M.N., & Dilgard, V.W. Psychological aspects of the care of children with cystic fibrosis. *American Journal of Disabled Children*, 1970, *119*, 424–432.

White, J. Screening programs for sickle cell disease. *Social Work*, 1974, *19*, 273–277.

Whitten, C., & Fischoff, J. Psychosocial effects of sickle cell disease. *Archives of Internal Medicine*, 1974, *133*, 386–391.

Wintrobe, M.M. Hemoglobinopathies and associated diseases. In *Clinical hematology*, (7th ed.). Philadelphia: Lea & Febiger, 1974.

Samuel LeBaron
Donald Currie
Lonnie Zeltzer

16

Coping With Spinal Cord Injury in Adolescents

Adolescence is a period of high risk for spinal cord injuries. In a sample population of 6000 such injuries (Young, Burns, Bowe, & McCutchen, 1982), approximately one third occurred during adolescence (see Table 16-1). The health care needs of youths combined with the special needs of any spinal cord—injured person, present a unique challenge to health care providers.

A spinal cord injury results in a dramatic transformation in the affected individual's life, regardless of age. In the period immediately following the injury a profound loss of function occurs as the patient is physically removed from familiar surroundings and moved to a hospital, where an entirely new world must be explored and assimilated. The duration of initial hospitalization ranges from only a few weeks to almost a year, with a median hospitalization of four months (Fig. 16-1).

Health care providers, such as physicians, nurses, rehabilitation therapists, psychologists, and social workers, are faced with an overwhelming array of complex problems in the treatment and management of these individuals. Spinal cord injured patients and their families must encounter and try to assimilate so much new information that they may react with apathy, depression, anger, or rebellion in order to cope. Still, decisions must eventually be made; there are many new problems to solve, including how to deal with increased financial burdens, home care for the injured family member, and his or her education.

Effects of the prolonged initial hospitalization are profound on some patients. Immobility and institutionalization have both been associated

Table 16-1
Age at Injury for Sample of Spinal Cord–Injured Patients (N = 6012)

Age	Frequency	Cumulative frequency	N
1–5	0.6	0.6	34
6–10	0.8	1.3	47
11–15	4.6	5.9	275
16–20	28.3	34.2	1699
21–25	21.5	55.7	1295
26–30	12.6	68.3	759
31–35	7.8	76.2	471
36–40	5.8	82.0	347
41–45	4.6	86.6	277
46–50	3.7	90.3	225
51–55	3.0	93.3	182
56–60	2.2	95.6	134
61–70	3.1	98.6	184
71–88	1.4	100.0	83

Data derived from Young, J.S., Burns, P.E., Bowen, A.M., & McCutchen, R. *Spinal Cord Injury Statistics,* 1982. These data presented with permission of the copyright owner, Good Samaritan Medical Center, Phoenix, Arizona.

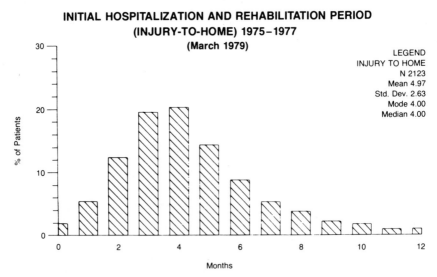

Figure 16-1. Median duration of initial hospitalization ranges from a few weeks to several months. (Data from Young, J. S., & Northup, N. E. (R. McCutchen, Ed.). *Statistical information pertaining to some of the most commonly asked questions about SCI.* Phoenix, Arizona: Good Samaritan Medical Center, 1979. With permission.)

with episodes of paranoia, panic, depression, disorientation, temporary diminution of cognitive function, and hallucinations (Wilson, 1972). Reviews and discussions of research related to sensory deprivation may be found in Zubek (1969).

Because the cost of hospitalization and treatment of spinal cord injuries is so high, it is imperative that health care systems be used in the most cost-effective manner. Young et al. (1982) presented estimates of annual charges for the initial hospitalization—based on 1981 figures—that ranged from $38,000 to $75,300, depending on the degree of disability. At that time, those authors also estimated that ongoing annual medical charges for hospitalization would range from $2,800 to $7,200.

The amount of physical assistance that spinal cord–impaired patients need throughout the years adds an additional financial and human burden to many families. Table 16-2 shows the percentage of cases by neurological category that required assistance in one large sample (Young, et al., 1982). Approximately one fourth of paraplegics and three fourths of quadriplegics required daily assistance; quadriplegics generally required assistance for twice as many hours daily as did paraplegics.

Since many spinal cord—injury patients are adolescents who have not yet finished their education or job training, considerable effort must be expanded to provide the support necessary to allow these patients to complete their education. Young et al. (1982) found that approximately three fourths of all spinal cord injuries occurred in individuals with a high school education or less. Many of these individuals cannot prepare for

Table 16-2
Physical Assistance Required Per Day in Follow-Up Years.

Neurological category	Cases requiring assistance	Mean hours/day	Median hours/day
Paraplegic			
Incomplete	16	3.3	1.9
Complete	28	3.1	1.9
All	23	3.1	1.9
Quadriplegic			
Incomplete	61	5.7	3.9
Complete	93	6.7	4.6
All	75	6.3	4.3
All cases:	50	5.6	3.7

Data derived from Young, J.S., Burns, P.E., Bowen, A.M., & McCutchen, R., *Spinal Cord Injury Statistics*, 1982. These data presented with permission of the copyright owner, Good Samaritan Medical Center, Phoenix, Arizona.

technical or professional employment unless they receive assistance in gaining access to educational resources.

Given the enormous medical, financial, and human resources that must be committed to the care of each spinal cord–injured adolescent, it seems only logical to pay particular attention to the one factor that will determine whether those resources are used in a cost-effective manner: the psychological adjustment of the spinal cord injured patient. A patient who is angry and overwhelmed by too much new information, or who feels that most decisions are made for him or her, is much less likely to comply with regimens for rehabilitation and management than is a patient who is able to organize and cope with new information and is given support in achieving early independence. The psychological aspects of spinal cord injury must be understood because they constitute an essential element of comprehensive health care, and they provide part of the basis for cost-effective medical treatment (Abramson, 1967; Roberts, 1972).

PSYCHOLOGICAL REACTIONS OF SPINAL CORD– INJURED PATIENTS AND THEIR FAMILIES

The Patient: A Personal Description

T.A. is a 17-year-old adolescent who has been a quadriplegic since she was involved in an automobile accident 18 months ago. Her loss of mobility and independence was compounded by the fact that she was a star athlete in her high school. Her life in the year and a half since her accident has been focused on medical management of her numerous physical problems. As her physical status has become more stable, T.A. has begun to express feelings of anger and hopelessness. However, a few of her physicians and therapists have helped her to persist in her efforts toward rehabilitation. One day, T.A. reflected upon some of her experiences:

I've thought a lot about what's helped me the most since the accident. It's all in one word: support. What does that mean? It's feeling that other people are standing behind me. I feel like there are only a few people who have stood behind me during all this time. They picked me up when I was down and gave me moral support. They never gave up, no matter how bad everything was. Some people gave me lectures. I really hate getting lectures. When people give me lectures I just ignore them. But if a doctor is trying to understand how I feel about something instead of lecturing, then I feel like I can have a conversation with him, and sometimes I come out learning something. You need to know people care.

Reaction Stages of Adolescents With Spinal Cord Injuries

Many clinicians who work with spinal cord–injured patients have noted a number of common features in their psychological reactions (Abramson, 1971). Various stages of adjustment may be observed in patients with spinal cord injuries (Fig. 16-2). Passage through the stages, the order in which they are experienced, and the duration of each stage varies widely among different individuals. One important determinant of the adolescent's passage through the various stages is his or her degree of physical, emotional, and cognitive development (Zager & Marquette, 1981). Indeed, these stages should not be viewed as a sequence to which patients need necessarily conform; rather, the progression of psychological adjustment should be viewed as a hypothetical construct that may help the clinician organize continuing observations of a given patient. Some clinicians have noted a progression of reactions, such as denial, despair, and grieving, followed by acceptance (Geller & Greydanus, 1979). As Figure 16-2 suggests, many clinicians observe patients responding to the initial crisis of a spinal cord injury with depression, hostility, a disturbed body identity, and a slowing of mental processes. Resolution of these problems can take months or years.

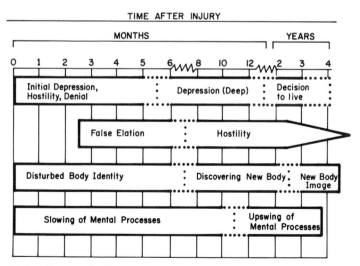

PSYCHOLOGICAL CHANGES AFTER
SPINAL CORD INJURY

Figure 16-2.   Stages of adjustment that may occur following a spinal cord injury.

The adolescent's reactions often include anger, both at the loss of function and at family and health care providers whose mobility and good health are bitter reminders of the adolescent patient's own physical limitations. For example, as one therapist left the hospital room of a quadriplegic adolescent after a friendly conversation, the patient called out "good night" in what sounded like an irritated tone. The therapist returned to the room and asked the adolescent if his tone of voice meant he was angry. The adolescent replied, "I was feeling so good visiting with you, but then when you were going, I thought of how you can go home to your family, or go anywhere you want whenever you want. I'm just stuck here, and it doesn't seem fair."

For some patients the spinal cord injury may seem to be a punishment. Not only is the patient confined and restricted from many pleasurable activities, but there are also numerous unpleasant events to which he or she is subjected, ranging from medical tests and surgery to an almost total loss of privacy and control. Adolescents who are obliged to depend on others to take care of their urine and bowel programs may feel as if they are forced to regress to an infantile dependency. This reaction is especially likely when parents assume the role of caring for all of the patient's personal hygiene.

Although the patient may express hostility by speaking angrily to the health care staff and family members or may show signs of depression by diminished speech, sleep, or appetite, these problems are manifested in other ways as well. Noncompliance may be a reflection of either hostility or depression. The adolescent who feels unable to participate in self-care often perceives noncompliance as a means for striking out at the world or for exercising some control. Physicians and nurses often try to "talk some sense into the patient's head" to no avail. If noncompliance is seen by health care providers as a challenge to overcome, the result is likely to become an escalating power struggle. During this period of denial, anger, or depression, those who care for the adolescent must be willing to tolerate these emotional storms, show kindness and consideration, and continue to manage the patient as well as possible. When the patient eventually accepts the reality of the condition, the staff will meet with more cooperation and participation from the patient in the rehabilitation process (Knorr & Bull, 1970).

Another reason for noncompliance is that much of the education for self-care and rehabilitation occurs simultaneously with a bombardment of unusual stimuli and new information. Rehabilitation is like going to school and attending many different courses; the patient is receiving verbal instruction in prevention and management of pressure ulcers of the skin, bladder management, wheelchair mobility, making transfers, equipment care and management, and new ways to carry out such activities of daily living as eating, dressing, personal hygiene skills, writing, and using a telephone. Usually, this information is presented in a piecemeal rather than an integrated sequence, which if utilized might enhance learning. Fragmented teaching makes learning and subsequent compliance more difficult to achieve. It is difficult for the patient to review and receive prompt feedback about his or her performance or intake of knowledge. An additional difficulty occurs when patients are depressed and do not care about self-rehabilitation. For example, even if patients are shown photographs of severe decubitus ulcers during their educational program, they cannot feel their skin and, thus, it is easy for them to think "that can't happen to me," since they have never had one. While such denial is a normal phase of adolescent development—Elkind (1976) calls it the "personal fable of immunity"—its consequences for the disabled may be life threatening. These patients may not care much whether they develop pressure sores if they feel as though life is not worth living from a wheel-chair. Noncompliance is usually based on more than one factor. It is important to identify the sources of noncompliance for any given patient in order to provide the best care possible.

Management of the adolescent with a spinal cord injury can be enhanced by sensitivity to the fact that the patient has very little choice about what is done and needs to reestablish control over aspects of his or her life. By first presenting only those tasks that are easily accomplished, one provides the adolescent with an opportunity to experience early success and to reestablish much needed control.

The patient at highest risk for serious problems is the one who has learned to hide any anger or depression he or she might be experiencing, for fear of increased "punishment," e.g., more examinations, lectures from the medical staff or family, medication, hospitalization, or restrictions.

Patients may react in this manner because they have always had difficulty in expressing anger. On the other hand, staff or family members may have unintentionally rejected them for expressing their feelings and thoughts honestly or rewarded them for wearing the pleasant mask of the "good patient." In any case, the patient who is unable or unwilling to express feelings of anger or despair should be considered at high risk for depression, noncompliance, or potentially, suicide. Adolescents who initially appear angry and uncooperative may later adjust well. The physician and other caretakers can facilitate the adjustment by allowing patients to express their anger and depression whenever they are ready. Such patience on the part of the physician is difficult because disabled teenagers are constant reminders of both human frailty and physician limitations in effecting cures.

Disturbed Body Identity and Slowing of Mental Processes

A spinal cord injury results in a variety of sensory deprivations (Harris, Patel, Greer, & Naughton, 1973). There is usually a loss of somesthetic perception and some loss of ability to interact somesthetically with the environment as well. During hospitalization, the patient is deprived of a varied, natural environment and is forced to exist (often for long periods) in a relatively unstimulating environment. This experience may result in a temporary decrement in judgment or cognitive abilities. Some patients may experience hallucinations. Spatial orientation may also decline with prolonged hospitalization, and some patients experience their bodies as foreign, useless, or repugnant (Zubek, 1964, 1969; Wilson, 1972). Management of hospitalized patients should include sensory stimulation from multiple sources, such as regular, brief conversations between the patient and the caretaker, and from radio or television.

External stimulation need not be a time-consuming venture. One example is of a depressed spinal cord–injured adolescent who had remained isolated in his room, refusing social contact for several days. His thinking and behavior gradually showed increased evidence of impaired perception and judgment. The process was reversed when a psychologist visited him for regular brief periods and simply held comic books up for him to see while the visitor read aloud. Many patients have expressed appreciation for a touch on an area of the body that still has sensation, such as the shoulder, face, or head.

Another serious concern relating to mental processes in spinal cord–injured patients is the possibility of brain damage. In one large sample (Young, et al., 1982) approximately 80 percent of the adolescents had sustained their spinal injury in a situation frequently associated with significant head trauma (e.g., automobile accidents, sports injuries, or falling objects). Even if abnormal neurological findings are absent in these patients, the possibility must be considered that the patient may have sustained mild brain injury resulting in sensory or perceptual sequelae, behavioral changes, or deficits in cognitive abilities (Boll, 1983; Klonoff, Low, & Clark, 1977). When such deficits are suspected, patients can be referred for formal neuropsychological testing; however, the range of useful tests is limited if the uppper extremities are paralyzed.

As Figure 16-2 suggests, patients may experience various combinations of mood and cognitive functioning. The actual progression of psychological adjustment is unpredictable and unique in each patient. It is important to note the various and sometimes contradictory responses in each youth. Many patients can be expected to require between two and four years before they begin to experience a sense of stability, identity, and readiness to actively seek a new role in society.

Interference With Normal Development

Human beings have the capacity for development throughout their entire life span; however, the rapid psychological and physical maturation that normally occurs during adolescence renders the sequelae of spinal cord injury unique for patients of this age group. The understanding of the accident and resulting injury will vary according to the level of the patient's pretrauma cognitive and emotional development. For example, the events may be perceived as magical for younger patients (e.g., "This injury is my punishment for thinking bad thoughts about my little brother"), and quite rational for older patients (e.g., "I have this injury because I wasn't careful"). Furthermore, the patient's need to be independent rather than dependent should be taken into consideration as the health care team formulates a discharge and rehabilitation plan.

Coping With a Spinal Cord Injury

Some of the factors that influence the adolescent's adjustment and ability to cope with a spinal cord injury are as follows (Knorr & Bull, 1970; Roberts, 1972; Zager & Marquette, 1981):

1. Neurological level and completeness of the spinal cord injury
2. Extent and severity of other physical injuries
3. Occurrence of additional complications
4. Pretrauma personality (e.g., degree of intelligence, impulsiveness, and adjustment to normal conflicts and stress)
5. Stage of physical, social, and emotional development
6. Educational level prior to the injury
7. Extent of emotional support available to the patient from family, staff, and friends

Patients who are perceived as fighters may be difficult in the early phases because they appear to the staff to be "pigheaded," obstinate, stubborn, and generally difficult to take care of. On the other hand, it is these same people who appear to cope best over the long term. The positive aspects of those qualities include perseverance and determination, which help the patient to keep going and to take risks of failing. The "model" patient is often one who maintains an acceptable appearance while unexpressed needs and feelings remain buried. In the long run, this type of patient often has trouble reintegrating into society. Other factors that appear to play an important role in a patient's psychological recovery from a spinal cord injury are intelligence and degree of family support. Support from a family includes not only sympathetic acceptance of the patient's problems, but also firm encouragement and a gentle push into attempting to meet appropriate goals.

REACTIONS OF HEALTH CARE PROVIDERS TO THE
SPINAL CORD–INJURED ADOLESCENT

The Health Care Provider

The rehabilitation personnel can provide valuable support by making honest, accurate information available to the adolescent patient as soon as it is requested. Failure to provide accurate information at the patient's request may prolong unrealistic expectations and hinder the process of grieving (Geller & Greydanus, 1979; Roberts, 1972). This does not imply that the physician and other staff members should not be optimistic; however, the optimism should reflect an accurate awareness of the adolescent's strengths and realistic views of the progress he or she can expect to make in rehabilitation.

The necessity for tolerance and support from the staff is obvious. Unfortunately, most medical center staff members are overburdened with responsibilities. While caring for an adolescent who appreciates support and responds gratefully is rewarding to staff members, treatment of an unresponsive, unappreciative adolescent may feel burdensome.

Those who provide care for the spinal cord–injured adolescent are reminded of the vulnerability of their own bodies and of the uncertainty of life. They may experience a mixture of reactions toward their patient, including anxiety, anger, avoidance, and denial that such a disaster could befall them. While working to help the adolescent patient cope with his or her feelings, the physicians, nurses, psychologists, and other professionals must work equally hard to examine and understand their own reactions (Geller & Greydanus, 1979).

An effort must be made to see the patient in the context of a lifespan, which includes the patient's history and potential for future development. Physicians and hospital staff often see teenagers with spinal cord injuries at their worst, when the patient is still struggling to cope with confusion, anger, loss resulting from the injury, and feelings of helplessness about the future. Unlike adults who may have a variety of well-established skills and close relationships from which they can draw comfort, many adolescents lack well-developed sources of support beyond their immediate family. It is precisely that close bond to the family that most adolescents have been working to sever. Health care professionals may have an image of the spinal cord–injured adolescent as an individual who is incapable of school, work, satisfactory social and sexual relationships, or even accepting the reality of the injury. Such professionals often face the spinal cord–injured adolescent with a show of cheerful optimism and jaunty reassurance. Knorr and Bull (1970) noted that ''it is not unusual to find that patient denial is supported by the staff immediately after injury to avoid the patient becoming overwhelmed with anxiety. This may lead to later distrust of the medical staff who, he feels, was not honest with him." Many spinal cord–injured adolescents describe how they learned to shut off their tears and keep strong feelings to themselves because they resented hearing from doctors and nurses such phrases as "I understand what you're going through" or "Come on, cheer up." What most injured adolescents want is a careful listener. One of the best ways to show genuine interest is to sit down while visiting the patient. This simple action tells the patient that the visitor is not in a hurry to leave. This also permits the patient and his visitor to be at the same eye level rather than for the visitor to be towering over the recumbent patient. One spinal cord injured patient put it this way:

I don't believe people when they say they care for me, but I can tell from their behavior whether they do or not. I can see it in the looks on their faces, and the way they listen shows how much they care. There was one doctor who came to see me when I was in the hospital who seemed to paste a smile on his face. His smile seemed to just represent a "doctor–patient relationship" but behind the smile he still seemed to have a cold look on his face. He asked me a lot of questions and I felt like he was prying. There are different ways of asking the same question that can make me feel like a doctor is or isn't prying. It's not the question that makes me feel like someone is prying; it's the way it's asked. This same doctor who seemed to paint a smile on his face frightened me. He would come into the room each time, and he would introduce himself and wouldn't give us a chance to get to know each other. He would just go about his business, asking questions and finding out what he needed to find out. He should have been able to learn a lot from my silence but he kept pressuring me when I was silent, and that made me feel even more like he was prying. When I was ready to be discharged from the hospital, he suddenly became very nice, and he seemed more genuine, and it made me wonder if maybe he didn't feel like he had to be my doctor anymore, and suddenly he seemed to become more relaxed and warm.

With most doctors there is seldom a chance to go outside of the usual doctor–patient relationship and get to know each other as people, but maybe most doctors don't have time. If a doctor wants to know me as a person, then I know he really wants to help me and care. I can tell quite quickly if a doctor really cares.

It is helpful for both those who care for spinal cord–injured adolescents and for the recently injured patients themselves to get to know adolescent patients who have graduated from the initial crisis to successful reintegration into society. This firsthand knowledge of the potential development of adolescents with spinal cord injury is important if one is to maintain an attitude that is realistic, but at the same time, optimistic and enthusiastic. By acquiring a realistic view of the patient's potential, the health care provider is better able to help him or her to establish and progress toward appropriate goals. A rehabilitation program that is too permissive and unstructured may be as harmful to the patient's development as one that is rigid and overcontrolling (Abramson, 1967).

Decubitus Ulcers: A Model for Integrating Medical and Psychological Management

The management of spinal cord injury in adolescents demands the simultaneous use of both medical and psychological treatment methods. Medical and psychological problems are inextricably interwoven for these patients, and the best care requires the expertise of a number of different professionals in order to address the great variety of problems and inspire the consistent participation of the patient. The following case illustrates a problem requiring this approach:

A 14-year-old male paraplegic adolescent had sustained complete T-9 paraplegia due to a motor vehicle accident two months previously. He was ready to begin sitting in a wheelchair, but almost immediately began to develop areas of skin irritation over his ischial tuberosities, although induration or frank ulceration had not yet occurred. He was a sociable boy who enjoyed joking with the nurses and visitors, but his joking demeanor barely masked his discouragement and depression regarding his injury. He was uninterested in all aspects of self-care, including skin care and hygiene. It was imperative that ischial pressure be relieved consistently in order to prevent the formation of frank pressure sores. The patient was asked several times to always use his wheelchair cushion while sitting in his wheelchair or any other chair, and to do a wheelchair pushup for 15 seconds every 15 minutes whenever he sat; he agreed to these measures. However, he consistently failed to carry out the instructions and frank ischial ulcers began to develop. The resident physicians and nursing staff became more impatient and angry and eventually began to avoid the patient.

One of the most common medical problems for spinal cord–injured patients is decubitus ulcers. Medical treatment of the condition involves bed rest if the ulceration is on the buttocks. Bed rest is necessary if the ulcer is to heal without surgery; often, however, this fails and plastic surgery followed by a minimum of three weeks in the prone position is required to allow the ulcer to heal sufficiently for the patient to sit again. The cost of hospitalization and doctor fees for treating decubitus ulcers can average $15,000 per ulcer—a costly problem both financially and personally, since it requires the patient to be removed from his or her routine life-style for a period of several weeks or even months.

The key to successfully managing decubitus ulcers is prevention. Beginning in the intensive care unit, measures must be taken to prevent their occurrence by provding proper pressure relief and rotation of pressure-bearing surfaces. However, prevention involves much more than mechanical manipulation. Patients must be educated in methods of leaning on the armrest of their wheelchair or, if strong enough, doing pushups out of the chair. In addition, the individual's motivation for participating in self-care must be evaluated, with particular attention paid to factors that could result in noncompliance. Some patients respond well to mechanical reminders, such as an inexpensive beeper that sounds every 15 minutes or so to remind them to relieve pressure. Others require a more elaborate behavioral plan implemented by the entire health care team. Thus, such an apparent medical problem is, in fact, both medical and behavioral. In spite of the best possible educational efforts regarding prevention of decubitus ulcers, compliance among adolescents with spinal cord injury is reported by many clinicians to be poor. Unfortunately, this new set of tasks is presented just at a time when the patient is likely to feel depressed and disorganized.

If the approach to spinal cord injury does not include a team concept, patients often do not initially receive the right equipment, the proper cushion, or the correct wheelchair adjustment for optimal pressure distribution. It is not unusual for preventive measures to fail in the intensive care unit, with the result that patients develop decubitus ulcers before they even get their first chance to sit. In the midst of acute medical lifesaving activities in the early stages after injury, when the patient, staff, and family are overwhelmed by other problems, decubitis ulcers tend not to command sufficient emphasis in patient education.

Developing a Problem List

The number and variety of mechanical, medical, psychological, and interpersonal problems involved in the care of spinal cord–injured patients may appear overwhelming to health care professionals, patients, and families alike. Many physicians have found it helpful to develop a problem list, which may be similar for all spinal cord–injured adolescents, but which can be individualized for each patient (see Table 16-3). An outline of function versus level of injury provides a useful supplement to the problem list (see Table 16-4).

Use of a problem list can assist the health care team not only in treating the injury but also in preventing those iatrogenic problems that result from not considering all of the potential problems sufficiently early. From a behavioral perspective, there is a variety of adaptations that encourage positive psychological readjustment. These include motor skills training and the use of transportation, self-care (such as eating, hygiene, and dressing), writing, using a telephone, and involvement in school, work, recreation, and social relationships.

Table 16-3
Problem List for Adolescents With Spinal Cord Injuries

Assess level of lesion and fracture
    Stability or instability of spinal fracture
    Spinal cord versus spinal nerve root damage
    Estimate prognosis*
    Assess sensory loss

Prevent further decrease in mobility
    Prevent contractures
    Encourage ambulation or standing
    Consider possibility of driving

Encourage maintainance of upper extremity function (use of mouthsticks for very high quadriplegia)
    Feeding
    Writing
    Dressing
    Personal hygiene
    Pushing wheelchair
    Using crutches
    Using telephone

Assess psychological stress
    Assess strength of patient
    Assess strength of support system
    Assist psychological adjustment of patient and family

Assess educational needs
    Carry out prevocational evaluation
    Provide counseling

Preventive management of skin problems and sores
    Medical management
    Education and behavioral reinforcement for proper care

Assessment and treatment of
    Spinal stability; scoliosis is much more frequent in adolesents than in adults with spinal cord injuries (Lancourt, Dickson, & Carter, 1981)
    Pulmonary dysfunction
    Prevention or treatment of deep venous thrombosis and pulmonary embolism
    Prevention or treatment of heterotopic ossification
    Neurogenic bowel dysfunction
    Neurogenic bladder dysfunction
    Sexual dysfunction
    Spasticity
    Prevention and treatment of joint and muscle contractions and deformities
    Osteoporosis and pathological fractures
    Orthostatic hypotension
    Autonomic hyperreflexia
    Pain
    Assessment of architectural barriers in patient's everyday life
    Assess development of social skills and facilitae social reintegration, including sexual function and sexuality

*See Table 4: Functional Expectations.

Table 16-4
Functional Expectations at Different Segmental Levels

	C-1-C-4	C-5	C-6	C-7	C-8-T-6	T-7-L-1	L-2-L-4	L-5-S-1	S-2-S-4
Walking (* = Crutches & braces)	–	–	–	–	–	*	*	*	+
Push wheelchair	–	±	±	+	+	+	+	+ or NA	NA
Transfers	–	–	±	±	+	+	+	+ or NA	NA
(Drive powered wheelchair)	±	+	+	+	+ or NA	+ or NA	NA	NA	NA
Drive car	–	–	±	±	+	+	+	+	+
Public transportation (* = Special)	*	*	*	*	*	*	* or +	+	+
Bed mobility	–	–	±	+	+	+	+	+	+
Feed self (* = Hand orthoses)	–	*	*	+	+	+	+	+	+
Kitchen independence	–	–	–	±	+	+	+	+	+
Dress self	–	–	–	±	±	+	+	+	+
Bathe & toilet	–	–	–	±	±	+	+	+	+
Writing, typing, telephone (* = Special adaptations)	*	*	* or +	+	+	+	+	+	+
Competitive employment	±	±	±	±	±	±	±	±	±

Adapted from Donovan, W. H., & Bedbrook, G. Comprehensive management of spinal cord injury. *CIBA Clinical Symposia* 1982, *34*(2). With permission.

Most of the problems listed in Table 16-3 require treatment combining medical and psychological components. For example, neurogenic bladder, infection from which was once the most common cause of death in spinal cord–injured patients, requires careful psychological management in addition to the obvious medical aspects of care. The management of urine involves numerous social conventions in nonhandicapped individuals. Dependency on adults for toileting is reminiscent of an infantile stage of development. Even more difficult is the loss of abilities such as eating and dresssing, which are learned very early in life. The loss of these abilities is perceived as a severe regression by the newly dependent teenager, who might prefer to be non–compliant and risk death rather than experience the painful loss of independence and the perceived regression to a more infantile state. Patients often feel dirty and degraded because of the loss of control over their bowel functions. The adolescent male especially may feel that his masculine identity is threatened by the loss of genital privacy. Unfortunately, the adolescent may confuse bowel functions with sexual functions and will assume that sexual relationships will never be possible. Following a spinal injury, patient, family, and friends are faced with the challenge of developing a new set of behaviors.

Paraplegic pain, a syndrome similar to phantom limb pain, is another problem that may require both medical and psychological management. Many patients eventually report a significant diminution of this pain when the health care team responds by focusing as little attention as possible on pain-related behavior, reassuring the patient that the sensations are common, and giving positive reinforcement (i.e., compliments or special privileges) for development of adaptive coping behaviors. More detailed discussion of the behavioral management of pain may be found in the work of Fordyce (1982).

Sexual dysfunction and anxieties regarding sexual capacity are to be expected in spinal cord–injured adolescents, although many of the these patients may be unwilling to consider these issues until others have been successfully mastered. Unfortunately, many health care professionals are reluctant to discuss sexual behavior with spinal cord–injured adolescents, so those teenagers who desire information and assistance pertaining to sexual adjustment may receive an inadequate response. Most women have normal ovulation and menstrual patterns and are capable of becoming pregnant. Reflex erections due to tactile stimulation of the penis occur in most males with intact sacral spinal cord reflexes, even with complete lesions. If a spinal cord–injured male has spasticity in the lower extremities, he usually can have reflex erections. Although ejaculation and seminal emissions usually do not occur in patients with complete lesions, they may occur in about one third of the males with incomplete upper motor neuron lesions. This explains the finding that most spinal cord–injured males are sterile but not impotent. With lower motor neuron lesions (those involving the sacral spinal cord, conus medullaris, or cauda equina), erection is unusual, although dribbling ejaculation may occur (Freed, 1982).

Birth control is complicated by the risk of deep venous thrombosis with oral contraception. An alternative means of birth control should be suggested. The type of birth control usually recommended is an IUD, but it has been criticized because of the risk of uterine perforations or infections, which the patient cannot feel, leading to peritonitis and even death. The use of condoms can help in the avoidance of such problems, although such use is not always within the patient's direct control. The physician must judge how compliant and motivated the patient is to practice birth control. The point to be emphasized is that birth control measures can and should be discussed with spinal cord–injured adolescents who may potentially have sexual involvement. If the female patient wants eventually to have a family she should be assured that she is physiologically competent, but that there will be many practical problems, such as physically taking care of her child, especially while it is an infant.

Approaching spinal cord–injured teenagers about sexuality is usually not difficult once the subject has been raised by the health care provider, but most adolescents will not initiate discussions on the topic. Requesting permission to ask some personal questions and then acknowledging that many people feel awkward discussing personal matters with a stranger is a good way for the health professional to start. It is important to assure the adolescent that personal information will be discussed only with other professionals and that requests to keep information confidential will be honored. The discussion may begin with questions about related, but less emotionally charged subjects such as plans for marriage or a desire to have children. It is important to let the patient ask questions, and to sit quietly for sufficiently long so as to allow him or her the chance to ask the questions being considered.

The four-stage "PLISSIT" (Annon, 1976) model helps one to determine the level of involvement of the sexual counseling process and to decide when referral to a professional psychotherapist is necessary. *P* stands for *permission* to talk about and be inquisitive about sexual matters, such as dating, being attractive although in a wheelchair, having children, and contraception. *LI* stands for *limited information* and usually refers to instruction about sexual function as well as matters of nongenital sexuality. Such instruction may be presented as general information in a group setting. *SS* stands for *specific suggestions* and is usually more individualized. Examples include instructions in what to do about catheters and personal cleanliness. *IT* stands for *intensive therapy*. This level implies a well-trained therapist working intensively with a patient, often for an extended period of time.*

Autonomic hyperreflexia is a syndrome that may occur if there is an intact stump of spinal cord remaining below the T-6 level following injury. This long stump of remaining spinal cord is cut off from the control of higher centers. Input into the stump may persist, particularly visceral input such as a distended bladder or bowel, which can cause sympathetic outflow, in turn resulting in vasoconstriction and hypertension. Centrally, the body attempts to adjust by parasympathetic outflow, which lowers the heart rate but still cannot significantly lower the blood pressure because descending fibers are blocked at the level of the injury. The patient may experience goose flesh, sweating, and nausea. As the blood pressure rises, the patient may become aware of his or her pulse and may experience a pounding headache. Autonomic hyperreflexia is a potentially dangerous condition that can result in a cerebral hemorrhage. The treatment of this syndrome can usually be accomplished without hypertensive medication by elevating the head of the bed as high as possible to lower intracranial pressure followed by quickly investigating the common causes of hypertension in this population. Most frequently it can be traced to a bladder that is distended, either from a plugged catheter or excessive fluid intake in a patient on intermittent catheterization or an overdistended bowel. Placing the patient in an erect position and emptying the bladder and bowel will almost always arrest an episode of autonomic hyperreflexia. If these measures fail, hypertensive medications are indicated. If a patient has recurrent episodes of autonomic hyperreflexia, chronic treatment with phenoxybenzamine can prevent exaggerated elevation of the blood pressure, usually without orthostatic hypotension or other complications. From a psychological point of view, it is important to be aware that these symptoms may be misinterpreted as an acute anxiety reaction, especially if the patient is already experiencing significant distress.

An extremely difficult problem for many spinal cord–injured adolescents is social reintegration. These individuals are no longer able to engage in many activities that normally facilitate peer interactions, development of social identity, and eventual development of intimate friendships. Even when the spinal cord–injured adolescent does begin to participate in activities, such as attending school or going to sporting events, he or she

---

*A very well written and humorous manual on sexuality for adolescents with a spinal cord injury may be obtained by writing to:
M. Scott Manley, Ed.D., Craig Rehabilitation Institute, 3425 S. Clarkson, Englewood, CO, 80110.

usually feels embarrassed or awkward and may even become angry at able-bodied peers. Social reintegration is a very slow, painful process. The sympathetic health care provider may be tempted to compensate by pushing the unwilling adolescent too quickly into new social situations or by trying to provide an intimate friendship within the rehabilitation setting (Cogswell, 1968).

For patients who are school-age, a member of the team (usually the psychologist or social worker) should attend a conference at school to help prepare for the student's return. A constant danger is that well-meaning teachers and administrators may arrange everything, in the belief that the student should not be presented with any problems in that setting. This usually creates resentment in the injured adolescents because they feel that their abilities and wishes are not respected.

Finally, unless they are included on an initial problem list, structural barriers that impede mobility are often forgotten until it is time for the patient to go home. Some patients have been discharged, only to find that they can not enter their home because there is no ramp. Brief, three to four hour passes home a few weeks prior to final discharge can be extremely helpful in identifying architectural barriers and any other problems that need to be remedied before final discharge.

CONCLUSION

Spinal cord injury is one of the most common causes of permanent paralysis in adolescents. These injuries present medical and psychological problems that can seem overwhelming to health care providers, patients, and family. Although the outlook for a return to normal life seems hopeless at first, many paraplegic and quadriplegic young people live healthy, happy, and productive lives if they receive adequate treatment, support from significant others, time to make the difficult adjustments, and the opportunity to prove themselves.

ACKNOWLEDGMENT

We especially thank Betty Sanchez, an adolescent with C5 quadriplegia who also became a friend. She taught us more about spinal cord injury than any book could have, and made many suggestions that we have incorporated into this writing. She died tragically in a house fire while we were writing this chapter.

REFERENCES

Abramson, A.S. Modern concepts of management of the patient with spinal cord injury. *Archives of Physical Medicine Rehabilitation,* 1971, 48, 113–121.

Annon, J. *The behavioral treatment of sexual problems:* Brief therapy. New York: Harper & Row, 1976.

Boll, J.J. Minor head injury in children - Out of sight but not out of mind. *Journal of Clinical Child Psychology,* 1983, 12, 74–80.

Cogswell, B. Self socialization: Readjustment of paraplegics in the community. *Journal of Rehabilitation,* 1968, 34, 11–13.

Donovan, W.H., & Bedbrook, G. Comprehensive management of spinal cord injury. *CIBA Clinical Symposia,* 1982, *34*, 2.

Elkind, D. Egocentrism in adolescence. *Child Development,* 1967, 38, 1028.

Fordyce, W.E. Psychological assessment and management. In F.G. Kottke, G.K. Stillwell & J.F. Lehmann (Eds.) *Krusen's handbook of physical medicine and rehabilitation, 3rd edition.* Philadelphia: W.B. Saunders, 1982, 124–150.

Freed, M.M. Traumatic and congenital lesions of the spinal cord. In F.J. Kottke, G.K. Stillwell & J.F. Lehmann (Ed.), *Krusen's handbook of physical medicine and rehabilitation, 3rd edition.* Philadelphia: W.B. Saunders, 1982, 643–673.

Geller, B. & Greydanus, D.E. Psychological management of acute paraplegia in adolescence. *Pediatrics,* 1979, 63, 562–564.

Harris, P., Patel, S.E., Greer, W. & Naughton, J.A.L. Psychological and social reactions to acute spinal paralysis. *Paraplegia,* 1973, 11, 132–136.

Klonoff, H., Low, M. & Clark, C. Head injuries in children: A prospective five year follow-up. *Journal of Neurology Neurosurgery Psychiatry,* 1977, 40, 1211–1219.

Knorr, N., & Bull, J. Spinal cord injury: Psychiatric considerations. *Maryland State Medical Journal,* 1970, 19, 105–108.

Lancourt, J.E., Dickson, J.H., & Carter, R.E. Paralytic spinal deformity following traumatic spinal cord injury in children and adolescents. *Journal of Bone and Joint Surgery,* 1981, 63A,47–53.

Roberts, A.H., Spinal cord injury: Some psychological considerations. *Minnesota Medicine,* 1972, 55, 115–117.

Wilson, L.M. Intensive care delirium: The effect of outside deprivation in a windowless unit. *Archives of International Medicine,* 1972, 130, 225–226.

Young, J.S., Burns, P.E. Bowe, A.M., & McCutchen R. *Spinal cord injury statistics.* Phoenix, Arizona: Good Samaritan Medical Center, 1982.

Young, J.S., & Northup, N.E. (R. McCutchen, Ed.). *Statistical information pertaining to some of the most commonly asked questions about SCI.* Phoenix, Arizona: Good Samaritan Medical Center, 1979.

Zager, R.P., & Marquette, C.H. Developmental considerations in children and early adolescents with spinal cord injury. *Archives of Physical Medicine and Rehabilitation,* 1981, 62, 427–431.

Zubeck, J.P. Effects of prolonged sensory and perceptual deprivation. *British Medical Bulletin,* 1964, 20, 38–42.

Zubek, J.P. (Ed.) *Sensory deprivation: Fifteen years of research.* New York: Appleton-Century-Crofts, 1969.

SUGGESTED READING LIST

General:

Burke, D.C., & Murray, D.D. *Handbook of spinal cord medicine*. New York: Raven Press, 1975.

Wheelchair prescription:

DeLisa, J.A., & Greenberg, S. Wheelchair prescription guidelines. American Family Physician, 1982, 25, 4, 145–150. *Modification and accessory analysis: Introduction to wheelchair prescription*. Camarillo, CA 93010: Everest & Jennings, Inc., 3233 E. Mission Oaks Blvd., January, 1979.

Pyschosocial & Sexual Aspects:

Thompson, D.D. Psychological, social, and sexual aspects related to spinal cord injury, I & II. (An annotated bibliography.) DHEW. Produced by the Virginia Spinal Cord Injury System, 1979.

Michael D. Resnick

17
The Teenager with Cerebral Palsy

Cerebral palsy (CP) does not refer to a single disease entity but rather to a group of conditions and disturbances characterized by disorders in the control of voluntary movement (Nielson, 1966). The condition was first reported in medical literature near the end of the 19th century, prior to which time it was known as *Little's disease* or *Little's syndrome* (Little, 1862).

Estimates of the incidence of cerebral palsy range from 1:500 (Anderson & Klarke, 1982) to 1:650 (Charles, 1981; Lansdown, 1980). Despite this variation, the incidence is judged to be declining (Anderson & Klarke, 1982; Charles, 1981). Its etiology is varied and includes prenatal factors, such as Rh incompatibility, intrauterine infection, nutritional disturbances, hypoxia, and prenatal and congenital infections. Contributing perinatal factors can include prolonged labor and birth injury; postnatal causes include head trauma and other neurological problems, kernicterus, and meningitis (Anderson & Klarke, 1982; Gordon, 1976; Lansdown, 1980). Heredity is discounted as an etiological factor by some authors (Anderson & Klarke, 1982) while others note that heredity is rarely a causal factor but is a possible cause if both parents are affected (Lansdown, 1980).

CP is classified according to three categories: tremor, rigid, and mixed. Those with tremor CP are characterized by shaking, similar to that which occurs with Parkinson's disease. The rigid group includes those whose muscles work slowly and stiffly, causing clumsiness, while mixed applies to those individuals with two or more of the entire range of designations

(Anderson & Klarke, 1982; Nielsen, 1966; Oswin, 1967; Yeadon & Grayson, 1979).

Additionally, CP is classified into three major forms: spastic, athetoid, and ataxic. Spasticity, which accounts for 75 percent of all CP, is associated with muscle spasms and exaggerated reflexes. Tremulousness and unsteadiness are also frequent, and rapid and coordinated movements are difficult. Damage is primarily to the motor cortex and associated areas. One or more limbs may be involved. It is estimated that 40 percent of those with spastic palsy have either diplegia or hemiplegia, and 40 percent have three limbs involved.

Athetosis is traced to damage of the basal ganglia and accounts for between 8 and 20 percent of the CP population. It is characterized by uncontrollable, involuntary movements that can be either rapid and jerky or quite slow. These movements increase during periods of emotional upset and stress. In its most mild manifestation, it may appear as generalized motor restlessness and difficulty in sitting, standing, or lying still. In more severe cases, considerable interference with movement is likely and often includes abnormal posturing. Many parts of the body can be affected, including arms, legs, facial muscles, lips, tongue, and throat. A lack of facial muscle control associated with drooling may be present, as may speech difficulty and loss of hearing. Mobility is frequently limited due to the presence of these involuntary movements.

Ataxia is the least common of the three forms of CP, comprising some 5 percent of individuals with the disorder. It is caused by damage to the cerebellum and results in problems of balance and coordination including difficulties with walking and standing. Depth perception is often distorted, speech may be slurred, and hearing is frequently impaired.

CP includes a range of disorders and often extends beyond motor disability. Individuals with CP frequently have multiple problems. In the approximately 750,000 Americans with CP, the following correlates are noted (Yeadon & Grayson, 1979):

Mental retardation (various degrees)—50–75 percent
Speech problems—70 percent
Convulsions—70 percent
Visual problems—35 percent
Hearing problems—20 percent
Mental abnormalities—20 percent
Abnormal or deformed joints—20 percent
Behavior disorders—20 percent
Learning disabilities—20 percent
Tremors, spasms, or seizures—20 percent
Paralysis of arms or legs—20 percent

Lansdown (1980) reports that while at least half of children with CP are educationally subnormal, the measured intelligence of one fifth of this group is average or higher.

INFLUENCE OF DISABILITY AND CHRONIC ILLNESS ON DEVELOPMENT

Leichtman and Friedman (1975) feel that the influence of chronic illness is primarily in the areas of independence from parents and the development of normal peer relationships. As problems of peer acceptance become heightened during midadolescence, dependency upon parents also increases, accentuating poor self-image, lowered self-confidence, fear of failure, and a generalized failure to develop normally throughout adolescence. Group activities that can mitigate the effects of isolation, such as sports participation and other social outlets, may be precluded by the nature of the illness. The authors note also that physical attractiveness may be affected, which can lead to further self-dislike and self-derogation. Academic performance can be interrupted by frequent bouts of illness or hospitalization, which could potentially affect occupational and professional options. The symbols of increasing independence that are so important during adolescence, such as cars, bicycles, use of public transportation, and other means of mobility, are often denied to adolescents afflicted with chronic illness or disability (Seidl & Altschuler, 1979). Indeed, in light of these threats to the development-promoting activities of youth, it comes as a wonder that development can occur at all among those deprived of such stimuli.

In adolescents with CP, Anderson & Klarke (1982) found a high level of dependency in many of the basic skills of living. Frequently, the study showed that teenagers aspired to a level of independence greater than that which parents felt they could allow. The majority of adolescents in their study indicated heavy reliance on parents for help with many of the activities of daily living. In her study of children with CP and their families, Podeanu-Czehofski (1975) found that 85 percent of the 65 children studied showed signs of development problems, particularly in relation to social isolation, teasing, and peer group rejection. Skellern (1979) described an exaggerated self-consciousness of adolescents with disabilities when compared with the normal self-obsession associated with physical appearance in adolescence. In light of this, adolescence may be the first time that the disabled individual experiences real depression, through comparing the imperfect physical self with the imagined physical perfection of peers and a dawning realization that the condition is irreversible and permanent. Finally, Chiles and Lipscomb (1979) summarized many of these developmental dilemmas in their case study of a 15-year-old boy with CP, noting his double burden of dealing with a physical handicap in addition to dealing with the developmental tasks that normally accompany adolescence:

While his age cohorts were arguing with parents over the length of their hair, he needed help washing his; while they were resisting doing assigned chores, he was unable to perform any; while they were battling curfews, he needed not only permission, but physical assistance in order to be out. Instead of sharing his peers' increased independence from parents and others, symbolized by mild acting out behaviors, this patient could merely fantasize his acting out, with his illness providing a constant reminder of his chronic dependent status.

It has been speculated that the greater the number of normal, healthy years a person has before he or she becomes disabled, the better off that person will be in terms of developmental achievement and psychological adjustment. Conversely, those who have experienced trauma or disability early in life will be at greater risk for adverse consequences. While those born with disability may be affected less by their actual disability and more by the psychological state or mindset that has developed as a result of the condition and society's reaction to it (Sandowski, 1979), adolescents with CP, who are thoroughly acquainted with their limitations from years of having lived with them, present a particular challenge in terms of the promotion and fostering of normal developmental change and growth.

While researchers have sought to document the impact of disability on development and psychological adjustment, relatively little is known about those everyday factors that promote or hinder optimal development of the disabled adolescent. As Roessler and Bolton (1978) note, the disability and personality literature generally supports three conclusions:

1. Specific disabilities are not associated with specific personality types.
2. There is no clear relationship between disability severity and degree of psychological impairment.
3. Individual reaction to disability is diverse; however, disabled people are more likely to report lower self-esteem than those without disability.

In his study of adolescents with CP, Minde (1978) found that those with intellectual impairment showed a higher incidence of behavioral difficulties than those without such impairment. However, Minde also noted that little is known about the long-term psychological development of children with CP—a statement that echoes the observations of Gliedman and Roth (1980)—so that there is a paucity of information on the social, psychological, and emotional development of disabled children in general. In a comparison of adolescents with CP or spina bifida with a normal control group, Anderson & Klarke (1982) found that 60 percent of the disabled group tended to worry "a lot," compared with 40 percent of controls; 30 percent of the parents of the disabled participants believed that their children experienced depression, compared with only 15 percent of controls. By self-report, 70 percent of the disabled group reported episodes of depression, compared with 50 percent of controls, and anxiety was reported twice as often in the former compared with the latter group. The authors noted that the disabled group had lower self-confidence and self-esteem, frequently worried about their handicaps and lack of skills, and frequently showed signs of unhappiness, depression, and misery. In summary, it was found that one-half of the disabled adolescents had satisfactory adjustment, while about one third showed marked problems. Those with the most severe handicaps were at highest risk, although psychological and developmental problems were not limited to those with severe limitations. Unstructured clinical impressions and studies based on samples of hospitalized patients are more likely to uncover psychopathology than are samples drawn from random community-based groups (Steinhaus, 1981). From such community-based samples as the Isle of Wight studies (Rutter, Tizard, & Whitmore, 1970), it has been found that the rate of psychiatric disorders among chronically ill and disabled children is twice as high as among healthy controls. Similar findings are derived from the Rochester Child Health Survey in the United States, which found a high risk of psychological maladjustment among chronically ill children (Pless & Douglas, 1971; Pless, Roghmann, & Haggerty, 1972). (For another perspective see Offer et al., Chapter 5, in this volume)

Conflicting data from other authors underscore the importance of looking at methodological differences among studies. Tavormina, Kastner, Slater, and Watt (1976) found that children with a wide array of conditions, such as asthma, diabetes, cystic fibrosis, and hearing impairments, showed psychological test profiles approximating norms. In a study of 104 physically disabled children and adolescents in West Germany, Steinhaus (1981) found that children and adolescents with disabilities, including CP, tended to have "impaired capability of emotional integration into the environment without conflict," as well as a greater tendency to withdraw than controls. In this context, visibility of the handicap is seen to play a major role in the young person's ability to cope with the condition. Other investigators remind us that psychological disturbances cannot automatically be equated with the presence of physical handicap (Podeanu-Czehofski, 1975). While common sense might indicate that the disabled enjoy their lives considerably less than do the able-bodied (Titley, 1969), comparative studies of handicapped, retarded, and normal persons (Cameron, Titus, Gnadinger, & Kostin, 1973) conclude that life satisfaction is generally equivalent among all groups.

Thus, although it is a conflicting picture regarding the risk or likelihood of psychopathology and developmental difficulties among youths with CP, the impression that such risks are greater for the disabled appears warranted. The task remains of identifying those psychological and sociological factors in the everyday life of youths that promote or inhibit healthy development.

SAMPLE STUDY

Description of the Study Population

In 1982, the author (Resnick) conducted a study with 60 adolescents with cerebral palsy. The purpose of the study was to examine the sociological and psychological factors in adolescents' everyday lives which promoted positive self-image and adaptation to physical disability. For inclusion in this sample study, individuals were required to have CP, to fall between the ages of 12 and 22, and to be of normal intelligence. Participants were solicited from the impaired programming divisions of the Minneapolis and St. Paul public schools and a summer camp for youth with CP. Completed interviews were obtained from 60 young people who met the study criteria.

Fifty-five percent of the participants were male, and 45 percent were female. Almost all of them were Caucasian (97 percent), and the mean age for the group was 16.7 years, with a mode of 16 and a median of 16.3. Over one third of the participants were age 15 or under, another third were between 16 and 18 years of age, and the remainder were between 19 and 22. The size of the community of residence of participants varied considerably. About 25 percent of the participants lived in communities of under 5,000; 20 percent from towns of 5,000 to 19,999 persons; almost 25 percent lived in communities of between 20,000 and 100,000, and the remainder of the sample resided in larger metropolitan areas.

Family social class status was computed using the Hollingshead Two Factor Index. This is a widely used method to obtain an objective, quantified score reflecting the place of an individual or family in the social stratification system. Computation is based on the assignment of points based on occupational and educational attainment, resulting in classification into class I (highest) to class V (lowest social class). For social classes 1 through 5, mean social class of the study group was 3.3, with a median of 3.6 and modal value of 4.0. Less than 10 percent of participants fell into either class 1 or 2; over 25 percent were in class 3; close to 50 percent were in class 4; and slightly under ten percent were in class 5.

Eighty-two percent, or 49 of the sample members, were currently enrolled in school. Of those, three were in a special education division of their public school, and two attended a residential school for the physically disabled. Fifty-four participants (90 percent) lived in their parents' home. Of the remainder, three lived in a residential school setting, one in a handicapped community-based residential setting, one in a college dormitory, and one lived independently, without special facilities, in the community.

In terms of physical condition, about half of the sample members were ambulatory; less than 20 percent used a motorized wheelchair; and the remainder used a manual wheelchair. Eight of the ambulatory participants had one or more leg braces, while the remainder ambulated unassisted. With regard to speech impairment, over one half had no identifiable impairment, about 20 percent had mild impairment, 13.3 percent had moderate difficulty in being understood, and 8.3 percent had severe impairment.

Methods

An extensive interview schedule was developed for this study. Forced choice and open-ended questions were designed to elicit information about the individual's activities, social relationships, family relationships, household responsibilities, and other contextual features of social life. Qualitative information was collected pertaining to the individuals' experiences with and perceptions of his or her physical disability, while qualitative measures of self-concept incorporated scales developed by Rosenberg and Simons (1972), Rosenberg (1965), and Klein (1975). These instruments were used to assess happiness, anxiety, body image, self-estimate of popularity, self-consciousness, and self-esteem. A scale measuring self-perceived parental protectiveness was derived using factor analytical methods, which replicated measures used by Klein (1975).

Given the premise that youth development is not a passive process and the fact that disabled and chronically ill adolescents often are unable to participate in the daily activities of living that promote healthy psychological and social development, this study attempted to investigate the extent to which activities of daily living affect various dimensions of self-concept and social psychological outcome. This chapter will offer findings relating to the use of discretionary time, peer and other nonfamilial social interaction, involvement in sports and athletics, and family dynamics, including participation in household activities and parental overprotectiveness.

USE OF LEISURE TIME AND PEER GROUP
INTERACTIONS: THE LITERATURE

Recent research supports the observation that the use of leisure time has an important socializing component and, thus, a major impact on the life of a youth. Together with the family, the peer group is central to the socialization process and frequently provides the structure for leisure time activities (Altman, 1981). It has been argued that the current generation of young people increasingly experience isolation from one another (Zimbardo, 1980), but qualitative studies of youths' use of discretionary time and their orientation toward peers do not support this contention. In their survey of 725 Minnesota high school youths, Hedin and Simon (1980) found that belonging, connections with others, and friendships were counted as the most important elements of their life. The quality-of-life study for adolescents done by Gage and associates (1980) similarly indicated that family and friends were the most important elements in a young person's life. Metropolitan youths tended to rank friendships above family, while the converse was true for rural youth. Hedin and Simon found that the centrality of peers in the use of leisure time included the fulfilling of three crucial roles: support and communication; companionship and conversation; and fun and socializing. Friends were viewed as central in the influencing of individual's decisions, including activities, behavior, thinking, and appearance, as well as use of leisure time.

While most studies of adolescent leisure time focus on what teenagers do, conclusions underscore the relation between the use of leisure time—particularly that time spent with peers—and the growth of social skills, competence, and sense of mastery over the external world. Peers are a major sociological reference group for adolescents and represent a social mirror as well as a context within which to experiment and play with new social skills. From peer interaction develops increased empathy and role-taking ability, as well as the mastery of social competencies that are prerequisites for the successful conduct of everyday adult life (Anderson & Klarke, 1982).

Leisure Time and Disabled Youths

The most important factors to be derived from the literature on leisure time are the context within which it occurs and the important socializing and developmental functions it serves. Brindley (1979) noted that in a culture that emphasizes work and productivity, the disabled are often faced with a lifetime of "obligatory leisure." Stressing the importance of the creative use of leisure time (O'Reilly & Elliott, 1971), schools are identified as particularly important in helping adolescents to learn creative and satisfying uses of time. In their discussion of chronic illness and adolescent development, Wolfish and McLean (1974) note the importance of the development of compensatory skills by those adolescents who are unable to participate in more typical leisure-time activities. They note, for example, the importance of substituting hobbies for athletic participation when the latter are not feasible. Adolescents should be encouraged to join groups or clubs for people with similar interests but not for people with similar disabilities. Creative use of leisure time is viewed not only as a remediating element in terms of what the disabled are unable to do, but as preparation for a satisfying life despite possible restrictions on the opportunity for meaningful work activities. Lancaster-Gaye (1973) reports the findings from an international conference in Sweden on sports and leisure for those with physical disabilities. The author notes specific cross-cultural examples of training for creative leisure, including special courses in dancing for the physically disabled in Czechoslovakia, a sports training program for the disabled in Indonesia, the organization of holiday activities for disabled children in the German Democratic Republic, and the formation of youth clubs for able-bodied and disabled children in France, Belgium, and the United Kingdom. In essence, the creative use of leisure becomes a vehicle for social integration.

The importance of socialization in the healthy development of disabled youths has been stressed by a number of authors in the United States and elsewhere. A variety of sociometric studies reveal the relative social isolation of the disabled from their immediate peer group, which results in diminished opportunities for social interaction, thereby impeding the development of social competence (Altman, 1981). As a consequence, limited social skills and capabilities compound the problems of the physical disability itself (Gottlieb & Budoff, 1973; Gottlieb & Davis, 1973; Goodman, Dornbusch, Richardson, & Hasdorf, 1963; Heber, 1956; Hunt, 1966; Johnson, 1950).

Detailed studies of disabled adolescents' use of time come from both Israeli and British investigators (eg. Anderson & Klarke, 1982; Egozi, 1976; Golan, 1977; Hen, 1974; Har Paz & Hadad, 1976). Recreational participation and other creative uses of leisure time have been advocated, not only as ways to foster social development but also to counteract the stultifying consequences of parental overprotection (Margalit, 1981) and family environment stimulus deprivation (Shere & Kastenbaum, 1966). To explore whether children with CP were being socially conditioned for a lifetime of passivity, Margalit compared the leisure activities of children with CP, both within and outside the home, with those of a healthy peer control group. For homebound activities it was found that the disabled children were much more likely to read books than were the controls; however, no differences were evident regarding watching television or listening to the radio. For outside activities, participation in youth centers was comparable for the two groups, although the able-bodied teens engaged in more diverse activities in those settings. Major differences were found in spontaneous social activities, such as visiting with a friend or going for a walk without a specific purpose. These were crucial aspects of normal children's self-reports but were extremely infrequent for the disabled. The children with CP also rarely went to movies, usually because they had no one to go with them. If they did attend films, they were more likely to go with a parent than were control group members. In fact, disabled children were less likely to go on any sort of excursion. In all, Margalit found that disabled children were more likely to engage in home- and family-based activities, while those in the able-bodied group were more likely to recreate with peers away from home. The activities of disabled children were planned and controlled by adults, such as teachers and parents, which permitted less exposure to peer culture. The range and variety of their activities was also more limited. The author concluded that the limited social experiences of children with CP, particularly with respect to peer culture and exposure, resulted in prolonged adult orientation and delayed social and emotional maturity.

Similar conclusions were reached by Minde and associates in their studies of children and adolescents with CP (1978, 1972). During their initial period of study, when participants were between five and nine years of age, peer-group isolation was the norm. In their follow-up five years later, most of the children had few meaningful relationships with nonhandicapped peers.

Other studies on the use of leisure time of disabled children and youths also indicate a high degree of social isolation (Dorner, 1977, 1976; Rowe, 1973). In his study of young adults with CP, Rowe found that 20 percent of participants had not been outside the house at all except to travel to their work center during two weeks prior to the study. Less than 40 percent had been out four times or more. Capacity to drive a car was a major factor in social integration. Over 60 percent said that they would like to be able to go out more frequently, citing problems with transportation and lack of architectural accessibility as their reasons for not doing so.

A frequent accompaniment to the relative social separation and isolation of disabled adolescents is the ubiquity of teasing at the hands of their peers. In her study of Danish children and youths with CP, ages 6–15, Nielson (1966) reported that all 40 participants had been teased by peers because of their disability. Anderson and Klarke (1982) found that adolescents with CP in ordinary schools were far more likely to report being the target of teasing and aggression from able-bodied peers than were their special school counterparts and the control group. Thus, social separation is reinforced by negative peer-group experiences, which cause the adolescent to focus on the disability as his or her primary characteristic.

Summing up their observations on the social life and experiences of disabled adolescents, Anderson and Klarke (1982) noted:

> Perhaps the most significant finding in our study was the extent of social isolation among the young people both in their school years and after. There was a clear relationship between social isolation and presence of psychological problems, and it is this issue we should particularly like to draw attention to, since it was our impression that their lack of social intercourse caused more distress and misery than any other factor, particularly for young people whose families were not very supportive.

Disabled adolescents typically lacked confidants and close friends, were less likely to have hobbies or developed interests, to read newspapers or books, and to follow sports when compared with their able-bodied peers. In short

> . . . the need to foster social outlets, also suggests that schools and colleges urgently need to develop education for living courses. The high rate of psychological disturbance revealed indicates a clear need for good counseling services.

To summarize their extensive findings, Anderson and Klarke (1982) note the high degree of dissatisfaction with social life during and after school; a perceived lack of control over their own life, coupled with little information about their disability or available services; limited choices available to those unable to find employment, with day-care providing limited opportunities and activities; and lack of preparation for everyday adult life, with little help offered during the transition period between school and adult life. According to the authors, the locus of remedy for these four areas lies with the disabled themselves and includes rejection of the low status conferred upon them by society and working actively to construct for themselves a satisfying life, despite the biological limitations inherent in their disability and the social handicap heaped upon it through societal reaction and stereotyping.

Use of Leisure Time—Findings*

Consistent with the findings and recommendations of other researchers, the author's study found that participation in activities that broaden the scope of the adolescent's social life had a positive impact on one or more dimensions of self-image.

Clubs

Less than half of the study participants (43 percent) belonged to a club or organized group. Regardless of whether these organizations were

---

*Statistical comparisons throughout this chapter are based upon chi-square, Fisher's Exact Test, and correlational analysis, depending on the variable's level of measurement.

exclusively for disabled individuals or for both able-bodied and disabled, participants who had CP described themselves as happier (p<.05) and more popular (p<.02) than their counterparts who did not have such affiliations.

Hobbies

Over 75 percent of participants said that they had some kind of hobby or activity in which they regularly engaged. Eighteen percent listed writing or drawing; 15 percent named participation in sports; 15 percent mentioned listening to music, radio, or records; 15 percent cited collecting objects; 10 percent mentioned sewing (all girls); 8 percent listed building models (all boys); 7 percent named riding bicycles; and 7 percent cited watching television. Like those in clubs and groups, those individuals with hobbies viewed themselves as more popular (p<.05) and happier (p<.05) than did those without hobbies.

After School or Work

We asked participants what they did when they got home from school or work. Thirty-eight percent said they watched television or listened to the radio, 15 percent would get together with friends, 13 percent would do their homework, 8 percent would eat and another 8 percent would spend time with family members. Seven percent mentioned being involved with their hobbies, 10 percent would go bicycle riding, and another 7 percent would talk on the phone with friends. Adolescents who typically spent time alone after coming home from school or work were significantly more likely to report low self-esteem than those who spent time with family members (p<.003) or other friends (p<.004) (Fisher's Exact Test).

PEER GROUP RELATIONSHIPS—FINDINGS

Friends

Whether the participant had a best friend was unrelated to any measure of social–psychological outcome. Eighty-two percent said they did have a best friend, but the likelihood of so reporting was found to be unrelated to the respondent's degree of physical limitation. The presence of other good friends (i.e., an extended peer network) was related to self-image, as was the disability status of those other friends. The actual number of other friends was irrelevant to this covariation. Over 80 percent of the respondents had other friends. Not surprisingly, they were more likely to view themselves as popular than were those without other friends (p<.02) and more likely to report higher self-esteem (p<.05). When other friends were able-bodied or when the respondents had both able-bodied and disabled friends, they were less self-conscious than those with only disabled friends (p<.05; p = .03 [Fisher's Exact Test]). Variations in self-consciousness were independent of disability severity. When the best friend of the disabled participant was also disabled, participants reported poorer body image for themselves than did those with able-bodied friends (p<.02). Again, this was not found to be related to severity of the respondent's disability.

This last point warrants some elaboration. Reviews of attitudinal studies regarding societal and individual response to disability (e.g. Resnick, 1983) indicate that, like their able-bodied counterparts, those with disability tend to internalize prevailing cultural values regarding beauty, wholeness, and the moral attributes that accompany those standards. Thus, stigmatization of the disabled by the disabled has been documented in studies of both children and adults. Our study members spoke clearly on this point, by expressing a dislike for being "overly associated" with only disabled peers. As one girl described it, "You start to feel like you're just some kind of freak if you only have people around you who are like you, and especially if they're worse off. You start to feel bad *if you can't do any better than that.*"

Having or not having a cross-sex friend paralleled findings pertaining to best or other friends. Having other friends (which by definition included having a best friend as well) was significantly related to positive self-image, while having a best friend was not. It could be speculated that having a cross-sex friend has the same underlying social–psychological dynamic of having a sense of belonging to, and similarity with, peers. Rather than one special or outstanding relationship (e.g., a best friend or going steady), it appears to be the more extended peer network and, therefore, less social isolation, that promotes positive outcomes for disabled youths. As the youth moves into late adolescence and early adulthood, however, it may be that the presence or absence of a more exclusive cross-sex relationship corresponds to self-image.

Cross-Sex Relationships

When researchers discuss cross-sex relationships, a relatively innocuous term is being used for an important kind of friendship among adolescents. Such relationships are a prelude and accompaniment to the development of intimacy, and they are a source of prestige and self-esteem in both males and females (Safilios-Rothschild, 1977). Since physical appearance is a pivotal consideration in adolescence, the opportunity to develop such friendships can be particularly problematic for those with physical disability.

Anderson and Klarke (1982) found that disabled teenagers had little experience with cross-sex relationships, although most worried about them. Only 25 percent of disabled adolescents in their sample had been on a date, compared with over 75 percent of the controls.

In the author's study, it was assumed that cross-sex relationships would be extremely important in terms of self-image, but problematic for most of the disabled adolescents. Adolescents with disability, as much as their nondisabled counterparts, are socially conditioned in a culture that places high value on romantic love, physical attraction and attractiveness, and sexual experience. Similar to Anderson and Klarke's findings, 28 percent of the participants in this study had been on a date. Seventeen percent said they were "going steady." However, neither dating nor having a steady relationship was related to variations in social psychological outcome.

Forty-three percent of the study sample reported that they did have a boyfriend or girlfriend. This was 50 percent greater than the proportion of respondents who had ever been on a date. Having a boyfriend or girlfriend was typically described as a less romantic or serious relationship than was going steady, and it seemed to be more like having a cross-sex companion or playfriend (depending on the age of the respondent). Those without such a cross-sex friend were significantly more likely to report higher anxiety levels than were their counterparts (p<.05).

FAMILY RELATIONSHIPS: THE LITERATURE

Parental and familial overprotectiveness is a frequent theme in literature concerned with family dynamics and relationships involving disabled adolescents and children. In an early study of mothers of children with CP, Boles (1959) characterized the mothers as overprotective of their children. In addition, these mothers were found to experience more marital conflict than were the mothers of nonhandicapped children. Parental attitudes are strongly linked to the socialization process between parents and child, which itself correlates to social behavioral outcomes in children. Studies of visually impaired children indicate that their degree of dependence can be systematically linked to parental overprotectiveness (Lairy & Harrison, 1973; Kemp, 1981). British investigators have reiterated this theme in the case of adolescents with CP, noting that some of these young people, especially those without siblings, spend too much time with adult friends and relations, as it requires too much effort to seek out contemporaries who may or may not understand their handicap: "Sometimes the parents themselves are responsible for the situation, being understandably reluctant to see their child rebuffed, and their constant companionship is an unconscious protection" (Oswin, 1967). This kind of overprotection, according to Oswin, in addition to other ways in which the child with CP is denied access to normal life experiences, retards social and psychological development.

Since parental overprotectiveness is described as an insidious socializing element with long-term consequences for self-concept and social competence, practitioners need to be aware of the factors that seem to promote overprotection in families with disabled children and adolescents. It is common for parents to deal with guilt feelings toward a disabled child by trying to do everything for the child; this only results in excessive overprotection (Sandowski, 1979) and reinforcement of the adolescent's traumatized self-concept. Parental overprotectiveness has been identified as a frequent cause or correlate of passivity and immaturity in disabled children. Explaining the origin of such parental response, Poznanski (1973) notes:

> Precisely because over-protection is such an issue, it is important to understand what lies behind it. Most obviously parents are helped to deny their feelings of anger, resentment and guilt by behaving as if they felt just the opposite emotions. The parents also were spared the pain of watching the child struggle with his limited capabilities, while they are once again reminded that the limitations exist. And, finally, over-protection allows the parents to 'make up' to the child for his disability—a need that springs apart from the parents' sense of guilt in 'giving' the child a defective endowment. Over-protection, thus, serves many purposes. It is deeply intertwined with the creating of the relative isolation for both parents and child.

Other researchers agree. Parents of chronically ill children are likely to retreat from their own relationships with their neighbors (Cummings, Bayley, & Rie, 1966), to infrequently take their disabled children on vacations or outings, and to discourage socializing by the disabled son or daughter (Poznanski, 1973).

Given the developmental lag that can occur in the face of overprotection in terms of social and interpersonal competence, individual self-confidence, and sense of mastery, researchers have emphasized the importance of encouraging parents to promote diverse forms of social activity in their adolescents, including recreation, peer involvement, and activity outside of the primary family. In her review of childhood chronic illness and its consequences for psychosocial adaptation, Mattson (1972) emphasized that undue restrictions and overprotection in the home and at school should be discouraged. She encourages fathers, in particular, to take active responsibility for child rearing and for promoting compensatory activities and interests. The relative uninvolvement of fathers in the daily lives, needs, and activities of disabled children and adolescents is frequently discussed in the literature (e.g. Anderson & Klarke, 1982). As a consequence, much of the discussion of overprotectiveness appears to center on the wife-mother, the family member who is most intimately responsible for making decisions about the health needs of other family members (Litman, 1974).

In their comparative study of disabled and nondisabled adolescents, Anderson and Klarke (1982) found that a much higher proportion of their disabled sample members viewed parents as *less* strict than average. Sixty percent of these adolescents said they never disagreed with parents about going out, in comparison with 36 percent of controls. Overprotection was assessed both in terms of the adolescents' perspective and that of the mothers. When mothers were asked whether they saw themselves as overprotective toward their children, about one quarter said yes. The greater the severity of handicap, the greater was the proportion of mothers who indicated that they were overprotective. The justification for overprotectiveness was frequently described as a function of time, i.e., for convenience or because of being in a hurry, they are unwilling to take the necessary time. Mothers frequently described their husbands as more likely than themselves to encourage their children to be independent, particularly if their children were attending ordinary schools. Six percent of parents reported marked friction and 19 percent reported some friction between themselves and their spouse over the issue of adolescents' independence. Most commonly, the father regarded the mother as overprotective and overly restrictive. These conflicts frequently occurred in relation to moderately handicapped teenagers.

When disabled adolescents were questioned on this issue, about two thirds believed parents did not try to do things for them when they thought they could manage themselves. Twenty percent believed their parents sometimes gave too much help, and 14 percent (19 percent of males and 9 percent of females) said they definitely gave too much help. Of particular interest was that over half of those severely handicapped thought their parents did too much for them, with no proportional difference between those with mild and moderate handicaps. The authors concluded that the term "overprotection" is frequently applied unfairly to parents of handicapped children. Second, they noted that the aspirations for independence on the part of disabled boys and those with severe handicaps is frequently misunderstood or not appreciated by parents. Commonly, those adolescents who felt their parents did too much for them also reported that they frequently argued with their parents on this subject. While the term "overprotectiveness" may be misapplied on occasion, the same study indicated that it did influence psychological adjustment. Among those adolescents with a mother who usually encouraged independence, 44 percent showed marked or some psychological problems, and 56 percent showed satisfactory adjustment. When mothers tended to give too much help, 70 percent showed marked or some problems, and only 30 percent demonstrated satisfactory adjustment.

Parental Relationships: Findings

For the purposes of this study, parental overprotectiveness was measured on the basis of adolescent self-report, which reflects the teenagers perceptions of the parenting experience. Adolescents who view themselves as overly restricted and protected by parents will respond to that situation behaviorally and psychologically as though it were, in fact, the real situation, regardless of objective criteria.

In the author's study the detrimental influence of parental overprotectiveness upon social–psychological outcome (as perceived by the adolescent) was clearly and consistently evident. For each of the social–psychological outcomes, with the exception of body image, the greater the perceived parental overprotectiveness, the poorer the outcome. Adolescents who considered their parents overprotective were significantly more likely than their counterparts to report lower happiness (p<.01), lower self-esteem (p<.05), higher anxiety levels (p<.02), lower self-perceived popularity (p<.01), and greater self-consciousness (p<.001). While Anderson and Klarke (1982) found a positive relationship between degree of physical disability and parental overprotectiveness, such was not the case in this study. In fact, self-reported overprotectiveness actually declined as level of severity increased (r = −.2039, p = .059), leaving those with lesser levels of severity more likely to describe parents as overprotective. In each instance, the significant relationship between overprotectiveness and adverse social–psychological outcome was unaltered when controlling for physical severity. In other words, severity of physical limitation is not an acceptable explanation for the relationship between overprotectiveness and adverse social–psychological outcome. The negative impact of perceived parental overprotectiveness existed for our sample participants regardless of limitations on physical ability.

Parental overprotectiveness was measured in terms of inappropriate parental attempts to shelter their adolescents from the stresses or demands of everyday life or to make decisions for them that the adolescents themselves felt capable of making. A qualitative analysis of interview data also revealed another form of overprotectiveness: a reinforcement by parents of the adolescent's inability. These parents, inadvertently through their words and actions, both conveyed and reinforced a negative self-concept on the part of the adolescent by reaffirming the belief that their son or daughter was unable to participate in many of the daily activities of living. Such parents acted on the assumption that their adolescent was incapable of doing much more than in fact that teenager believed himself or herself capable of. This is particularly important because of the influence of parental expectation on adolescent behavior and self-concept. One respondent's comments were particularly illustrative of this point:

> My dad thinks I'm shit! Right before camp he said I'd never be able to earn money like my brother, and I'll have to live off the government. It makes me feel like I'm so much less than he is! If I had a different father, I would think better of myself. I probably would have done more things than I did because he led me to believe I couldn't do things. You name it—going out, doing work, everything! He wouldn't let me drive the tractor. When I was fourteen, my brother-in-law let me drive the tractor, so since I was sixteen *I* have been doing over half the farmwork—but he won't let me drive [a car]. He doesn't think I'm worth a damn. Now that I've proved I can, he thinks I can do *that* but I can't do *this* so he just keeps on going like this. I can drive the pickup to work, but not for enjoyment or alone. It doesn't make sense to me that I can't drive like that. If I can do fieldwork, why can't I drive a car and get a license?

Such overprotectiveness and negative parental attitudes deny the teenager the opportunity for greater independence and positive self-concept. When parental definitions of, and responses to, physical disability assume overtly negative forms, the development of a positive sense of self as competent and capable is jeopardized (Mattson, 1972). The emotional development and social competencies of the disabled youth depend far more on the way in which parents and family relate to the disabled child than do the actual physical limitations (Bentovin, 1972).

SPORTS, EXERCISE AND PHYSICAL ACTIVITY: THE LITERATURE

Athletic participation and exercise have long been advocated as important components of healthy development of the child and the adolescent. In the past decade, increasing attention has been directed to the importance of physical activity, exercise, and sports participation in youths with CP. In his review of issues related to physical fitness and CP, Brown (1975) noted a number of complications of CP that limit athletic participation. These include lack of flexibility, endurance, strength, balance, and vitality. After puberty, there is also a high incidence of obesity among those with CP. While some youth with CP are too limited physically to partake in fitness activities, others stand to benefit considerably from such participation. Severely handicapped individuals can undertake limited exercise routines, and tremendous benefit has been found to accrue for individuals who engage in such exercise, even on psychological grounds alone (Brown, 1975).

From a review of cross-cultural evidence, the author concludes that the motor inefficiency found in children with CP was due in part to the condition itself and in part to their general conditions of daily living, in which exercise was not encouraged or even considered. When physical training programs realistically bear in mind the physiological limitations of the individual, a number of beneficial effects can accrue in both the physical and psychological domains. Brown's suggestion for health professionals is that "these children must not be treated like china dolls. We need to be fully aware of the tremendous physical and psychological benefits which accrue from exercise."

Similarly, Berg (1970) has observed that fatigue frequently accompanies CP. Such adaptive measures as electric wheelchairs, hydraulic beds, transportation services, and electric typewriters require a minimum muscular movement and energy expenditure. Such an environment can reduce the general level of physical output that a child with CP will experience. On the other hand, Berg (1970) found that a structured training program was helpful in raising the activity level and along with it, the disabled youth's sense of well-being on the social–psychological level. Analogous gains in body coordination and movement were reported by Mauser and Reynolds (1977) in an eight-week developmental activity training program for children between 4 and 12 years of age who had perceptual–motor deficits. Little change in positive self-concept was reported in these cases, however.

In addition to physical fitness training programs, strong support has been expressed for organized competitive sports activities for CP adolescents. Huberman (1976) views the 1970s as the decade in which organized sports for those with CP and related conditions truly emerged. He notes that while the need for competitive sports activities for disabled individuals is recognized, in practice the majority of such activities are recreational. Despite such advocacy, participation of adolescents with CP in organized sports activities and concomitant fitness training programs is infrequent and directly related to the availability of such organized activities in the adolescents' community. In their comparison of adolescents with CP and age-matched nondisabled controls, Anderson and Klarke (1982) found that relatively few of the disabled teenagers reported any involvement in either indoor or outdoor sports outside of the school setting. This diminished their opportunity for physical exercise and lost them the opportunity of interacting with both disabled and nondisabled friends outside of school.

Sports and Physical Exercise—Findings

Study participants were interviewed extensively about their athletic involvement and participation. The majority (70 percent) currently participated in some kind of sports activity, including organized sports at school, with other agencies, and on an informal basis at home with friends and acquaintances. In the school setting these were usually adapted sports and physical education activities, including hockey, basketball, baseball, gymnastics, soccer, swimming, and bowling. Participation was found to be unrelated to degree of severity of disability.

No differences in social–psychological outcomes were found between those who were and those who were not currently involved in sports or athletic activities. Rather, it was whether or not the individual had played sports when he or she was younger that correlated with the various levels of outcome. Those involved in athletic activity when they were younger described themselves as happier (p<.02) and less self-conscious (p<.05) than did their counterparts. Qualitative analysis of the participants' comments revealed that a key issue in playing sports at a younger age was the sense of involvement each individual felt with his or her peers and with others. As one put it, "I would often modify the situation rather than not play. The most important thing to me was to have the time to be with my friends, do something with them together. Mostly they would bend the rules for me a little bit so I could just be part of the group. That's what really felt good." Others described the sense of disappointment experienced over not being able to join in with their peers. One noted,

> I felt like a freak, and it got worse as we got older 'cause the girls would come and I would sit at the sideline and feel apart from everyone.

Another said,

> It really used to bother me. It used to make me feel that I was just an outsider and that I'd feel like that all my life. After a while I got adjusted to it. You have to face that you have a disability. For when you're younger, it's really hard to be standing on the outside looking in. Alone.

Those adolescents who were asked to join in and play with their peers when they were younger reported a higher self-esteem than those adolescents who were left on the sidelines to sit and watch but not get involved (p<.05). And notably, it was the way in which the adolescent defined the experience of playing games and being in sports that coordinated with current self-image.

Disabled adolescents were asked to describe what it was like to participate in sports while they had CP. Over half of the sample involved in sports noted few differences from able-bodied sports: "It's essentially the same. It just takes a little longer than it would otherwise." "It's not really different. We just can't go as fast as other people, or maybe our chairs get in the way, but essentially it's all the same. The feeling is the same." "We just have to make adaptations. The sport is the same with just a few changes or modifications." One sports enthusiast described the experience this way:

> The physical play is different for the handicapped but the feeling about play-
> ing sports is the same, including the ups and downs. Just because these legs
> don't work as well as walking people's legs do, it doesn't mean I'm different.
> It's a rush; it gets frustrating at times, but I play all kinds of sports. Look,
> in bowling I have a high game of 38 and a lot of time I'll get all gutter balls
> and score zero. It's the process, not the score, that makes all the difference.

Conversely, there were others who focused more on their disability than on the process of active involvement with others. Interestingly, the degree of disability was unrelated to the attitude toward athletic involvement. For one third of those who participated in sports, physical limitations became the focus of their attention and reaction to the experience; not surprisingly, it was these individuals who reported lower self-esteem than those individuals with CP who defined participating in sports as essentially the same as for able-bodied individuals ($p<.001$).

The diminished sense of self was clearly reflected in the comments of those who defined sports participation as just another of many areas in their lives in which difference from others was accentuated. One adolescent bitterly reflected on his own experiences:

> For me playing sports or doing just about anything with the kids is a rotten
> experience. It was sort of 'Let's all be nice to the gimp'—like I would go out
> there like some of kind of spaz and act like I could play ball or run or something
> like that and everybody would stand around and wait for me and then I would
> just stop right there in the middle of what I was doing and look around and realized
> that everybody had their eyes on me waiting for me to fall or something. It's really
> stupid to pretend you're like other people when you're not like them. They're
> trying to be nice to you, but deep down you know you're just making an ass out
> of yourself, so that's why I don't do that sort of thing anymore. I've just got to
> accept the fact that I'm different and I'm not good.

Sports can be viewed as activities that help normalize the lives of children and youths with disabilities. Reflecting on their younger days (which with this sample population meant anywhere from childhood to early adolescence), teenagers frequently commented on the lessening of their sensitivity; they also noted an increase in their ability to shrug off and disregard the negative social aspects of physical disability. Belonging was still identified as a key life issue, but many seemed to be developing an inner resource that could be called upon in those times when previously they had felt themselves buffeted about by the unkind winds of peer injustice. This positive attitude, however, was missing from that subgroup of adolescents who evidenced both lower self-esteem and lower happiness levels, in whom there remained that sense of nonaffiliation with their age mates:

> When other kids would start playing some game, I would just watch. Sometimes somebody would ask me if I wanted to play, but I knew that they were just feeling sorry for me, and I wasn't going to play that kind of bullshit game. They were just trying to be nice and I didn't want their pity. I don't want it now. I don't expect much to change, so I'll have to deal with it, won't I? Nothing changes. It's this (indicating leg brace) that screws everything up, and gets in the way of everything.

CHORES AND HOUSEHOLD RESPONSIBILITIES: THE LITERATURE

Responsibility, accountability, and participation in household activities and decision making are all important social skills needed by individuals, both for the present and in preparation for their future as independent adults. Skill in decision making and the exercise of responsibility are also important developmental accomplishments related to the achievement of independence. These skills are learned in the home and practiced and negotiated with adults as a prelude to self-sufficiency. Anderson and Klarke's (1982) study of physically disabled adolescents and their families indicated that some severely physically impaired teenagers held positions of high responsibility in the household. The authors concluded that "many could and should have been doing more in this respect." The authors did not relate the presence or type of household responsibilities held by the disabled adolescent to social–psychological outcomes; however, it was seen by these investigators as an important component of independent decision making, increasing movement toward responsible and accountable behavior, and therefore, a significant developmental experience for teens. The authors concluded that it was unfortunate that so many adolescents in their study had no chores, or only one minor or major chore in the household (68 percent). Seventeen percent of the disabled adolescents had two or more minor chores, and 15 percent had two or more major chores. Characteristically, boys did less than girls, which would appear to be consistent with general sex-role expectations.

Chores and Household Responsibilities: Findings

In the author's study, the majority of adolescents described themselves as having a chore or special job at home (83.3 percent). This was unrelated to age of the adolescent. The remaining participants had no household chores or responsibilities whatsoever. For the purpose of classification, chores were divided into three categories: self-care activities, such as getting dressed and washing; minor responsibilities, including cleaning one's own room, feeding a household pet, and occasionally doing dishes; and major responsibilities, including any routine, frequent activity in the house outside of the adolescent's room and self-care, such as taking out garbage, house cleaning, cooking, regular dishwashing, and farming chores.

The relationship between social–psychological outcome measures and participation in household chores was first examined for those who did or did not report any such responsibilities. Adolescents with any kind of household responsibilities beyond self-care reported higher self-esteem (p<.05) and higher body image scores (p<.05). Variations in self-esteem and body image were not evident across different categories or types of chores. It was also found that the presence or absence of household responsibilities as well as the kinds of responsibilities assigned to the adolescent were consistently related to the severity of the disability. In other words, much as in Anderson and Klarke's (1982) sample, youths with severe physical limitations were found to carry out major household responsibilities and tasks as well as those with a lower degree of physical disability. In fact, those with the most severe physical limitation were the most likely to report having household chores (94 percent). These adolescents were also most likely to report responsibility for major household tasks (67 percent), significantly more so than the less severely disabled (p<.05). Commenting on this, one respondent noted:

A lot of my friends bitch and moan about having to do things around the house. I don't mind it as much probably because I am in this thing (indicating his electric wheelchair). My folks have always pushed me to do the best I could, given that I can't do a lot in some areas. So this makes me feel I am contributing my fair share to the house, which is important to me, because the only way you are not going to feel like a cripple when you look like I do, is not to act like one, and not think that you're one. I guess that is what I do.

Another respondent observed:

My mom told me that I better start thinking of myself like other kids instead of being different from other kids, because the world wasn't going to bend and change just 'cause I walk funny and couldn't talk right. She said that if I wanted the privileges that went along with being treated like any other kid, I had to take some of the responsibility. So, I guess that is why I wash dishes, take out the garbage and stuff like that because it is all part of being just like everybody else.

From these young persons' comments, the link between self-esteem, positive body image, and household responsibility becomes clearer. The assignment of chores and household duties serves as one means of normalizing intrafamilial interaction and of involving the adolescent in the

daily rhythms and routines of the household, rather than setting him or
her apart from it.

OBSERVATIONS AND CONCLUSIONS

The relating of individual activities, behaviors, and social involvement
to social–psychological outcomes is important in the development of a
generalized understanding of the factors that influence disabled adolescent's satisfaction with self and with everyday life. The specific activities
discussed, including use of discretionary time, presence of hobbies and
outside-of-the-home involvements, and same- and cross-sex friendships,
and the overprotectiveness of parents are related to several of the generic
developmental milestones necessary for optimal adolescent growth and
evolution into adulthood. These include the development of a sense of
competence, mastery, identity, and capability as part of a generalized outlook on the world and one's view of self. Anderson and Klarke (1982)
describe the experiences that are associated with optimal development
on the part of disabled adolescents:

1. Having a confidant
2. Gaining a sense of mastery rather than playing a dependent passive role
3. Having successful experience in the development of self-esteem
4. Having someone in one's life with personal meaning and significance, particularly during times of stress
5. Having the ability to discuss stressful or potentially stressful situations with others facing such difficulties
6. Having available an adult other than a close relative for advice
   and support
7. Knowing where to go for support
8. Having the opportunity to engage in activities outside the home
   that confirm the adolescent's identity as an emerging adult
9. Having the opportunity to develop one's own inner resources,
   such as interests and leisure pursuits

The author's own findings concur with most of these observations.
The relatively lesser importance of disability severity to self-image in
comparison with societal and significant-others' response to the disability
(Goldberg, 1977) indicates that increasing the exposure of even the most
severely disabled adolescent to normal daily activities is a fundamentally
important consideration in the promotion of optimal development. This
must be accompanied by the instruction of family members as to how
their actions and attitudes facilitate (or impede) such development. If social

and interactional limitations persist in the disabled adolescent's everyday milieu, a lag in the development of social and interpersonal competence will most likely result (Oswin, 1967). With fewer opportunities to share, to engage in reciprocal helping behavior, and to use affection, the limited social contacts that characterize the lives of many children with CP can affect their ability to communicate and develop a sense of belonging and identity outside the setting of the primary family. Indeed, it is the absence of a peer group and the lack of friends that are identified as the most serious problems facing a brain-damaged disabled adolescent (White, 1978).

The author's study has sought to demonstrate that the promotion of a positive self-image and developmental capability in disabled adolescents does not require extraordinary measures or methods. Rather, it is the content and quality of daily life—with family, friends, age mates, and strangers—that determines the development of competency and capability in all adolescents, including both the disabled and the able-bodied. It is in this direction that practitioners' attentions should be directed.

ACKNOWLEDGMENTS

The author would like to express his appreciation to the following people: Robert Blum, Tom Norris, Melissa Hamp, Tommy Wells, Judy Brady, Bruce Johnson for participating in interviews for this study; Bob Polland at Camp Courage, who made the interviews possible; Richard Owen at the Sister Kenny Institute, our adult "key informant" panel; and Michael Baizerman who participated in those initial explorations. A heartfelt thanks is given to project assistant Anne Damon, who fully participated in this project from conceptualization through interviewing, content analysis and coding, and providing humor and insight when both were badly needed.

This research was supported in part by Bio-Medical Research Support Grant #507RR05448, Division of Research Resources, National Institutes of Health, and by a University of Minnesota Graduate School Grant-in-Aid of Research.

REFERENCES

Altman, B.M. Studies of attitudes towards the handicapped: The need for a new direction. *Social Problems*, 1981, *28*(3), 321–337.
Anderson, E.M., & Klarke, L. (B. Spain, Collaborator). *Disability in adolescence*. London & New York: Methuen, Inc., 1982.

Bentovin, A. Emotional disturbances of handicapped pre-school children and their families—attitudes to the child. *British Medical Journal*, 1972, *3*, 579.

Berg, K. Effective physical training of school children with cerebral palsy. *Acta Paediatrics Scandinavica*, 1970, *204*(Suppl.), 27–33.

Boles, G. Personality factors in mothers of cerebral palsied children. *Genetic Psychology Monographs*, 1959, *59*, 159.

Brindley, A *Special education: Forward trends*, 1979, (Sept), *6*(3), 26.

Brown, A. Review: physical fitness and cerebral palsy. *Child: Care, Health and Development*, 1975 (March/April), *1*(2), 143–152.

Cammeron, P., Titus, D., Gnadinger, J., & Kostin, M. The life satisfaction of non-normal persons. *Journal of Consulting Clinical Psychology*, 1973, *41*(3), 207–214.

Charles, M. Stark reality. *Nursing Mirror*, *153*(16), Clinical Forum 10, IV–VI, 1981.

Chiles, J., Lipscomb, P. Cerebral palsy in early adolescence: A developmental crunch. *Psychiatric Opinion*, 1979, *16*(9), 29–32.

Cummings, S.T., Bayley, H.C., & Rie, H.E. Effects of the child's deficiency on the mother: A study of mothers of mentally retarded, chronically ill and neurotic children. *American Journal of Orthopsychiatry*, 1966, *35*(4), 595–608.

Dorner, S. Psychological and social problems of families of adolescent spina bifida parents: A preliminary report. *Developmental Medicine and Child Neurology*, 1976, *15, 29*, (Suppl.), 24–27.

Dorner, S. Sexual interest and activity in adolescents with spina bifida. *Journal of Child Psychology and Psychiatry*, 1977, *18*, 229–237.

Egozi, M. *Survey of youth leisure activities ages 10–18*. Jerusalem: Israel Ministry of Education (Hebrew), 1976.

Gage, G., Stoeckler, H., & Thibault, B.J. Minnesota youth share their views. *Quality of life studies series* (Miscellaneous publication 4, 1980). Agricultural Experiment Station, University of Minnesota, Center for Youth Development.

Gliedman, J., & Roth, W. *The unexpected minority: Handicapped children in America*. New York: Harcourt Brace Jovanovich, Inc., 1980.

Golan, H. *Patterns of free time activities of adolescents of Eastern and Western communities*. Unpublished thesis for Master degree, Tel Aviv University (Hebrew), 1977.

Goldberg, R.T. Rehabilitation research on disability. *Journal of Rehabilitation*, 1977, *42*, 14–18.

Goodman, N., Dornbusch, S., Richardson, S., & Hasdorf, A. Variant reactions to physical disabilities. *American Sociological Review*, 1963, *28*, 429–435.

Gordon,N. *Paediatric neurology for the clinician*. London: Heineman, 1976.

Gottlieb, J., & Budoff, M. Social acceptability of retarded children in nongraded schools differing in architecture. *American Journal of Mental Deficiency*,1973, *78*, 15–19.

Gottlieb, J., & Davis, J.E. Social acceptance of EMRs during overt behavior interaction. *American Journal of Mental Deficiency*, 1973, *78*, 141–143.

Har Paz, H., & Hadad, M. Studies, employment and leisure activities among young people. *Researches and Surveys* (No. 50). Tel Aviv: Tel Aviv Municipality (Hebrew), 1976.

Heber, R.F. The relation of intelligence and physical maturity to social status of children. *Journal of Educational Psychology*, 1956, *47*, 158–162.

Hen, M. Similarities and differences in leisure patterns in Israel. *Megamot*, 1974, *13*, 2 (Hebrew).

Hollingshead, A.B. *Two Factor Index of Social Position*, 1965 Yale Station, New Haven, Connecticut, 1957.

Huberman, G. Organized sports activities with cerebral palsied adolescents. *Rehabilitation Literature*, 1976 (Apr.), *37*(4), 103–106.

Hunt, P. *Stigma: the experience of disability*. London: Geoffrey Chapman, 1966.

Johnson, G.O. Social position of mentally handicapped children segregated in the regular grades. *American Journal of Mental Deficiency*, 1950, *55*, 60–89.

Kemp, N.J. Social-psychological aspects of blindness: a review. *Current Psychological Reviews*, 1981, *1*, 69–89.

Klein, S. *Chronic kidney disease: Impact on the child and family and strategies for coping.* Unpublished doctoral thesis, University of Minnesota, Aug. 22, 1975.

Lairy, G.C., & Harrison, C.A. The blind child and his parents: Congenital visual defect and the repercussion of family attitudes in the early development of the child. *Research Bulletin of the American Foundation for the Blind*, 1973, *25*, 1–24.

Lancaster-Gaye, D. What about leisure? *International Rehabilitation Review*, 1973, *24*(2), 6–11.

Lansdown, R. *More than sympathy: The everyday needs of sick and handicapped children and their families.* London & New York: Tavistock Publ., 1980.

Leichtman, S., & Friedman, S. Social and psychological development of adolescents and the relationship to chronic illness. *Medical Clinics of North America*, 1975 (Nov.), *59*(6), 1319–1328.

Litman, T. The family as a basic unit in health and medical care: A social behavioral overview. *Social Science and Medicine*, 1974 (Sept.), *8*, 495–519.

Little, W.J. On the influence of abnormal parturition, difficult labours, premature birth and asphyxia neonatorum on the mental condition of the child, especially in relation to deformities. *Tractus of the Obstetrical Society of London*, 1862, *3*, 293–345.

Margalit, M. Leisure activities of cerebral palsied children. *Israeli Journal of Psychiatry and Related Sciences*, 1981, *18*(3), 209–214.

Mattson, A. The chronically ill child: A challenge to family. *Medical College of Virginia Quarterly*, 1972, *8*, 171.

Mattson, A. Long term physical illness in childhood: A challenge to psychosocial adaptation. *Pediatrics*, 1972, *50*(5), 801–809.

Mauser, H.J., & Reynolds, R.P. Effects of a developmental physical activity program on children's body coordination and self-concept. *Perceptual and Motor Skills*, 1977, *44*, 1057–58.

Minde, K.K. Coping styles of 34 adolescents with cerebral palsy. *American Journal of Psychiatry*, 1978 (Nov.), *135*(11), 1344–1349.

Minde, K.A., Hackett, J.D., Killou, D., & Silver, S. How they grow up: 41 physically handicapped children and their families. *American Journal of Psychiatry*, 1972 (June), *128*(12), 104–110.

Nielsen, H.H. *A psychological study of cerebral palsied children.* Copenhagen: Munksgaard, 1966.

O'Reilly, S., & Elliott, D. The future of the cerebral palsied child. *Developmental Medicine and Child Neurology*, 1971, *13*, 635–640.

Oswin, M. *Behavior problems amongst children with cerebral palsy.* Bristol: John Wright & Sons, Ltd., 1967.

Pless, I.B., Roghmann, K.J., & Haggerty, R.J. Chronic illness, family functioning, and psychological adjustment: A model for the allocation of preventive mental health services. *International Journal of Epidemiology*, 1972, *1*, 271–277.

Pless, I.B., & Douglas, J.W.B. Chronic illness in childhood. Part I. Epidemiological and clinical characteristics. *Pediatrics*, 1971, *79*, 351–359.

Podeanu-Czehofski, I. Is it only a child's guilt? Aspects of family life of cerebral palsied children. *Rehabilitation Literature*, 1975 (Oct.), *36*(10), 308–311.

Poznanski, E.O. Emotional issues in raising handicapped children. *Rehabilitation Literature*, 1973 (Nov.), *34*(11), 322–326.

Resnick, M.D. The social construction of disability and handicap in America. In R. Blum (Ed.), *Chronic illness and disabilities in childhood and adolescence.* New York: Grune & Stratton, Inc., 1983.

Roessler, R., & Bolton, B. *Psychosocial adjustment to disability.* Baltimore: University Park Press, 1978.

Rosenberg, M. *Society and the adolescent self image*. Princeton: Princeton University Press, 1965.

Rosenberg, M., & Simmons, R. Black and white self esteem: The urban school child. *Arnold M. and Caroline Rose Monograph Series*. Washington: American Sociological Association, 1972.

Rowe, B. *A study of social adjustment in young adults with cerebral palsy*. Unpublished B.M.Sc. dissertation, University of Newcastle-on-Tyne, 1973.

Rutter, M., Tizard, J., & Whitmore, E. *Education, health and behaviour*. London: Longman, 1970.

Safilios-Rothschild, C. *Love, sex and sex roles*. Englewood Cliffs, NJ: Prentice-Hall, Inc., 1977.

Sandowski, C.L. The handicapped adolescent. *School of Social Work Journal*, 1979, *4*(1), 3–13.

Seidl, A.H., Altschuler, A. Interventions for adolescents who are chronically ill. *Children Today*, 1979 (Nov-Dec), 16–19.

Shere, E., Kastenbaum, R. Mother–child interaction in cerebral palsy: Environmental and psychosocial obstacles to cognitive development. *Genetic Psychology Monographs*, 1966, *73*, 244–335.

Skellern, J. The self-concept of children and adolescents and the effects of physical disability. *The Australian Nurses' Journal*, 1979 (Dec-Jan) *8*(6), 36–38.

Steinhause, H.C. Chronically ill and handicapped children and adolescents: Personality studies in relation to disease. *Journal of Abnormal Child Psychology*, 1981, *8*(2), 291–297.

Tavormina, J.B., Kastner, L.S., Slater, P.M., & Watt, S.L. Chronically ill children: A psychologically and emotionally deviant population? *Journal of Abnormal Child Psychology*, 1976, 99–110.

Titley, R.W. Imaginations about the disabled. *Social Science and Medicine*, 1969, *3*, 2938.

White, R. *Special child: A parents' guide to mental disabilities*. Boston & Toronto: Little, Brown & Co., 1978.

Wolfish, M.G., & McLean, J.A. Chronic illness in adolescence. *Pediatric Clinics of North America*, 1974 (Nov.), 1043–1049.

Yeadon, A., & Grayson, D. *Living with impaired vision: An introduction*. American Foundation for the Blind, New York, 1979.

Zimbardo, P. The age of indifference. *Psychology Today*, 1980 (Aug.), 70–76.

Sarah O. Colwell

18

The Adolescent with Developmental Disorders

Defining disorder as *a derangement of function* and development as *the whole process of growth and differentiation by which the potentialities of a zygote, spore, or embryo are realized* (Webster's Third New International Dictionary, 1966), the adolescent with a developmental disorder could be one with any condition that interferes with the realization of potential. This could include cognitive disorders, motor handicaps, sensory defects, language impairments, and disorders of social functioning.

This broad range of disorders can be due to a variety of factors that might occur at any time in an individual's life cycle. Genetic influences include chromosomal disorders, such as trisomy 21 or fragile-X syndrome; inborn metabolic defects, such as Phenylketonuria and mucopolysaccharidoses; and the possible polygenic inheritance of some learning disabilities. Prenatal events, including congenital infections, bleeding, poor maternal nutrition, and toxic substances such as alcohol may also cause developmental difficulties. Perinatal sources of problems include prematurity, birth asphyxia, and jaundice. In childhood, infections such as encephalitis or meningitis, serious trauma, abuse, starvation, or poisonings, such as with lead, can all adversely affect the future adolescent's development. Failure to reach full potential can also be due to problems with parents or society. Parents who are themselves adolescents, for instance, may be unprepared for the role; there may be family stresses secondary to divorce; economic pressures may overwhelm a family's capacity to cope; and society may not accept or provide useful niches for each individual. From this diverse range of problems, two of the most common

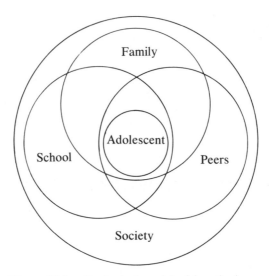

Figure 18-1. Ecological model of functioning.

are learning disorders and mental retardation. Both are diverse in their own right. There is no archetypal learning disabled or retarded adolescent. Each individual is different, with different strengths, weaknesses, and ways of interacting with their surroundings.

Using an ecological model, such as that outlined by Bronfenbrenner (1979a), adolescents can be viewed as existing in a variety of environments (including their family, school, and peer group), which in turn are embedded in the macrosystem of the society and culture to which they all belong (see Figure 19-1). All of these environments interact with and affect one another and the individual adolescent. A developmental disorder will change these interactions; this change will in turn have repercussions on the adolescent's development.

The issues and developmental tasks facing the adolescent who has a developmental disorder are the same as those faced by any other teenager. The adolescent must develop a sense of self, of identity, and an integrated body image. There should be growth toward independence and separation from family. School imparts knowledge and preparation for employment in addition to acting as a social environment for the adolescent. Peers form an increasingly important system of support and a milieu for the expression of sexuality. Finally, the adolescent has to find his or her place in society. The presence of a disability can influence how all of these issues are approached and resolved.

THE ADOLESCENT

The child enters adolescence with a set of characteristics derived from genetics, prenatal and postnatal events, and interactions with family, friends, and society. As the adolescent develops an identity and a sense of self, all of these factors will play a role. A certain amount of cognitive ability is needed to be able to look at one's self as a separate entity and to understand and incorporate the rapid physical changes that come with maturation. Interactions and feedback from family and peers play a large role in the development of self-esteem and the feeling of being in control. The adolescent with a developmental disorder must adjust to being different at a time when he or she most wants to be like others.

The Adolescent With Learning Disorders

Learning disorders affect from 5 to 20 percent of school-aged children at a male:female ratio of 6–8:1. These disorders have been described as the "high-incidence–low-severity" handicaps of childhood (Levine, Brooks, & Shonkoff, 1980). Although these disorders may be considered of low severity when compared perhaps to retardation, they have a great range of severity, type, and impact. The whole concept of learning disabilities is a relatively new one, and in many ways these disorders are still being characterized and defined. One definition in common usage is that outlined by the National Advisory Committee on Handicapped Children (1968):

"Specific learning disability" means a disorder in one or more of the basic psychological processes involved in understanding or in using language, spoken or written, which manifest in disorders of listening, thinking, talking, reading, spelling, or arithmetic. Learning disabilities *include* conditions referred to as perceptual handicaps (auditory or visual), brain injury, minimal brain dysfunction, dyslexia, and developmental aphasia, etc. Learning disabilities *do not include* problems due primarily to visual, hearing, or motor handicaps, mental retardation, emotional disturbance, and environmental disadvantage.

Although this definition is designed to describe the child of normal intelligence who is not doing as well as expected in school because of a presumed processing difficulty, it is important to remember that the child with the excluded disorders may have a learning disorder in addition to his or her primary handicap. By adolescence, it is often particularly hard to determine which came first—an emotional problem causing poor functioning in school or years of academic failure causing a secondary emotional problem.

There are multiple areas of development that appear to be important for school functioning. These include visual–spatial skills, sequencing abilities, memory, language, fine and gross motor skills, and appropriate selective attention (Levine et al., 1980). Weakness in any of these areas, and particularly in multiple areas, can lead to specific academic problems, such as poor reading, math, and writing skills. Poor selective attention and the associated symptoms of distractibility, impulsiveness, failure to complete tasks, and frequent excessive motor activity (especially in the younger child) can have a pervasive effect on school functioning. This constellation of symptoms has been most recently labeled the attention deficit disorder (DSM-III, 1980).

The controversy over the etiology of learning disorders is reflected in the multitude of terms used to label children with school failure. These have included minimal brain damage, minimal brain dysfunction, hyperactivity, dyslexia, specific learning disability, and many others. The problems have been viewed as secondary to brain injury, lags in neurodevelopmental maturation, or variations in brain "wiring" or neurotransmission. The high incidence of affected males and the evidence of positive family histories suggest that genetics may play a role in some cases of learning disabilities. It has been shown that some children with sex chromosomal anomalies have an increased incidence of learning disabilities. Girls with Turner's syndrome (45, X), for example, have an increased incidence of visual–spatial problems, leading to difficulties with writing, math, and finding their way around, while both males and females with an extra X chromosome (47, XXY and 47, XXX) commonly have more language difficulties (Pennington, Bender, Puck, Salbenblatt, and Robinson, 1982; Ratcliffe, 1982). For most children, however, the probability is for a polygenic inheritance with a sex difference in expression (Morrison & Stewart, 1973; Pennington & Smith, 1983). There certainly exists a multitude of possible etiologies that can "alter brain development through a large number of different pathways, including interaction between a specific genetic change in a particular environment" and thus cause a learning disorder (Pennington & Smith, 1983). These multiple causes manifest themselves in a wide variety of expressions; with the expanding taxonomy of syndromes, a descriptive approach may be the most useful in the effort to understand and help the learning-disordered child.

Many learning disorders present early in childhood or when the child begins elementary school. By adolescence, effective remediation of the problem may have allowed some students to learn basic skills well enough to apply them to the more complex tasks of junior high and high school. Other adolescents may have residual problems but have developed bypass strategies to handle the work. Yet others will have experienced years of school difficulties and chronic academic failure.

Certain learning disorders go unrecognized until adolescence, when the changing demands of school overcome coping abilities that were adequate for elementary school. The adolescent with a high IQ score may be significantly underachieving, yet be able to remain at grade level through elementary school, until he or she presents in junior high with academic problems, lowered self-esteem, withdrawal and depression (Faigel, 1983). The greater demands for written output in the higher grades may make keeping up more difficult for the adolescent with inefficient processing abilities combined with weaknesses in fine motor skills, rapid visual retrieval, expressive language, and attention, leading to what has been termed "developmental output failure" (Levine, Oberklaid, & Meltzer, 1981). There is a danger that the problems arising in junior high and high school will go unrecognized and that the adolescent will be moralistically labeled lazy or poorly motivated.

Attention deficits are a common cause of school problems in the early elementary school years and are frequently associated with other learning disorders and excessive motor activity. By adolescence, there is generally a decrease in the level of motor activity with approximately half showing marked improvement, and the other half equally divided between those showing minimal and moderate improvement (Mendelson, Johnson, & Stewart, 1971). Although no longer motorically overactive, the student may show persistent problems with attention, distractibility, and concentration, and may need continued pharmacological counseling and educational intervention (Feldman, Denhoff, & Denhoff, 1979). It is important, therefore, to review the early history of the adolescent with a suspected attention deficit for evidence of a persistent problem.

The long-standing academic and social problems of the learning-disordered adolescent all contribute to the increased incidence of poor self-esteem, frustration, depression, and acting-out behaviors—the emotional consequences of chronic failure. These difficulties may form part of the increased risk for school avoidance, truancy, dropping out, and delinquency in these youths.

The Mentally Retarded Adolescent

Mental retardation affects from one to three percent of the population, with a slight male predominance. Retardation is defined by the American Association on Mental Deficiency (AAMD) as "significant subaverage general intellectual functioning existing concurrently with deficits in adaptive behavior and manifesting during the developmental period" (Grossman, 1977a). The modifying effect of considering adaptation accounts in part for the variation in prevalence figures. Mildly handicapped preschool children and adults may function well and, therefore, not be

considered retarded, although the demands imposed by school would uncover their deficits and lead to the diagnosis of retardation.

There is a wide range in severity of retardation; in general, the more
severe levels can be diagnosed at a younger age. Current DSM-III (1980)
terminology distinguishes four subtypes of retardation, using IQ measures:

1. Mild (IQ level 50–70)
2. Moderate (IQ level 35–49)
3. Severe (IQ level 20–34)
4. Profound (IQ level below 20)

Children falling into the 71–84 IQ range are classified as having borderline intellectual functioning. They may need special educational intervention but are not considered retarded.

Adaptive behaviors can have an important modifying effect on the
functioning of individuals with a given IQ score. Adaptive behavior factors
have been defined as "intellectual, affective, motivational, social and motor abilities" (Grossman, 1977b) and have generally been measured using
the Vineland Social Maturity Scale or the AAMD Adaptive Behavior Scale.

Children with mild retardation make up the majority (approximately
75–80 percent) of the retarded population. These children are described
as *educable* and may achieve an academic level of up to the sixth grade.
Many will be self-supporting and independent in adulthood. Associated
medical problems are much less likely than in the more severely retarded.
As noted, these children are frequently not identified as retarded at all
until school age (only 25 percent are diagnosed in the preschool period)
and about two thirds lose the label when they become adults (Tarjan,
Wright, Eyman, & Keeran, 1973). There is an overrepresentation of children from socioeconomically deprived families in this group, indicating
the potential effect of a disadvantaged environment on intellectual functioning.

Those who are moderately retarded make up 12–15 percent of the
retarded population. These people are described as *trainable*. Some are
capable of achieving a second-grade academic level, and they can often
be taught vocational skills that allow for employment in a sheltered workshop. Daily living skills can be developed and used in a group home setting
where supervision is available.

The severely and profoundly retarded make up the smallest group,
generally eight percent and less than one percent, respectively, of the
handicapped population. They need constant supervision, and frequently
they require total care. The severely retarded may learn some self-care
skills but, generally, can learn no academic skills and will develop only
limited speech.

There is a much higher probability of finding an identifiable cause for retardation in the moderately and severely affected. The possible causes include a multitude of chromosomal anomalies, metabolic disorders, malformations, congenital viral infections, toxins, perinatal factors (including a history of prematurity and birth asphyxia), and childhood trauma, abuse, infections, and poisonings. Associated medical conditions are also much more common in the severely retarded. Such things as seizure disorders, cerebral palsy, sensory handicaps (including hearing difficulties and visual disturbances), hydrocephalus, and other forms of brain dysgenesis are common. All socioeconomic classes are equally represented in this more severely affected population.

By the time the retarded child enters adolescence, the fact and degree of his or her retardation is usually well known. In those few adolescents who sustain a severe head trauma, stroke, or infection during this period, the extent of damage and degree of retardation must be determined and the difficult adjustment to a handicap made by the child and family.

Emotional problems are much more common in the retarded population. Between 30 and 50 percent show significant behavioral and psychiatric problems; the range is broad and includes hyperactivity, psychosis, personality disorders, neuroses, and antisocial behavior (Corbett, 1976). In one study (Eaton & Menolascino, 1982) of retarded children and adults referred for psychiatric evaluation, the most common diagnoses were:

1. Organic brain syndromes with behavioral or psychotic reactions (29.8 percent)
2. Personality disorders (27.1 percent)
3. Adjustment reactions (21.0 percent)
4. Schizophrenia (21.0 percent)

These disturbances probably have a multifactorial etiology. Important factors include the organic brain damage that could be causing the retardation, temperamental characteristics (including impulsiveness, poor attention, and difficulty with new situations), peer isolation and rejection, poor language skills (making communication difficult), family stresses caused by having a retarded child, and the effects of poor institutional care (Corbett, 1976).

THE FAMILY

An important issue for any adolescent is separation from the family and development of a new, mature relationship with parents and siblings. This task becomes possible as new connections are made with peers for support, and as identity as a separate individual, capable of economic independence, is developed. The ability of the adolescent with a learning disorder or retardation to negotiate this issue is dependent on both the nature and the severity of the handicap and on past family relationships.

Family can be defined as biological parents, who have a genetic and prenatal influence on the child; siblings; and, for some, adoptive family members and the significant adult caretakers and peers in foster homes, group residences, and institutions. All play an important role in providing the family environment in which the adolescent develops. This environment is not static but is formed by the changing characteristics of parents and siblings and by the ongoing interactions with the child, schools, and society.

During adolescence, the child goes through changes, becomes physically larger and perhaps more difficult to control, develops secondary sexual characteristics, and at times, falls further from parental expectations. Parents of adolescents are generally middle-aged and may be facing their own mid-life developmental issues. An increasing awareness of their own mortality may make them more anxious about their child's future. With the current high divorce rate and the strain a disability places on a marriage, family stress may be increased due to parental separation, divorce, or single parenting. In group home and institutional settings, frequent staff turnover may also make supportive relationships difficult to establish. Siblings are also growing up and moving away from the family. Older siblings may be able to take more responsibility for the adolescent with a disorder, but at the same time, they may resent this increased burden and the time spent by parents dealing with their handicapped sibling.

The Adolescent With Learning Disorders

The type and severity of learning disorder and the possible presence of an attention deficit will affect how the family adjusts to and handles the problem. The child who is impulsive, nonreflective, insatiable, distractible, and motorically overactive from early childhood may leave parents feeling exhausted, frustrated, inadequate, angry, and guilty. By adolescence, parents of these children may have had years of experience in dealing with professionals and school programs, whereas other parents may be taken by surprise if their adolescent develops school problems in junior high after a successful elementary school career.

Parental expectations for school achievement may significantly change the impact of a learning disorder. A reading disorder may cause more stress in a family that places a high value on academics than it does in a family where most knowledge is received from television and neither of the parents completed school.

The school experiences of the parents will also affect their view of the problem. There is an increased incidence of history of hyperactivity in parents of hyperactive children. This may lead either to feelings of guilt about "causing" the condition or to an understanding and acceptance of the child's difficulty. The painful memory of a grade retention may make a parent much less accepting of this remediation option.

An increased rate of psychiatric illness may also adversely affect family functioning. Cantwell (1972) found an increased prevalence of alcoholism and sociopathy in male relatives, and hysteria in female relatives, of hyperactive children.

In their longitudinal study of the children of Kauai, Werner and Smith (1979) showed that the interaction of perinatal stresses and family instability led to a high risk for developing learning problems. The majority of learning disabilities persisted from age 10 to 18, with continued academic underachievement, truancy, and acting-out behavior. The factors of parental understanding, involvement, and emotional support, along with the development of an internal locus of control in the child, correlated with improvement of learning and behavior problems during adolescence.

Siblings of the adolescent with a learning disorder may be another source of support or conflict. The nondisabled child may resent the increased involvement of parents with their troubled sibling and the frequent double standard in parental treatment. It can be difficult when a younger sibling surpasses the often hard-won academic achievements of the child with a learning disability. Finally, siblings, like peers, may be less tolerant of the adolescent who is different.

The role of parents in the life of the learning-disabled child appears to be one of advocacy, especially during adolescence when services are less often available. Parents also provide opportunities for learning and support for the development of a positive self-image. During adolescence, this parental support must be balanced with a "letting go" and allowance of more independence.

The Mentally Retarded Adolescent

The effect of mental retardation on a family depends to a great extent on the severity of the handicap and the child's skills and behaviors. The more severe the disorder, the earlier it becomes evident to the family. When parents first learn of their child's retardation, they will encounter feelings associated with any loss: shock, disbelief, denial, anger, and guilt. They have lost their hoped for "perfect child," and they grieve for him or her. Over time, these feelings are often joined by loneliness, isolation, and exhaustion.

Parents of the retarded are frequently overprotective. This may result from uncertainty about the child's abilities, guilt over feeling that they caused the condition, and feeling that it is easier and faster to "do it themselves" (Gayton, 1975). The continuing dependence of the moderately and severely retarded adolescent on the family is a strain, as are worries about the mildly retarded adolescent and whether he or she will be able to function independently. Frequently, there are also ongoing financial stresses associated with medical difficulties, extra expenses for adaptive equipment, respite care, and providing for the future of the retarded adolescent.

Over time, the reality of the retarded child's problems becomes clear. Parents often come to accept the child, although they may not accept the child's condition. Frequently, parents develop what has been termed "chronic sorrow," characterized by periodic recurrence of sadness, guilt, shock, and pain (Wikler, Wasow, & Hatfield, 1981). These recurrences often happen at times of stress and are frequently precipitated by the child's deviance from normal developmental patterns at specific crisis points. For adolescents, these developmental crisis points include the onset of puberty, the retarded child's 21st birthday, discussion about placement outside the home, and arrangement of guardianship and care for the disabled individual after the parents die (Wikler, et al., 1981).

Parents must balance the needs of their handicapped child against the needs of the rest of the family. Over time, the retarded child effectively becomes the youngest sibling. The adjustment of other siblings is often dependent on the overall coping abilities of the family. Brothers and sisters may be embarrassed by their sibling, may be angry at their own increased responsibilities, or may neglect their sibling and feel guilty for that. During adolescence, many siblings may worry that they will have to take over as permanent caretakers, or they may become concerned about their own reproductive risk.

Multiple supports are often needed to help the family adjust to a mentally retarded adolescent. Parent groups can often decrease the family's sense of isolation and offer the opportunity to share ideas. The availability of family counseling services may aid the adjustment of parents and siblings to the handicapped child. Respite care is another important aspect of family coping. Families of handicapped children who were surveyed about the use of respite care indicated that it was important for relief time, vacations, special events, and covering for family and medical emergencies. However, they also indicated that many of the severely handicapped were excluded from respite care and there was a great variation in community availability (Upshur, 1982). The community, therefore, must develop respite care services for families and adequate living situations for the retarded adult, in order to support a movement toward independence that is comfortable for the retarded adolescent and his or her family.

THE SCHOOL

School plays many roles in the life of the adolescent. It is a place where academic skills are taught, knowledge about the world is imparted, and preparation is made for future employment. It is also a social system of peers and nonparent adults. By the end of the school career, the average child will have spent 15,000 hours in school.

Michael Rutter (Rutter, Maughan, Mortimore, & Ouston, 1979) has shown that schools have a significant impact on their students' behavior, academic performance, attendance, and delinquency. In a study of London school children, factors that were not associated with school outcome included available resources, class and school size, amount of punishment, and organizational structure. Positive effects, however, were derived from the intellectual balance of students and from a number of "school processes," including the amount of praise given students, the physical appearance and comfort of the school environment, opportunities for student responsibility and participation, academic emphasis, positive role models provided by teachers, style and efficiency of classroom teaching, and cohesiveness of the approach to curriculum and discipline.

Certainly, the skills and intelligence a child brings to school are important factors in determining his or her academic success, but schools play an important role. For the adolescent with a developmental disorder, attending school can be like trying to fit a square peg into a round hole—full of frustrations. Since the passage of the Education for All Handicapped Children Act (Public Law 94-142, 1975), schools are mandated to serve all children with disabilities, to utilize individualized educational programs, and to serve them in the least restrictive environment feasible. The law also stresses parental participation and periodic review. This allows schools to help the handicapped adolescent by modifying both the "peg" and the "hole" (see Reynolds, Chapter 6).

The Adolescent With Learning Disorders

Early and appropriate remediation is probably the key to helping the learning-disabled adolescent, although what constitutes effective intervention is still not clear. An accurate description of the child's strengths and weaknesses may pinpoint the areas in need of remediation and what skills can be used to devise bypass strategies. For example, a child may have poor handwriting because of poor visual–spatial skills and fine motor problems. Work with matching tasks, puzzles, and drawing may help improve visual–spatial perception and integration, while a handwriting program to overlearn the fine motor control needed for letter formation may also be of benefit. Learning to type can be an effective way to produce clear, legible output. Decreasing writing demands and allowing the child to present material as a class presentation or tape recorded report can be another effective bypass strategy.

With the recognition of learning disorders, and programs mandated by Public Law 94-142, a variety of levels of educational intervention are now possible. In ascending order, these include special education monitoring (for example, of a child with an attention deficit and no academic difficulties), Title I tutoring, varying amounts of resource-room time, a substantially separate classroom with limited mainstreaming, and finally, placement in a special school for learning-disabled children. The severity and type of the child's disorder, behavioral–emotional factors, and at times, the parents' abilities to advocate for their child can all influence the educational setting and program.

By adolescence, many children whose learning problems surfaced earlier have developed the skills needed for continued adequate academic functioning and do not require services. Others may need help in developing basic survival skills in reading and math. Some adolescents may need programs to develop organizational skills, particularly in the stressful new environment of junior high school. Here the new exposure to changing classes, multiple teachers, and increased homework demands may overwhelm the coping capabilities of the child. Remediation of individuals in this age group is often further complicated by the adolescent's denial of being "different," or of having a problem.

Another important intervention strategy for the learning-disabled adolescent is vocational training. Learning a nonacademic skill may provide a new sense of mastery to the child who has experienced little academic success, and simultaneously leading to possible future employment opportunities.

For the adolescent who wants to continue education past high school, it is now possible to take the Scholastic Aptitude Tests in both untimed written and oral formats. Some colleges have also shown an interest in providing special programs for the learning disabled.

Despite the parental involvement outlined by Public Law 94-142, there has been a gradual isolation of the school from the family and community. This appears to be occurring because of the centralization of education, with the closing of neighborhood schools, an increase in family mobility, and working parents who are not available for interaction with the school. Bronfenbrenner (1979b) suggested that

> the alienation of children and youth and its destructive developmental sequelae reflect a breakdown of the interconnections among the various segments of the child's life—family, school, peer group, neighborhood, and the beckoning, or all too indifferent or rejecting, world of work.

The Mentally Retarded Adolescent

Educational programs for the mentally retarded adolescent demand flexibility and multiple components. These components include mainstreaming with normal peers, academics, life skills and activities of daily living, vocational and work training, appropriate social skills, sensory stimulation, and respite care for families.

Mildly retarded adolescents need a program with a strong academic focus to develop their skills in this area to their fullest potential. For some, this is up to a sixth-grade level, which would allow adequate reading of a daily newspaper. Many, however, will attain a much lower grade level. Skills needed in daily living should also be stressed. Learning about time, how to handle money, balance a checkbook, write letters, fill out applications, and read cookbooks and food labels would all be of use. A *family living* curriculum is another aspect of education necessary for this group. Important topics would include sexuality, decision making, relationships, and child rearing and development. Vocational training programs also play a vital role in the education of the mildly handicapped. These programs can prepare them for paying jobs, which will allow them to achieve financial independence as adults. Most of the academic teaching is done in a special education classroom, but mainstreaming into the regular classroom with nonhandicapped peers is frequently possible for other subjects. This allows for decreased isolation and more social contacts with the peer group. Some mildly retarded adolescents will also have learning disorders, making academics difficult despite relative intellectual strength. Bypass strategies and drill in basic skills may be effective in helping them cope to the best of their ability.

The school program for the moderately retarded adolescent usually stresses social and self-help skills. Activities of daily living include instruction in grooming, dressing, toileting, eating at a restaurant, and using home appliances. Academic tasks for this group include learning a reading vocabulary of important survival words (such as stop, go, exit, and danger), counting, identifying coins, and reading a digital clock. Some may be able to learn simple arithmetic. Vocational training to prepare the moderately retarded adolescent for a sheltered workshop position is also an important educational component.

In severe and profoundly retarded adolescents, educational efforts are directed primarily at sensory stimulation and socialization. Vocational training is usually not possible in this group, and the primary goal is to maximize their participation in feeding, dressing, and toileting tasks. An important component of the educational program of the severely and profoundly handicapped adolescent is the respite care it provides families.

PEER RELATIONSHIPS

The adolescent also lives within a network of peers developed from school, various activities, the neighborhood, and the community. With the move away from the family toward a new independence, relationships with peers become increasingly more important. These relationships include the development of friendships, formation of cliques, and exploration of romantic and sexual relationships.

There is typically a need to be liked by friends and age-mates and also to be like them, leading to a frequent uniformity of dress, language, and style. The latest fad quickly becomes a widespread phenomenon and is viewed as necessary for acceptance. Although the adolescent years are a time of idealism, there can be an intolerance of those who are different. Erikson (1963) views this as a defense against identity confusion. Adolescents with learning disorders and many of the mildly and moderately retarded do not appear to be different at first glance, but their behavior and social interactions may mark them to their peers and cause them difficulties.

The success of the handicapped adolescent in handling the issue of peer relationships depends on the nature of his or her handicap, its visibility, and the practice the adolescent had in making and keeping friends as a younger child. The self-esteem generated by successes in some areas of functioning and by a supportive family during childhood is also of help. Integration into school and the community is important to decrease the isolation of the adolescent who is different.

The Adolescent With Learning Disorders

The great variability in areas of strength and weakness that characterize those with learning disorders make generalizations difficult. On the one hand, these are invisible handicaps; this may make it harder for peers to understand the nature of the problem and empathize. On the other hand, these disorders are not as threatening to peers as a more obvious handicap; and this perhaps allows for a more complete integration.

Levine (Levine et al., 1980) has outlined multiple factors that can lead to "social failure" in learning-disordered children. These include:

1. Impaired feedback
2. Difficulty predicting social consequences
3. Gross motor problems
4. Behavioral disorganization

5. Physical unattractiveness
6. Stigmatization and bad reputation

Perceptual and language problems may make it difficult for these individuals to interpret the social cues present in peer interactions. The impulsiveness of those with attention deficits can be disruptive and irritating to others and can render them socially unattractive. Some even accentuate their problems and try to fit in by becoming the class clown.

Gross motor skills can be another source of humiliation, or for some individuals, can be a way of gaining acceptance. There is a higher incidence of clumsy children among the learning disordered, probably based on perceptual difficulties, poor sensory organization and, especially by adolescence, a lack of practice (Dare & Gordon, 1970). Always being the last picked for a team, banished to right field, and carrying the label *spaz* can have a detrimental effect on self-esteem and feelings of success and effectiveness. In contrast, the adolescent who does well in sports may be able to use those skills to develop relationships with peers. Although he or she may continue to have difficulty with the academic parts of school, the value placed on gross motor prowess can act to bolster feelings of self-worth. Even those who are awkward may improve their self-esteem, body sense, and skills by participation in individual sports, such as swimming, running, and hiking. Soccer and many of the noncompetitive "new games" can also encourage interaction and cooperation with peers.

The reputation of the adolescent depends on prior and current functioning. The history of a grade retention may be remembered for years by the adolescent, as well as by his or her classmates. The actions of the adolescent, and even the fact of receiving special services, can cause peers to apply such labels of "weirdo," "mental," or "retard" (Levine et al., 1980). Once outcast and negatively labeled, some adolescents may become alienated and drift into groups, in which their impulsiveness and disregard for consequences is considered an asset, leading to vandalism and delinquency.

Intervention in this process requires early and appropriate remediation of the learning disorder. Areas need to be found in which the adolescent can succeed. Contact with peers in a variety of settings apart from the stressful school situation may help. Examples include involvement in clubs, scouts, sports programs, and other available community projects. Peer counseling groups and supportive therapy may help the adolescent with poor social skills develop improved sensitivity to social cues and thus improve relationships. Finally, teachers may be able to develop increased awareness of and sensitivity to learning disorders among their students.

The Adolescent With Mental Retardation

The retarded adolescent, as well as his or her family, tends to be isolated from peers. Parents may have been more protective of their mentally handicapped child and thus decreased the child's chances for interaction in the neighborhood and community. The child who made friends in elementary school may find these friends becoming distant as they move into adolescence and become uncomfortable with their handicap. Often, the retarded adolescent has had little contact with a wide variety of agemates; even with mainstreaming, more time is spent in the isolated special education programs. Opportunities for practicing social skills and developing relationships are therefore limited. The appearance and behavior of some mentally retarded students can also impair their acceptance. They suffer from the effects of peer labeling and the realization of being different.

In mainstreaming programs for the mildly retarded, the retarded students generally were found to have a relatively low social status. Several classroom factors were found to influence this. For example, cohesiveness of the class, more time in teacher-taught groups, positive social interactions with the teacher, and structured group activities that stressed cooperative behavior all had a positive influence (Semmel & Cheney, 1979).

The development of social skills and peer relationships has an effect on the handicapped adolescent's self-esteem, which in turn may influence the emergence of psychological problems and future success at employment. The social skills that seem to be important for eventual successful job placement include personality, self-esteem, absence of antisocial behavior, and an appropriate supervisor–worker relationship (Foss & Peterson, 1981).

Leisure activities can be important to the development of self-esteem and peer relationships in the retarded. For younger children and adolescents, involvement in programs such as Special Olympics can be an arena for success and involvement with a group of peers with similar handicaps. For older adolescents, leisure activities can help integrate them into the community. This may be best approached by programs that promote personal friendships with nonhandicapped peers in an individualized way, concentrating on everyday activities (Salzberg & Langford, 1981).

SOCIETY

The society and culture in which the adolescent and his or her more immediate surrounding environments are embedded also play an important role in the adolescent's development. There is great variation between societies existing at the same time, as well as in the same society over time. The whole notion of childhood has changed through the centuries and varies from one society to another. Adolescence itself is seen as a cultural invention of more complex societies, in which there is a delay in the granting of adult status beyond the time of biological maturation (Stone & Church, 1975).

The prevailing view toward handicapping conditions can affect the attitude of parents, schools, peers, and even of the developmentally disordered individual. In many cultures in the past, severely handicapped children were killed in infancy. Even now, there is a higher incidence of child abuse of children with developmental disorders, ranging from those with hyperactivity to those with severe handicaps. This abuse may be the result of the handicap and the stress and emotional strain on the family; abuse can, in turn, cause a handicap (Solomons, 1979). In general, however, there has been a recent expanding acceptance of the child who is different, with a growth of community-based programs for education, work, and living.

The Adolescent With Learning Disorders

The concept of learning disorders is a relatively recent one. In years past, the higher illiteracy rate, lack of compulsory education, and multitude of valued occupations in agriculture and trades that did not require reading and writing skills, obviated the need for such an idea. The adolescent who was not academically inclined had a variety of options leading to financial independence and respect within the community. With the current practice of more standardized and mandatory education and the high value placed on academic pursuits in our society, the adolescent with academic problems faces fewer alternative opportunities. Learning disorders have been used to explain the etiology of the adolescent falling short of his or her potential. The negative effects of what is still a poorly understood label can be seen to be offset by the benefits of increased services to children, greater understanding by parents and teachers of the behaviors shown, and the support provided by such groups as the Association for Children with Learning Disabilities (Rist & Harrell, 1982).

Legally, adulthood for the learning disordered adolescent comes at 18 years, the age of majority. Life often becomes much easier for the learning-disabled child and adolescent in adulthood. There is much more freedom in what can be done and what can be avoided. If survival reading and math skills are attained, the adult can function in society, using radio and television to keep current instead of newspapers and books. Success will then depend on whether the adolescent has had adequate preparation for jobs and appropriate vocational counseling and placement.

The Mentally Retarded Adolescent

The severely retarded have probably been identified in all cultures, while the more mildly retarded may, like those with learning disorders, have found useful roles in earlier or more nontechnological societies. In his study of China, Robinson (1978) found that mild retardation was not viewed as a problem in that culture. Schools stressed group learning with large doses of repetition and drill, and part of each school day was spent in a work environment. Socialization was "exceptionally consistent from home to school to peer group," allowing full participation of the slow child. The cultural expectations for adolescents and young adults to live at home, the supports of the community, and the availability of work for all made integration of the retarded adult much smoother.

In America, the mentally retarded were at one time cared for at home. In the early 1900s, large-scale institutional care of the retarded and handicapped became more prevalent. This, in turn, has been followed by the recent trend toward resettling the retarded in smaller group residences in the community. This societal move toward deinstitutionalization and recognition of the rights of the retarded has resulted in greater visibility of the handicapped in the community and legal mandates for appropriate educational programs. Advocacy groups, such as the Association for Retarded Citizens, have been influential in promoting care of the retarded and providing support for families.

The attainment of adult status is a more difficult issue for the retarded. At age 18 years, the question of their competency to handle their legal rights and property must be addressed. If some form of continued supervision is needed, the level required must be determined. This can range from guardianship, by either an individual or the state, to more informal supervisory arrangements that preserve the retarded individual's civil rights.

One of the civil rights maintained in a less restrictive supervisory relationship is that of marriage. This, coupled with the increased recognition of the right to sexual expression and the greater freedom of living in community residences, makes marriage and childbearing now more likely in the retarded population. This places additional demands on society to provide adequate supports for parents with limited intellectual abilities and appropriately stimulating environments for their children, who are frequently of normal intelligence.

CONCLUSIONS

In order to realize the full potential of the adolescent with a developmental disorder, early identification of the problem, without pejorative and harmful labeling, is necessary. Families need supports, including accurate and complete information about their child's difficulties, respect for being the experts on their child, services such as schooling and respite care, and emotional support for parents and siblings (Featherstone, 1980).

Educational services must be appropriate and available. Early intervention may decrease the incidence of problems, particularly in the "culturally" retarded and the learning disordered. In adolescence, a wide range of programs, including vocational training and skills of daily living, must be offered.

Integration of the adolescent into peer groups and the community is also vital. There must be a new understanding of those who are different and acceptance of each as an individual of inherent worth.

REFERENCES

Bronfenbrenner, U. *The ecology of human development: Experiments by nature and design.* Cambridge: Harvard University Press, 1979a.

Bronfenbrenner, U. Contexts of child rearing: Problems and prospects. *American Psychologist,* 1979b, *34*(10), 844–850.

Corbett, J. Mental retardation-psychiatric aspects. In M. Rutter & L. Hersov (Eds.), *Child psychiatry: Modern approaches.* Philadelphia: J.B. Lippincott, 1976, 829–855.

Dare, M.T., & Gordon, N. Clumsy children: A disorder of perception and motor organization. *Developmental Medicine and Child Neurology,* 1970, *12*, 178–185.

DSM-III. *Diagnostic and statistical manual of mental disorders* (3rd ed.). Washington, D.C.: American Psychiatric Association, 1980.

Eaton, L.F., & Menolascino, F.J. Psychiatric disorders in the mentally retarded: Types, problems, and challenges. *American Journal of Psychiatry,* 1982, *139*(10), 1297–1303.

Erikson, E.H. *Childhood and society.* New York: W.W. Norton, 1963.

Faigel, H.C. Learning disabilities in adolescents with high IQ scores. *Journal of Developmental and Behavioral Pediatrics,* 1983, *4*(1), 11–15.

Featherstone, H. *A difference in the family—life with a disabled child.* New York: Basic Books, 1980.

Feldman, S.A., Denhoff, E., & Denhoff, J.I. The attention disorders and related syndromes: Outcome in adolescence and young adult life. In E. Denhoff & L. Stern (Eds.), *Minimal brain dysfunction: A developmental approach.* New York: Masson, 1979, 133–148.

Foss, G., & Peterson, S.L. Social-interpersonal skills relevant to job tenure for mentally retarded adults. *Mental Retardation,* 1981, *19*(3), 103–106.

Gayton, W.F. Management problems of mentally retarded children and their families. *Pediatric Clinics of North America,* 1975, *22*(3), 561–570.

Grossman, H.J. (Ed.) *Manual on terminology and classification in mental retardation.* Washington, D.C.: American Association on Mental Deficiency, 1977a.

Grossman, H.J. Mental retardation. In M. Green & R.J. Haggerty (Eds.), *Ambulatory pediatrics II.* Philadelphia: W.B. Saunders, 1977b, 271–283.

Levine, M.D., Brooks, R., & Shonkoff, J.P. *A pediatric approach to learning disorders.* New York: John Wiley, 1980.

Levine, M.D., Oberklaid, F., & Meltzer, L. Developmental output failure: A study of low productivity in school-aged children. *Pediatrics,* 1981, *67*(1), 18–25.

Mendelson, W., Johnson, N., & Stewart, M.A. Hyperactive children as teenagers: A follow-up study. *Journal of Nervous and Mental Disorders,* 1971, *153*(4), 273–279.

Morrison, J.R., & Stewart, M.A. Evidence for polygenic inheritance in the hyperactive child syndrome. *American Journal of Psychiatry,* 1973, *130*(7), 791–792.

National Advisory Committee on Handicapped Children. *Special education for handicapped children.* Washington, D.C.: First Annual Report United States DHEW, 1968.

Pennington, B.F., Bender, B., Puck, M., Salbenblatt, J., & Robinson, A. Learning disabilities in children with sex chromosome abnormalities. *Child Development,* 1982, *53*(5), 1182–1192.

Pennington, B.F., & Smith, S.D. Genetic influences on learning disabilities and speech and language disorders. *Child Development,* 1983, *54*(2), 369–387.

Ratcliffe, S.G. Speech and learning disorders in children with sex chromosome abnormalities. *Developmental Medicine and Child Neurology,* 1982, *24*(1), 80–84.

Rist, R.C., & Harrell, J.E. Labeling the learning disabled child: The social ecology of educational practice. *American Journal of Orthopsychiatry,* 1982, *52*(1), 146–160.

Robinson, N.M. Mild mental retardation: Does it exist in the People's Republic of China? *Mental Retardation,* 1978, *16*(4), 295–298.

Rutter, M., Maughan, B., Mortimore, P., & Ouston, J. *Fifteen thousand hours: Secondary schools and their effects on children.* Cambridge, MA: Harvard University Press, 1979.

Salzberg, C.L., & Langford, C.A. Community integration of mentally retarded adults through leisure activity. *Mental Retardation,* 1981, *19*(3), 127–131.

Semmel, M.I., & Cheney, C.O. Social acceptance and self-concept of handicapped pupils in mainstreamed environments. *Education Unlimited,* 1979, *1*(2), 65–68.

Solomons, G. Child abuse and developmental disabilities. *Developmental Medicine and Child Neurology,* 1979, *21*(1), 101–108.

Stone, L.J., & Church, J. Adolescence as a cultural invention. In A.H. Esman (Ed.), *The psychology of adolescence: Essential readings.* New York: International Universities Press, 1975, 7–11.

Tarjan, G., Wright, S.W., Eyman, R.K., & Keeran, C.V. Natural history of mental retardation: Some aspects of epidemiology. *American Journal of Mental Deficiency,* 1973, *77*(7), 369–379.

Upshur, C.C. Respite care for mentally retarded and other disabled populations: Program models and family needs. *Mental Retardation,* 1982, *20*(1), 2–6.

Webster's Third New International Dictionary. P.B. Gove (Ed.), Springfield, MA: G&C Merriam, 1966.

Werner, E.E., & Smith, R.S. An epidemiologic perspective on some antecedents and consequences of childhood mental health problems and learning disabilities: A report from the Kauai Longitudinal Study. *Journal of the American Academy of Child Psychiatry,* 1979, *18*(2), 292–306.

Wikler, L., Wasow, M., Hatfield, E. Chronic sorrow revisited: Parent vs. professional depiction of the adjustment of parents of mentally retarded children. *American Journal of Orthopsychiatry,* 1981, *51*(1), 63–70.

RESOURCES

Association for Children with Learning Disabilities
    4156 Library Road
    Pittsburgh, PA 15234
Association for Retarded Citizens
    2709 Avenue E East
    Arlington, TX 76011

Mary Ella Pierpont
Bonnie S. LeRoy
Shari R. Baldinger

19
Genetic Disorders

Thousands of conditions affecting adolescents have a proven genetic or familial etiology. In addition, there are many other conditions that may have a genetic etiology. The discussion of genetic disorders in this chapter will, therefore, be limited to some examples that present in adolescence and those with medical problems significant in adolescence. Finally, a discussion of genetic counseling techniques and case examples is included.

GENETIC DISORDERS THAT COMMONLY PRESENT IN ADOLESCENCE

Disorders of Sexual Differentiation

Puberty and subsequent sexual maturation are aspects of development that are important to each and every adolescent. In almost all cases, individual sex and gender role have long been established by the time of adolescence. It is a time when many physiological processes are occurring within the adolescent body. These changes include rapid growth, change in external genitalia, synthesis of sex hormones, and menarche in females. All of these processes are under genetic control, and consequently, many disorders of sexual differentiation can be traced to a genetic basis. Many genetic forms can be identified long before adolescence because they commonly present with ambiguous genitalia (e.g., congenital adrenal hyperplasia, an autosomal recessive condition). However, there are many

CHRONIC ILLNESS AND DISABILITIES IN CHILDHOOD AND ADOLESCENCE ISBN 0-8089-1635-1

genetic disorders of sexual differentiation that are most commonly identified in adolescence, among which are chromosomal abnormalities and
gonadal dysgenesis.

Chromosome Abnormalities

Turner syndrome (45, XO).   Turner syndrome is a relatively common
cytogenetic disorder affecting as many as 1 in 1000 female live births. The
syndrome can usually be identified after puberty because the female has
primary amenorrhea. It was first described by Turner in 1938, long before
its chromosomal basis was understood. Physical characteristics of the
original female patient included sexual infantilism, short stature, webbed
neck, and cubitus valgus (Crawford, 1979). In 1944, it was discovered that
streaks of stromal tissue without follicles replaced ovaries in these patients.
Thus, the condition became known as gonadal dysgenesis.

The chromosomal basis for Turner syndrome (45, XO) was established
by the end of the 1950s (Nyhan, 1983). Although this is the most
common karyotype, many cytogenetic variations have been described,
including individuals with one normal X chromosome and the second X
affected by various deletions, isochromosomes, and ring abnormalities.
Sometimes, mosaicism (45, XO/46, XX) is encountered, indicating a
postzygotic error of nondisjunction. It is possible that 30 percent or more
of all Turner females are mosaics, with two or more cell types (Nyhan,
1983).

Ideally, this syndrome may be recognized at birth and its cytogenetic
basis established. However, the patient is usually not diagnosed until after
the age of puberty, when amenorrhea becomes obvious. Clinical features
that may aid in diagnosis are:

1. Lymphedema, although this usually resolves by one year of age
2. Coarctation of the aorta or aortic stenosis, seen in 15 percent
   of cases
3. Hypoplastic nails
4. Cystic hygroma
5. Ureteropelvic stenosis
6. Low birth weight
7. Short fourth metacarpals
8. Shield-shaped chest with wide-set nipples
9. Multiple pigmented nevi that appear at puberty
10. Retarded bone maturation or osteoporosis
11. Recurrent otitis media

Patients with Turner syndrome should be distinguished from those
with Noonan syndrome. Noonan syndrome affects both sexes; individuals

have short stature, unusual facies, and neck webbing. It is thought to be an autosomal dominant condition with normal chromosomes. Patients often have mental retardation and pulmonic stenosis (Collins & Turner, 1973). Somatic features of Turner syndrome are sometimes seen with mixed gonadal dysgenesis (45, XO/46, XY). Identifying these patients by chromosomal analysis is essential because they have a high risk (15–20 percent) of gonadoblastoma. Preventive surgical intervention is advised (i.e., removal of streak gonadal tissue) (Simpson & Photopulos, 1976a).

Management of patients with Turner syndrome may include plastic surgery for prominent webbing. Because most Turner patients have no ovarian follicular components, plasma gonadotropins are in post menopausal ranges by age 11 (Peress, Sosnowski, Mathur, & Williamson, 1982). Cyclic hormone replacement can be initiated in adolescents to induce menses, promote secondary sexual characteristics, and maximize height, which rarely exceeds five feet (Park, Bailey, & Cowell, 1983). Various complications involving different degrees of cellular dysplasia have been reported in patients receiving such supplementation; therefore, benefits must be weighed against risks when using hormonal therapy in adolescents.

Growth hormone supplementation has been considered for Turner females. Although some of these females have lower growth hormone levels than normal females, all patients with supplementation experienced an increased growth rate (Wilson, 1983). The ultimate potential of this mode of therapy has yet to be determined, but such supplementation has some potential for inducing disorders of carbohydrate metabolism (Nielson, Sorensen, & Sorensen, 1981).

Two other problems potentially facing the adolescent patient with Turner syndrome are dental malocclusion and poor posture (Crawford, 1979). Normal intelligence is the rule, although patients may have problems with spatial relations. Turner females have succeeded in highly academic vocations, unlike patients with most other chromosomal abnormalities.

The vast majority of cases are sporadic and are unassociated with maternal age. This is in contrast to other meiotic nondisjunction anomalies. Amniocentesis is available for prenatal diagnosis in families who wish reassurance that no chromosomal abnormalities have occurred. As many as 99 percent of 45, XO conceptions are spontaneously aborted. The 45, XO karyotype is the most common chromosomal abnormality found in first trimester spontaneous abortions (Crawford 1979).

Until the 1960s, all Turner syndrome patients were counseled that they were sterile. However, in 1960, the first report of a pregnancy in "gonadal dysgenesis" appeared (Kable & Yussman, 1981). Several other cases of pregnancy have been reported over the past two decades in both mosaic and apparently nonmosaic 45, XO females with Turner syndrome (Kohn, Yarkoni, & Cohen, 1980; Nielson, Sillesen & Hanson, 1979; Wray,

Treeman, & Ming, 1981). However, 45, XO women have an increased risk of stillbirths, spontaneous abortions, and chromosomally abnormal offspring if conception takes place. The aforementioned exceptions should be reviewed when providing counseling regarding menses, possible fertility, and genetic amniocentesis, as well as plans for long-term hormone supplementation and management.

In the author's experience, adolescent females with Turner syndrome are most concerned with having menstrual periods "like other girls," and with the development of secondary sexual characteristics. In addition, they are concerned with achieving a good height, although even when they are small, they do not have dwarfism. As older adolescents and adults, they frequently require psychological counseling because of their sterility and the anxieties that this generates.

Klinefelter syndrome (47, XXY). In 1942, Klinefelter described a syndrome characterized by gynecomastia, azoospermia, small testes, and elevated levels of follicle-stimulating hormone in an adult male phenotype. In 1959, the 47, XXY karyotype was demonstrated in these patients. The frequency appears to be approximately 1–2 in 1000 live male births (de Grouchy & Turleau, 1977; Wu, Bancroft, Davidson, & Nicol, 1982).

Klinefelter males appear to be normal at birth (Humphrey, Posen, & Casey, 1976), and due to the absence of dysmorphic features, the diagnosis is often not made until puberty or adulthood. In childhood, the testes are normal in appearance and histology. Around the time of puberty, the seminiferous tubules are irregular in arrangement, and atrophic with hyaline tissue. The testes fail to mature into adult size and function. Sterility is usually the rule with these patients; however, there are reports of Klinefelter patients producing spermatozoa (Foss & Lewis, 1971; Futterweit, 1967). Testosterone levels are usually below normal when compared with age-matched controls (Raboch, Mellan, & Starka, 1979; Sorensen, Nielsen, Wohlert, Bennett & Johnson,1981).

Adolescents with Klinefelter syndrome often are tall and eunuchoid, with an upper to lower body-segment ratio of less than one. There is a tendency toward gynecomastia, especially in overweight patients. Acute nonlymphocytic leukemia has been reported to occur at a higher than expected incidence in Klinefelter males, suggesting an association between the two disorders (Geraedts, Mol, Briet, Hartgrink-Gronevald & den Ottolander, 1980; Mamunes, Lapidus, Abbott, & Roath, 1961; Muts-Homsma, Muller, & Geraedts, 1981; Penchansky, & Krause, 1982).

Most often, Klinefelter males are normal in intelligence (Nielson et al, 1981), although verbal IQ scores tend to be lower than normal, and some patients have language difficulties (Ratcliffe, Bancroft, Axworthy, & McLaren, 1982; Salbenblatt, Bender, Puck, et al., 1981; Tolksdorf, Gutezeit, & Munke, 1981). Personality problems are common, with a tendency toward shyness, withdrawal, underachievement, and compulsive aggressive behavior (Harkulich, Marchner, & Brown, 1979). These problems sometimes can be resolved by family and individual patient counseling, including supportive and educational guidance in school. Early counseling of parents may help to decrease feelings of guilt and anxiety and improve the parent–child relationship. Adolescents raised in a stable home environment with open communication will have fewer adjustment problems on reaching adulthood. The combination of low testosterone levels and the usual personality characteristics in these males contributes to retarded sexual development. Sexual interest is typically lower than normal (Raboch et al., 1979).

Hormone treatment (testosterone) is usually initiated between 12 and 13 years of age; in many patients, testosterone replacement therapy brings on normal pubertal changes and improves the behavioral problems associated with this disorder. In some, however, hormonal therapy elicits a minimal response, suggesting variable sensitivity of each patient to the supplementation (Nielson et al., 1981; Wu et al., 1982).

Cytogenetic studies of males who exhibit the Klinefelter phenotype usually have 47 chromosomes, with an extra X chromosome in all cells. There are reports of other rare cytogenetic constitutions in some patients. Mosaicism including 47, XXY/46, XY cell lines, 48, XXYY, and even 46, XX karyotypes have all been demonstrated in the Klinefelter phenotype (Nicolis, Hsu, Sabetghadom, Kardon, & Chernay, 1972; Parker, Mavalwala, Melnyk, & Fish, 1970; Schlegel, Aspillaga, Neu, & Gardner, 1965). Patients with 48, XXXY karyotype may have some features of Klinefelter syndrome, but mental retardation is likely, and hypogonadism is more severe (de Grouchy, 1977).

Gonadal Dysgenesis

Hypogonadism at puberty is sometimes caused by gonadal dysgenesis. Usually, affected individuals have streak gonadal tissue and female phenotype. Most cases of gonadal dysgenesis are caused by the 45, XO karyotype, or other structural rearrangements of the X chromosome. However, there are cases of adolescents with gonadal dysgenesis who have normal karyotypes (Simpson, Christakos, Horwith, & Silverman, 1971).

XX Gonadal dysgenesis.   Over 150 cases of XX gonadal dysgenesis have been reported. These adolescent females have sparse pubic hair, minimal breast development, and amenorrhea. They usually are of normal height and do not exhibit other clinical characteristics of 45, XO females (Simpson, 1979a). Identification of these females is important so that hormonal therapy can be initiated and also because this appears to be an autosomal recessive condition (i.e., siblings may be affected) (Simpson, 1979b).

XY Gonadal dysgenesis. In cases of XY gonadal dysgenesis, the adolescent has a female phenotype but a normal male karyotype (46, XY). XY gonadal dysgenesis is composed of a heterogeneous group of clinical expressions (Simpson, Blagowidow, & Martin, 1981). In the "pure" form (to be discussed here), individuals have streak gonads, amenorrhea, and lack of somatic features of Turner syndrome. This form is believed to be determined by an X-linked gene; familial clusters of affected individuals have been reported (Espiner, Veale, Sands, & Fitzgerald, 1981).

The most significant medical problem in individuals with XY gonadal dysgenesis is that they have a 20–30 percent chance of developing dysgerminoma or gonadoblastoma in the streak gonadal tissue (Simpson & Photopulos, 1976b). This may occur even in the first or second decade. Since this condition is commonly recognized only after puberty, surgical removal of streak gonadal tissue should be performed as soon as the diagnosis is confirmed. Other possible medical problems include any of several forms of renal disease (congenital nephrotic syndrome, renal failure), which may be evident in adolescent years (Gertner, Kauschansky, Giesker, Siegel, Breg, & Genel, 1980; Harkins, Haning, & Shapiro, 1980).

Understanding why these individuals have a female phenotype is possible through a review of embryological differentiation of gonadal tissue (Simpson, 1980). It is believed that the Y chromosome normally controls testicular differentiation. Somehow, perhaps by H–Y antigen (Jones, Rary, Rock, & Cummings, 1979; Wachtel 1980), a Y chromosome product influences the indifferent embryonic gonad to transform into a testis. The testis can then synthesize testosterone (Wolffian stabilization), dihydrotestosterone (genital virilization) and müllerian inhibiting factor (regression of female structures). Without these hormones, female genital, structural, and phenotypical differentiation ensues.

In the case of XY gonadal dysgenesis, one of several abnormalities may be present. Y chromosome production may be inhibited or, alternatively, receptors of the indifferent gonad may be insensitive to the Y product. Finally, another gene locus (perhaps on the X chromosome) may be responsible for suppression of the Y product for testicular differentiation (Simpson, 1980; Wachtel, 1980).

Genetic counseling of individuals with XY gonadal dysgenesis should include a thorough discussion of embryology of gonadal tissue as well as an explanation of X-linked inheritance. Female offspring of females who may be carriers should undergo early chromosomal study. Psychological problems may occur in adolescent females affected by XY gonadal dysgenesis, and they may require long-term counseling.

Single Gene Disorders

Over 3000 known medical disorders are due to single gene alterations. The patterns of inheritance include autosomal dominant, autosomal recessive, and X-linked. Since autosomal recessive and X-linked conditions usually manifest before adolescence, this section will concentrate on conditions with autosomal dominant inheritance.

Marfan Syndrome

The Marfan syndrome, an autosomal dominant disease, has many manifestations that cause significant medical problems in adolescence. The major clinical features involve the eye (ectopia lentis, myopia, retinal detachment), skeleton (dolichostenomelia, pectus excavatum, joint laxity, scoliosis), and cardiovascular system (aortic root dilatation, mitral valve prolapse).

Most individuals with the Marfan syndrome have been diagnosed by the time they reach adolescence because of their physical appearance, ophthalmological status, or cardiac manifestations. As many as 85 percent of the cases are familial, with only 15 percent sporadic cases or new mutations (Pyeritz & McKusick, 1979). The expressivity of the Marfan dominant gene is highly variable, however, and not every patient with Marfan syndrome has all of the features (Pyeritz, Murphy, & McKusick, 1979).

At least two of the characteristic features (family history and ocular, skeletal, or cardiovascular involvement) should be present for diagnosis. Individuals with one or two clinical features (for example, scoliosis and mitral valve prolapse) may be classified as forme frustes of Marfan syndrome. However, a study of relatives of 18 patients with severe aortic disease resembling Marfan syndrome did not detect any others with classic Marfan features (Emanuel, Ng, Marcomichelakis, Moores, Jefferson, MacFaul, & Withers, 1977). For this reason, care must be taken to obtain the correct diagnosis, especially since accurate genetic counseling depends upon it.

For adolescents with the Marfan syndrome, there are significant chronic medical problems that require special care. Each patient, for instance, should be under the regular care of an ophthalmologist. When dislocation of lenses occurs it is usually bilateral (Cross & Jenson, 1973). Although it may not be possible to correct the lens problems, other, treatable complications, such as glaucoma and retinal detachment, commonly occur during the second decade of life. Rapid diagnosis and management of these treatable conditions may be essential to the preservation of vision.

In adolescence, the development of scoliosis is a serious complication of Marfan syndrome. Scoliosis may progress rapidly during the adolescent growth spurt. Consequently, frequent examination of adolescents with Marfan syndrome is advisable (Robins, Moe, & Winter, 1975). Other skeletal manifestations that could cause significant medical problems in adolescence include joint hypermobility and instability, and pectus excavatum. Pectus excavatum may be especially unpleasant for the adolescent, who may be self-conscious about this deformity. The major indication for surgical repair of pectus excavatum has been cardiopulmonary compromise, which may manifest in adolescence.

Cardiovascular manifestations constitute a significant medical problem. In fact, previous reports have documented that the shortened life span of individuals with the Marfan syndrome is usually due to cardiovascular complications (Pyeritz & McKusick, 1979; Roberts & Honig, 1982). The most common cardiovascular complications are aortic root dilatation and mitral valve prolapse (Phornphutkul, Rosenthal, & Nadas, 1973; Pyeritz & McKusick, 1979). Progressive aortic root dilatation occurs over many years and can lead to aortic insufficiency in adolescence. Aortic dissection and rupture usually do not occur in adolescence, but they have been known to occur. All patients with the Marfan syndrome should have frequent cardiovascular examinations. If aortic dilatation becomes severe, elective prophylactic repair of the ascending aorta (Pyeritz, Gott, McDonald, Achuff, Brinker, Haller, & Hutchins, 1982) with prosthesis is indicated, even in childhood or adolescence. Other recommendations include prophylactic propranolol (Pyeritz & McKusick, 1979), which is not fully proven to be of benefit, and antibiotic prophylaxis to prevent bacterial endocarditis.

The cardiovascular aspects of this disease also necessitate restriction of the life-style of the adolescent. Contact sports, isometric exercise, lifting weights, and exhaustive physical activities should be avoided. In addition, those with serious cardiovascular disease should avoid any significant physical exertion. Affected females should avoid pregnancy because of the increased risk of vascular rupture. In addition, significant psychological problems may result from having to face this chronic potentially lethal disorder; the knowledge that it is inherited and can be passed on with 50 percent risk may also contribute to emotional disturbance in adolescents.

Neurofibromatosis

Classic neurofibromatosis, or von Recklinghausen disease, is one of the most common disorders produced by a single gene mutation. Approximately 75,000 people in the United States are affected by this disorder, including individuals of all races and ethnic backgrounds. Onset of symptoms usually occurs in childhood or adolescence.

The disorder involves cells of neural crest origin, thus, it affects all areas of the neurological system and the skin (Riccardi, 1980). Marked variability in expression of this disease is usually present, even within the same family (Carey, 1979). Neurofibromatosis tends to be progressive.

Understanding this and the potential scope of systemic involvement is important to the diagnosis, management, and counseling of affected individuals and their families.

Cafe au lait spots are present in well over 99 percent of all patients with neurofibromatosis (Riccardi, 1981a, 1981b). Crowe, Schull, and Neel (1956) specified six spots larger than 1.5 cm in diameter as a criterion for defining the disorder. Some families have affected members with only multiple cafe-au-lait spots. This may present a counseling and diagnostic dilemma; these cafe au lait spots may be insufficient to diagnose neurofibromatosis.

Cafe au lait spots are often present at birth and tend to increase in size and number throughout the first decade of life. The main concerns of adolescent patients with respect to their cafe au lait spots include cosmetic appearance and self-image, since the spots themselves represent no medically significant threat. They may even be found in the fundus of the eye (Cotlier, 1977).

Other diagnostic clinical features that aid in defining the disorder are axillary freckling, Lisch nodules or iris nevi (94–97 percent), areolar tumors in postpubertal females (86 percent), and cutaneous neurofibromas, 5–10 percent of which undergo malignant transformation (Knight, Murphy, & Gottlieb, 1973; Riccardi, Kleiner, & Lubs, 1979). These manifestations tend to exacerbate with puberty, use of oral contraceptives, and pregnancy, all three of which commonly occur in adolescence (Riccardi, 1981a, 1981b).

Of great importance in diagnosing and counseling is a positive family history. However, it appears that 40–50 percent of all cases are new mutations, giving this gene one of the highest mutation rates (Riccardi, 1981a, 1981b). Other clinically significant manifestations of the disorder are listed in Table 19-1.

Besides the classic form, neurofibromatosis has a genetically distinct form that affects only the central nervous system (Eldridge, 1981). The hallmark features of central neurofibromatosis are bilateral acoustic neuromas. Unlike the more common peripheral form, the central form is rarely associated with pigment changes, malignant transformation, or other skin

Table 19-1
Clinical Features of Classic
Neurofibromatosis

Cafe au lait spots	Pseudarthrosis
Lisch (iris) nodules	Pheochromocytoma
Axillary freckling	Delayed puberty
Cutaneous nodules	Scoliosis
Areolar neurofibromas	Mental retardation
Central nervous system tumors	Malignant tumors

Table 19-2

Comparison of Characteristics of Peripheral and Central Neurofibromatosis

Characteristic	Peripheral neurofibromatosis	Central neurofibromatosis
New mutations	40–50%	Few
Inheritance	Autosomal dominant	Autosomal dominant
Multiple cafe au lait spots	75%	0%
Malignancy	5–10%	Rare
Skeletal changes	Common	Rare
Acoustic neuromas	5%	90%
Variable expression	High	Low
Prevalence	1 in 3000	1 in 10^6
Onset of symptoms	First decade	Second decade

lesions. However, symptoms of hearing loss, tinnitus, headaches, and visual changes are common in the central form and are secondary to the characteristic neuromas. Onset of symptoms usually occurs in the second or third decade. The central form is not marked by the high variability of expression of peripheral neurofibromatosis.

Both forms of neurofibromatosis are inherited as autosomal dominant traits, and males and females are equally affected (Table 19-2, Eldridge, 1981). In each pregnancy, affected individuals have a 50-percent risk of having a child with neurofibromatosis. With the peripheral form, it is difficult to provide accurate counseling because of the wide range of expression; mildly affected individuals sometimes have difficulty understanding that they may have severely affected offspring. It is important to thoroughly explain this concept, which is characteristic of many autosomal dominant traits, so that there is an accurate appreciation of potential burden (Knudson, 1981).

Both the potential health risk and the cosmetic changes involved in neurofibromatosis tend to isolate and stigmatize the patients and their families. Fear of the unknown is best dealt with by full explanation of the natural history of the disorder. Adolescents are especially fearful of the potentially disfiguring aspects of this disease. Peer support groups and genetic counseling are extremely helpful in long-term management.

Tuberous Sclerosis

Tuberous sclerosis was first reported by von Recklinghausen in 1863. The classic form of the disease includes moderate to severe mental retardation (60–83 percent), epilepsy, and adenoma sebaceum (86 percent) (Berberich & Hall, 1979; Lagos & Gomez, 1967; Monaghan, Krafchick, MacGregor, & Fitz, 1981). It was not until 1942 that the term "tuberous sclerosis complex" was employed in view of the hamartomatous nature of the disorder (Moolten, 1942).

Tuberous sclerosis is of interest because of the problems in evaluating and counseling the patient and family. Among the most critical to appreciate are high variability of presentation within a family, lack of penetrance and apparently high percentage of new mutations or sporadic cases (80–90 percent) (Monaghan et al., 1981), and the unpredictability of the clinical course. Although autosomal dominant inheritance is the rule, modifier genes have been suggested to explain the variations (Berberich & Hall, 1979).

Tuberous sclerosis is more common than was originally believed; the incidence estimates are approximately 1 in 30,000 births. The disorder usually is slowly progressive in its clinical course and begins in infancy or early childhood. The central nervous system symptoms tend to be most prominent. In addition to mental retardation, epilepsy, and adenoma sebaceum, tuberous sclerosis may include any or all of the following:

1. Infantile spasms
2. Hypopigmented lesions (15–85 percent)
3. Shagreen patches (20 percent)
4. Intracranial calcifications
5. Retinal phacomas
6. Ungual fibromas at puberty (17 percent)
7. Cafe-au-lait spots (7 percent) (Boesel, Paulson, Kosnick, & Earle, 1979; Roth & Epstein, 1971)

In some cases, there is neither apparent mental retardation (Kofman & Hyland, 1959) nor epilepsy, and onset of neurological symptoms may be abrupt.

Sometimes, only after neurosurgical procedures will some subtle skin lesions be noted and renal hamartomas discovered (O'Callaghan, Edwards, Tobin, Basab, & Mookarjee, 1975). Hydrocephaly and hypothyroidism are occasionally associated with tuberous sclerosis. In its fully developed form, the disease is multisystemic (Table 19-3); patients so affected rarely live beyond 25 years of age (Reece, Gimovsky, & Petrie, 1981). Consequently, during adolescent years, there may be substantial debilitation. In addition, difficulties may be encountered in diagnosing and evaluating the incomplete cases and their family members who are at risk.

The minimal recommendations for testing all family members interested in genetic counseling include the following:

1. Establishment of the diagnosis in the proband
2. Obtaining a detailed family pedigree for all possibly affected individuals, including possible incomplete presentations

Table 19-3
Manifestations of Tuberous Sclerosis

Brain	Intracranial calcifications
	Mental retardation
	Seizures
Skin lesions	Adenoma sebaceum
	Hypopigmented lesions
	Shagreen patches
	Cafe au lait spots
	Ungual fibromas
Eye	Retinal phacoma
Lungs	Cystic changes
Heart	Rhabdomyomata
Bones	Sclerotic changes
	Osteoblastic changes

3. Physical examination with Wood's lamp to detect any hypopigmented skin lesions
4. Ophthalmological examination to rule out retinal hamartomas
5. Computerized axial tomography of brain
6. Ultrasound of kidneys
7. Chest x-rays in females over the age of 35

Included in this evaluation should be all first degree relatives of the proband.

Affected individuals should be counseled that there is a 50 percent
risk of affected offspring for each pregnancy; they should be informed of
the concept of variable phenotypical expression. Both sexes are affected
equally, and the disorder shows no racial predilection.

Osteogenesis Imperfecta

Osteogenesis imperfecta, or hereditary bone fragility, is a connective
tissue disorder. A wide variety of phenotypical features have been reported
in association with the major symptom of bone fragility. The marked heterogeneity observed in patients with osteogenesis imperfecta allows for
separation into at least four distinct syndromes—osteogenesis imperfecta
I, II, III, and IV (Sillence, Senn, & Danks, 1979b; Sillence, Rimoin, &
Danks, 1979a). This classification is based on mode of inheritance, age
of onset, presence or absence of progressive deformity, blue sclerae, defective dentition, and hearing loss.

Types II and III are congenital forms that are fatal in the neonatal
period (II), or progressive and severely deforming (III). These will not be

Table 19-4
Incidence of Manifestations in
Osteogenesis Imperfecta—Type I

Bone fragility	90–95%
Blue sclerae	100%
Presenile deafness	40–60%
Loose joints	25%
Dentinogenesis imperfecta	50%

discussed further in this chapter. By far the most common, with a frequency of approximately 1 in 30,000 live births (Sillence, 1981) and accounting for about two thirds of all cases is osteogenesis imperfecta I. Previously, this disorder was also known as *dominantly inherited osteogenesis imperfecta* and was associated with deeply blue sclerae and osteogenesis imperfecta tarda. Affected individuals have fragile bones, hypermobile joints, blue sclerae, variable skeletal deformities, otosclerosis with variable progressive deafness, and dentinogenesis imperfecta (Table 19-4). The disease can be quite mild, although as with many other dominant disorders, there can be marked variability within a given family.

An adolescent with this disease has already learned to make many adjustments in life-style. These include avoidance of sports or hazardous recreation that might produce fractures. In spite of this avoidance, trauma-free fractures may occur in childhood but tend to occur less frequently after puberty. Fractures again become a significant problem at menopause in females and with advanced age in males. Other potential clinical considerations in the osteogenesis imperfecta patient are osteosarcoma, pseudarthrosis, kyphoscoliosis, and aortic insufficiency (Sillence et al., 1979a, 1979b).

Osteogenesis imperfecta type I is an autosomal dominant condition with complete penetrance of the blue sclerae and over 90 percent penetrance of bone fragility (Lubs & Travers, 1981). About ten percent of all cases occur without family history and may represent new mutations. Most critical in counseling of osteogenesis imperfecta patients is to establish the correct diagnostic form (I, II, III, or IV). Apparently isolated cases should be confirmed by parental x-ray to rule out mild parental cases (decreased bone density) (Sillence,1981; Sillence et al., 1979a, 1979b).

Counseling these patients and their families must go beyond the need to impress upon them the risks of recurrence. Parents of affected children often greatly overprotect their offspring in order to avoid fractures. This causes tension within the family and emotional problems for the child. In the teenage years, even when symptoms abate, overprotective attitudes often persist. Awareness of family attitudes and a clear understanding by the family of complications, burden, clinical variability, and course of the disease are essential to patient management. Reproductive options should be discussed and should include information pertaining to the possibilities of adoption or artificial insemination (depending on which parent is affected). Affected adolescents who are nearing reproductive age should receive similar counseling, since each pregnancy represents a 50 percent risk of an affected offspring. Prenatal diagnosis by ultrasound or fetogram, although usually used in the severe congenital form (II), may rarely be useful for identification of a very severe neonatal presentation of type I.

Other Disorders

Two other conditions that may present in adolescence are the Prader-Willi syndrome and the fragile-X syndrome. They are both associated with unique chromosomal features.

Prader-Willi Syndrome

The Prader-Willi syndrome frequently is not identified until adolescence. At that time, the cardinal features of obesity, hypogenitalism, short stature, and mental retardation may be recognized as suggestive of the diagnosis. Though many of these features are often present long before adolescence, the obesity may become extreme in early adolescence due to food obsession and thus, the diagnosis may be more apparent (see Story, Chapter 7).

First described in 1956 (Prader, Labhart, & Willi, 1956), it was long considered a sporadic condition. Recently, however, the frequent association of this syndrome with an interstitial deletion of part of the proximal long arm of chromosome 15 (Ledbetter, Riccardi, Airhart, Strobel, Keenen, & Crawford, 1981) has been established. Figure 19-1 illustrates several pairs of chromosome 15 in two patients with Prader-Willi syndrome. Of each pair, there is one normal chromosome 15 and one with a deleted sequence.

The prevalence of obesity in adolescence often brings these patients to attention and diagnosis. In addition to obesity, scoliosis (Holm & Laurnen, 1981) may be a serious medical problem and often requires bracing or surgery. Diabetes may develop and usually requires treatment (Laurance, Brito & Wilkinson, 1981). Life span may be significantly shortened for individuals with this syndrome, especially for those with massive obesity.

Treatment of the obesity may be of benefit in increasing the life span. Careful weight-reduction plans can be instituted, particularly those with behavior modification aspects (Holm & Pipes, 1976; Thompson, Kodluboy, & Heston, 1980). There is some evidence to suggest that a decline in IQ of Prader-Willi patients with age may be prevented by weight control

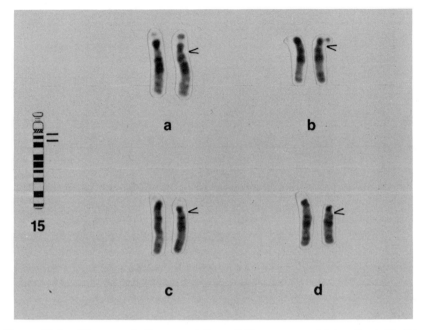

Figure 19-1. Diagramatic Representation of Chromosome 15 (on the left). The bars delineate the area involved in the Prader-Willi deletion, with breakpoints at q 11.2 and q 13. On the right are four pairs of chromosome 15 from different metaphases. The normal chromosome is on the left of each pair and the deleted chromosome is on the right. Pairs *a* and *b* are from patient 1, while *c* and *d* are from patient 2. Photo courtesy of D. Arthur and D. W. Ball, University of Minnesota. (From An International System for Human Cytogenetic Nomenclature —High Resolution Banding (1981). Basel, S. Karger, for the March of Dimes Birth Defects Foundation, *Birth defects: Original article series*, 1981, *17*(5):1–23. With permission.)

through behavior modification techniques of caloric-intake control (Crnic, Sulzbacher, Snow, & Holm, 1980).

Counseling of families of a Prader-Willi adolescent includes discussion of their hypogenitalism and the unlikely chance for reproduction. In addition, recurrence risks (low unless familial translocation is involved) should also be discussed.

Fragile-X Syndrome

For many years it has been known that there is a preponderance of males with mental retardation and more than one clinical form of X-linked mental retardation. One of these forms, the fragile-X or marker-X syndrome, is more often apparent in adolescence or at an older age. The name of the syndrome relates to a fragile site or secondary constriction, which can be demonstrated at Xq27 or 28 in some males with mental retardation (Carpenter, Leichtman, & Say, 1982; Lubs, 1969; Martin, Lin, Mathies, & Lowry, 1980). Expression of the fragile-X site is inhibited by folic acid, thymidine, and folinic acid (Sutherland, 1979), and therefore, lymphocytes must be cultured in a medium deficient in these factors for fragile-X sites to be observed.

In addition, it has been found that some males with mental retardation and fragile-X chromosomes have postpubertal macro-orchidism (Carpenter et al., 1982; Martin et al., 1980; Turner, Gill, & Daniel, 1978), although not all retarded males with macro-orchidism have fragile-X chromosomes (Carpenter et al., 1982; Jacobs, Mayor, Rudak, Gerrard, Ives, Shokeir, Hall, Jenninger & Hoehn, 1979). Other clinical features of the fragile-X syndrome, although highly variable, include preseverative speech patterns, prominent supraorbital ridges, prognathism, and large ears. The syndrome is more frequently detected in adolescence because the enlarged testes become evident at that time.

Females can be heterozygous for the fragile-X chromosome; some of these females are dull or have mild mental retardation (Carpenter et al., 1982). The reason for the occasional occurrence of retardation in a heterozygous female is presumably related to X-inactivation (Lyon hypothesis) of the normal X chromosome. Heterozygous females are usually normal but can transmit the fragile-X chromosome to one half of their sons, as is seen in X-linked conditions. Prenatal diagnosis of fragile-X males has been accomplished (Shapiro, Wilmont, Breholl, et al., Leff, Martino, Harris, Mahoney, & Hobbins, 1982; Sutherland & Jacky, 1982).

One aspect of fragile-X syndrome may be very significant for adolescents and other age groups affected by the disorder: this is the possibility for treatment. Some affected individuals have developed improved performance with folic acid supplementation (Lejeune, 1982). Currently, trials of this treatment are underway, and demonstration of beneficial effects may be forthcoming. It will be important to review these results because it has been estimated that the fragile-X syndrome affects 30–50 percent of families with X-linked mental retardation (Turner et al., 1978).

GENETIC DISORDERS WITH SIGNIFICANT MEDICAL PROBLEMS IN ADOLESCENCE

In this section, examples of genetic disorders with major medical management problems are discussed. The chosen conditions represent several kinds of genetic inheritance.

Duchenne Muscular Dystrophy

Duchenne, or pseudohypertrophic muscular dystrophy, is the most common type of muscular dystrophy. It occurs in 1 of 3000 live male births (Brooke, 1978; Emery, 1980). It is inherited in an X-linked fashion, and carrier females rarely show any clinical symptoms. Approximately one third of all cases represent new mutations. Clinically, the disease usually becomes evident between three and five years of age, with gait difficulty and proximal muscle weakness. The calves appear large and muscular, even though by this time muscle wasting has taken place. Toe-walking, difficulty in climbing stairs, and problems keeping up with other children are usually the first symptoms noticed by parents of affected youngsters. An affected child usually becomes wheelchair dependent by adolescence and frequently death occurs in the late teens to early twenties. At present, there is no definitive treatment available to alter the course of the disease. Physical therapy to prevent contractures (Scott, Hyde, Goddard, & Dubowitz, 1981) and cardiovascular management of the cardiac failure common in these boys are important (Hunsaker, Fulkerson, Barry, Lewis, Leier & Unverferth et al., 1982).

This is a chronic, progressively debilitating disease that can produce significant psychological problems. Mental and emotional disabilities vary from child to child. In general, these boys are found to have a lower than average IQ (Brooke, 1978; Leibowitz & Dubowitz, 1981). Depression is not uncommon, especially around the time the child becomes wheelchair bound. Families, who are themselves often unable to fully accept the disease, frequently have difficulty in helping the child to accept and cope with his clinical course. Teachers and friends at school who may not understand the disorder may add to his emotional problems. Early adolescence is difficult for any child, but when this time includes a progressive debilitating disorder and confinement to a wheelchair, and therefore exclusion from most "normal" adolescent activities, extra support is needed.

When involved with the care of a child with Duchenne muscular dystrophy, it is important to remember that the whole family is affected in some way. Psychosocial counseling should always be made available to the entire family, including siblings. From a genetic standpoint, not only are parents at risk for having another affected child, but female siblings and other female relatives on the maternal side of the family may also be at significant risk of being carriers.

Due to X-chromosome inactivation in females (Lyon hypothesis), carrier status can be determined with 70–80 percent accuracy. Various methods are used for carrier testing, including serum enzyme assays, muscle biopsies for abnormal histology, electromyography (EMG), and electrocardiography studies. The most widely used test is the serum creatine kinase (CK). Between 70 and 80 percent of known carriers have elevated serum CK levels (Lane & Roses, 1981; Muir, Knoke, Martin, Vignos & McErlean, 1983). Testing should be performed on two or three separate occasions, one week apart and following a 24-hour period of limited physical activity (Brooke, 1978; Emery, 1980). Abnormalities in muscle histology and EMG studies have been described, but may not yield more information than the serum CK levels. Carrier detection in pregnant females is unreliable (Zatz, Karp, & Rogatko, 1982).

Prenatal diagnosis of an affected fetus is currently not available with consistent reliability (Emery, 1980). It is, however, possible to determine fetal sex with cytogenetic studies on cells obtained through amniocentesis. Carrier females at risk for having an affected child should be made aware of this option. Often, this is not a popular option with families because it does not specifically identify affected males, but rather all males. However, it is an option that should be fully discussed since the alternatives are a 50 percent risk of bearing an affected son or making the decision not to have children at all. These alternatives may be significantly worse for some individuals. Birth control counseling for any sexually active female who may be a carrier should be available.

Phenylketonuria

Phenylketonuria (PKU) was first described by Folling in 1934. This autosomal recessive disease was previously the most common of all metabolic causes of mental retardation. In the 1950s, the affected population of PKU patients represented one percent of all residents of institutions for the retarded. Since mass screening was begun in the 1960s, dietary treatment has all but eliminated PKU-related retardation (Levy, 1973). Dietary therapy usually is continued until age five or six years, although some patients may not discontinue the special diet until the adolescent years. Scattered reports have shown a decrease in IQ and learning disability upon termination of dietary therapy. One collaborative study found subtle changes in cerebral function in PKU children who have discontinued the diet (Koch, Azen, Friedman, & Williamson, 1982).

Classical PKU is caused by the inability to convert phenylalanine to tyrosine, due to lack of the enzyme phenylalanine hydroxylase. Treatment consists of a strict diet limiting intake of phenylalanine. The diet consists of a basic milk or artificial substance supplemented with natural foods low in protein. In terms of maintaining optimal performance, dietary control may be as important in the adolescent PKU patient as it is in the diabetic.

The striking observation of mental retardation in non-PKU offspring of mothers with PKU was first noted in 1957 by Dent (Levy, 1973). Furthermore, as more treated PKU females have reached childbearing age, a high incidence of microcephaly, retardation, and congenital heart disease has been found in their offspring (Lenke & Levy, 1982; Levy, Lenke, & Crocker, 1979). Recent studies suggest that the pregnant PKU patient should be on a phenylalanine-restricted diet throughout pregnancy; in addition, it is suggested that if this diet is to be effective, the mother must follow it before conception. Perhaps females with PKU should begin the diet at birth and never discontinue it. In those who have discontinued the diet, a similar low phenylalanine diet should be reinstituted to prevent toxic elevation of phenylalanine. At present, fetal levels of 10 mg/dl are considered safe. Due to the fact that phenylalanine concentrates on the fetal side of the placenta, the maximal maternal levels should not exceed 5 mg/dl. Pregnant PKU patients may have difficulty maintaining their pregnancies because the low-protein diet may not permit normal fetal growth.

Counseling of families should involve a discussion of the preceding problems. There are at least 100 PKU treatment centers to aid physicians in patient management. Carrier parents should be apprised of the 25 percent recurrence risk in each pregnancy. Since there is presently no reliable carrier detection available, other family members who are potential carriers should also receive counseling. Any offspring of potential carriers or known carriers should have a serum phenylalanine screen at two weeks postpartum, in addition to the neonatal screen. Prenatal diagnosis is not possible at this time.

As mentioned, early diagnosis and treatment can largely prevent the mental retardation associated with untreated PKU. This applies to the classic phenylalanine hydroxylase deficiency and not to the recently defined tetrahydrobiopterin-deficient PKU. Infants with the latter disorder are likely to experience progressive neurological deterioration when treated only by diet (Matalon, Michals, Lee, & Nixon, 1982).

THE GENETIC COUNSELING PROCESS

A good definition of genetic counseling is the following, offered by McKusick in 1975:

Genetic counseling is a communication process which deals with the human problems associated with the occurrence, or the risk of occurrence, of a genetic disorder in a family. This process involves an attempt by one or more appropriately trained persons to help the individual or family to 1) comprehend the medical facts, including the diagnosis, probable course of the disorder, and the available management; 2) appreciate the way heredity contributes to the disorder, and the risk of recurrence in specified relatives; 3) understand the alternatives for dealing with the risk of recurrence; 4) choose the course of action which seems to them appropriate in view of their risk, their family goals, and their ethical and religious standards, and to act in accordance with that decision; and 5) to make the best possible adjustment to the disorder in an affected family member and/or to the risk of recurrence of that disorder.

Although this is a broad definition, it clearly outlines goals for the genetic counselor. Communication is the key word: to be effective, the necessary information must be communicated at the adolescent's level, at a time when the adolescent is ready to hear the information and is in an environment in which he or she feels safe.

Adolescents are capable of understanding most of the medical facts concerning their disorder. Free and open discussions among the adolescent, the parents, and the physician can provide needed answers. This will reduce fear of the unknown and will help the patient to feel safe enough to ask questions and, hopefully, to accept their condition.

Adolescence is a time for setting future goals. Often one of these goals includes planning a family. Understanding their disease process and the genetics involved will help the adolescent choose realistic goals.

Discussing the genetics of their disorder may be difficult, due to the technical information involved. In many cases, high school biology classes provide a good basis for understanding. Examples of common physical traits such as eye color, hair color, or things such as blood type may help take away the adolescent's feeling of abnormality when discussing a genetic disorder. The risk of having affected offspring is viewed differently, depending upon personal experience with the disease. It is sometimes surprising to discover that one adolescent may view a 50 percent risk as being acceptable while another may view even a one to ten percent risk as too high. The adolescent can be assisted to understand the options available, including adoption, artificial insemination when appropriate, and prenatal diagnosis. Birth control methods should be discussed before an unplanned pregnancy occurs.

There is much information available on the psychosocial aspects of genetic disorders (Kessler, 1979; Reed, 1980). One thing common to all genetic disorders is that the entire family is in one way or another affected—either with the disease itself, with guilt for having "caused" the disorder, or with the fear of developing or passing on the disease. Education pertaining to medical facts and genetic aspects can alleviate guilt and fear, but the patients and family must still face day to day obstacles, especially when the disease results in a physical or cosmetic handicap. Support systems within the family, school, and peer group can make all the difference in self-image. The family often needs help in locating outside support systems for themselves and for the adolescent. In many cases, national and local support groups hold meetings and publish newsletters. The family should always be made aware of these resources and encouraged to participate.

Following are two case histories that illustrate adolescents with genetic disorders. Discussion of counseling issues is provided.

A 17-year-old female was referred due to suspected neurofibromatosis. Ms. A presented to a dermatologist for removal of several moles from the back of her neck, which pathology reports revealed to be neurofibromas. A referral was made to a genetics unit.

Physical examination revealed multiple cafe au lait spots of varying sizes over the trunk and extremities. Multiple small to moderate-sized neurofibromas were found on the trunk and upper extremities, and a few were found on the neck. A large plexiform neurofibroma was present on the anterior left thigh area and on the lateral right hip. Axillary freckling was present. Lisch nodules were not seen. The remainder of the physical examination was normal. CT scan revealed normal optic foramina and auditory canals. Pelvic radiographs were normal. Femoral radiographs revealed a large neurofibroma in the lower right femur. The patient's medical and developmental histories were unremarkable.

Ms. A. gave the following family history: Both parents were alive and well. Her mother had an adrenal tumor removed several years ago. The patient had three brothers and two sisters, all healthy and without nodules or spots on their skin. One sister had her appendix removed at ten years of age. The patient had one maternal first cousin who was mentally retarded, cause unknown, and two other maternal first cousins who were born with heart defects. The remaining family history was negative.

Medical records were obtained regarding the adrenal tumor of the patient's mother and regarding her sister's appendectomy. The patient's mother had a pheochromocytoma, which was surgically removed. The patient's sister had a carcinoid tumor of the appendix. After surgery, neither the mother nor the sister had further complications or stigmata of neurofibromatosis.

The final assessment was classic neurofibromatosis (NF). In this case, as in all such cases, it was essential to communicate to the patient and her family the natural history of the disorder and its autosomal dominant mode of inheritance. Implicit in this, is the 50 percent risk of recurrence for all pregnancies of affected individuals. It is important that the counseled families gain a meaningful appreciation of the intrafamilial variability as discussed in this chapter. To do this effectively, all at-risk family members should be examined to rule out a mild presentation of NF.

To a young female, it is important to communicate the problems pregnancy may create in excerbating the course of the disease. This will involve a discussion of birth control, including recommendation of the best methods for a female with NF. However, of primary concern to a teenage female will be the fears of deformity and possible malignancy. Close medical follow-up by physicians is imperative, and an annual visit to a genetics clinic for discussion and support is encouraged.

An 18-year-old female was referred for chromosome analysis due to primary amenorrhea. Ms. H had previously seen her gynecologist with complaints of no menstrual periods and sparse secondary sexual characteristics. Gynecological examination revealed a normal vaginal canal, small cervix, and small uterus. The patient had sparse pubic hair and small breasts. The cause of the primary amenorrhea could not be determined at that time. A referral was made to a genetics unit.

The patient was a normal healthy female, with a height of five feet ten inches and a weight of 158 pounds. With the exception of amenorrhea, the patient's medical and developmental history was normal. The family history was noncontributory. Blood was drawn for chromosomal analysis. The chromosome studies revealed a 46, XY karyotype. The patient underwent laparotomy and removal of streak gonadal tissue.

Since the final assessment in this case was XY gonadal dysgenesis, important counseling for this patient included a detailed explanation of the chromosomal and genetic basis for sexual development. Through counseling, an appreciation is gained for where the "error" occurred in the normal sequence of gonadal development. This is essential to maximize the patient's identity as a female. One way to help communicate this concept is to explain that male sex is dependent upon an active and working Y chromosome. Therefore, the presence of the Y chromosome in this patient does not detract from her "femaleness," nor does it tamper with her sexual identity. Of course, the need for preventive gonadectomy, as well as the natural course of this condition should be explained. Of special concern regarding this most sensitive sexual disorder is to aid the patient to deal openly and honestly with her feelings of being different from other women and to realize that such a difference does not make her a "freak." One must also address the obvious concerns regarding marriage, sterility, and reproductive alternatives. It is important to communicate to the patient that a normal life is possible. Plans for ongoing psychological counseling should be made if necessary. Follow-up visits with the patient to evaluate pyschological adjustment are highly recommended.

REFERENCES

Berberich, M.S., & Hall, B.D. Penetrance and variability in tuberous sclerosis. *Birth Defects,* 1979, *15* (5), 297–304.

Boesel, C.P., Paulson, G.W., Kosnik, E.J., & Earle, K.M. Brain hamartomas and tumors associated with tuberous sclerosis. *Neurosurgery,* 1979, *4* (5), 410–417.

Brooke, M.H. *A clinician's view of neuromuscular diseases.* Baltimore: Williams & Wilkins, 1976, 95–107.

Carey, J.C., Laub, J.M., & Hall, B.D. Penetrance and variability in neurofibromatosis: A genetic study of 60 families. *Birth Defects,* 1979, *15* (5), 271–281.

Carpenter, N.J., Leichtman, L.G., & Say, B. Fragile X-linked mental retardation. *American Journal of Diseases in Childhood,* 1982, *136,* 392–398.

Collins, E., & Turner, G. The Noonan syndrome—a review of the clinical and genetic features of 27 cases. *Journal of Pediatrics,* 1973, *83,* 941–950.

Cotlier, E. Cafe-au-lait spots of the fundus in neurofibromatosis. *Archives of Ophthalmology*, 1977, *95*, 1990–1993.

Crawford, J.D. Management of children with Turner's syndrome. *Progress in Clinical & Biological Research*, 1979, *34*, 97–109.

Cross, H.E., & Jenson, A.D. Ocular manifestations in the Marfan syndrome and homocystinuria. *American Journal of Ophthalmology*, 1973, *75*, 405–420.

Crowe, F.W., Schull, W.J., & Neel, J.V. *A clinical, pathological, and genetic study of multiple neurofibromatosis*. Springfield, Illinois: Charles C. Thomas, 1956.

Crnic, K.A., Sulzbacher, S., Snow, J., & Holm, V.A. Preventing mental retardation associated with gross obesity in the Prader-Willi syndrome. *Pediatrics*, 1980, *66*, 787–789.

de Grouchy, J., & Turleau, C. *Clinical atlas of human chromosomes*. New York: John Wiley & Sons, 1977, 242–245.

Eldridge, R. Central neurofibromatosis with bilateral acoustic neuroma. *Advances in Neurology*, 1981, *29*, 57–63.

Emanuel, R., Ng, R.A.L., Marcomichelakis, J., Moores, E.C., Jefferson, K.E., MacFaul, P.A., & Withers, R. Formes frustes of Marfan's syndrome presenting with severe aortic regurgitation: Clinicogenetic study of 18 families. *British Heart Journal*, 1977, *39*, 190–197.

Emery, A.E.H. Duchenne muscular dystrophy genetic aspects, carrier detection, and antenatal diagnosis. *British Medical Bulletin*, 1980, *36*, 117–122.

Espiner, E.A., Veale, A.M.O., Sands, V.E., & Fitzgerald, P.H. Familial syndrome of streak gonads and normal male karyotype in five phenotypic females. *New England Journal of Medicine*, 1970, *283*, 6–11.

Folling, A. Uber Ausscheidung von Phenylbrenztraubensaure in der Harn als Stoffwechselanomalie in Verbindung mit Imbezillitat. *Hoppe-Seyler Zeitschrift fuer Physiologische Chemie*, 1934, *227*, 169–176.

Foss, G.L., & Lewis, F.J.W. A study of four cases with Klinefelter's syndrome showing motile spermatozoa in their ejaculates. *Journal of Reproduction & Fertility*, 1971, *25*, 401–408.

Futterweit, W. Spermatozoa in seminal fluid of a patient with Klinefelter syndrome. *Fertility & Sterility*, 1967, *18*, 492–496.

Geraedts, J.P.M., Mol, A., Briet, E., Hartgrink-Groneneveld, C.A. & denOttolander, G.J. Klinefelter syndrome: Predisposition to acute non-lymphocytic leukaemia? *Lancet*, 1980, *1*, 774.

Gertner, J.M., Kauschansky, A., Giesker, G.W., Siegel, N.J., Breg, W.R. & Genel, M. XY gonadal dysgenesis associated with the congenital nephrotic syndrome. *Obstetrics & Gynecology*, 1980, *55*, 665–695.

Harkins, P.G., Haning, R.V., & Shapiro, S.S. Renal failure with XY gonadal dysgenesis: Report of the second case. *Obstetrics & Gynecology*, 1980, *56*, 751–752.

Harkulich, J.F., Marchner, T.J., & Brown, E.B. Neurological, neuropsychological, and behavioral correlates of Klinefelter's syndrome. *Journal of Nervous & Mental Diseases*, 1979, *167*, 359–363.

Holm, V.A., & Laurnen, E.L. Prader-Willi syndrome and scoliosis. *Developmental Medicine & Child Neurology*, 1981, *23*, 192–201.

Holm, V.A., & Pipes, P.L. Food and children with Prader-Willi syndrome. *American Journal of Diseases in Childhood*, 1976, *130*, 1063–1067.

Humphrey, T.J., Posen, S., & Casey, J.H. Klinefelter's syndrome experiences with 24 patients. *Medical Journal of Australia*, 1976, *2*, 779–782.

Hunsaker, R.H., Fulkerson, P.K., Barry, F.J., Lewis, R.P., Leier, C.V. & Unverfertl, D.V. Cardiac function in Duchenne's muscular dystrophy. Results of a 10 year follow-up study and noninvasive tests. *American Journal of Medicine*, 1982, *73*, 235–238.

Jacobs, P.A., Mayer, M., Rudak, E., Gerrard, J., Ives, E., Shokeir, M., Hall, J., Jenninger, M. & Hoehn, N.H. More on marker chromosomes, mental retardation, and macroorchidism. *New England Journal of Medicine*, 1979, *300*, 737–738.

Jones, H.W., Rary, J.M., Rock, J.A., & Cummings, D. The role of the H-Y antigen in human sexual development. *Johns Hopkins Medical Journal*, 1979, *145*, 33–43.

Kable, W.T., & Yussman, M.A. Pregnancy in mosaic Turner patients: Case report and a guide to reproductive counseling. *Fertility & Sterility*, 1981, *35*, 477–479.

Kessler, S. *Genetic counseling, psychological dimensions*. New York: Academic Press, 1979.

Knight, W.A., Murphy, W.K., & Gottlieb, J.A. Neurofibromatosis associated with malignant neurofibromas. *Archives of Dermatology*, 1973, *107*, 747–750.

Knudson, A.G. A geneticist's view of neurofibromatosis. *Advances in Neurology*, 1981, *29*, 237–243.

Koch, R., Azen, C.G., Friedman, E.G., & Williamson, M.L. Preliminary report on the effects of diet discontinuation in phenylketonuria. *Journal of Pediatrics*, 1982, *100*, 870–875.

Kofman, O., & Hyland, H.H. Tuberous sclerosis in adults with normal intelligence. *Archives of Dermatology*, 1959, *81*, 43–48.

Kohn, G., Yarkoni, S., & Cohen, M.M. Two conceptions in a 45, X woman. *American Journal of Medical Genetics*, 1980, *5*, 339.

Lagos, J.C., & Gomez, M.R. Tuberous sclerosis reappraisal of a clinical entity. *Mayo Clinic Proceedings*, 1967, *42*, 26–49.

Lane, R.J.M., & Roses, A.D. Variation of serum creatine kinase levels with age in normal females: Implication for genetic counseling in Duchenne muscular dystrophy. *Clinica Chimica Acta*, 1981, *113*, 75–86.

Laurance, B.M., Brito, A. & Wilkinson J. Prader-Willi syndrome after age 15 years. *Archives of Diseases in Childhood*, 1981, *56*, 181–186.

Ledbetter, D.H., Riccardi, V.M., Airhart, S.D., Strobel, R.J., Keenen, B.S. & Crawford, J.D. Deletions of chromosome 15 as a cause of the Prader-Willi syndrome. *New England Journal of Medicine*, 1981, *304*, 325–329.

Leibowitz, D., & Dubowitz, V. Intellect and behavior in Duchenne muscular dystrophy. *Developmental Medicine and Child Neurology*, 1981, *23*, 577–590.

Lejeune, J. Is fragile X syndrome amenable to treatment. *Lancet*, 1982, *1*:273–274.

Lenke, R.R., & Levy, H.L. Maternal phenylketonuria. Results of dietary therapy. *American Journal of Obstetrics and Gynecology*, 1982, *142*, 548–552.

Levy, H.L. Genetic screening for inborn errors of metabolism. *Advances in Human Genetics*, 1973, *4*, 1–106.

Levy, H.L., Lenke, R.R., & Crocker, A.C. Maternal PKU. *Proceedings of a conference*. DHHS Pub No (HSA) 81-5299, 1979, 1–90.

Lubs, H.A. A marker-X chromosome. *American Journal of Human Genetics*, 1969, *21*, 231–244.

Lubs, H.A., & Travers, H. Genetic counseling in osteogenesis imperfecta. *Clinical Orthopaedics & Related Research*, 1981, *159*, 36–41.

Mamunes, P., Lapidus, P.H., Abbott, J.A., & Roath, S. Acute leukaemia and Klinefelter's syndrome. *Lancet*, 1961, *2*, 26–27.

Martin, R.H., Lin, C.C., Mathies, B.J., & Lowry, R.B. X-linked mental retardation with macro-orchidism and marker-X chromosomes. *American Journal of Medical Genetics*, 1980, *7*, 433–441.

Matalon, R., Michals, K., Lee, C.L., & Nixon, J.C. Screening for biopterin defects in newborns with phenylketonuria and other hyperphenylalaninemias. *Annals of Clinical Laboratory Science*, 1982, *12*, 411–414.

McKusick, V.A. Genetic counseling. *American Journal of Human Genetics*, 1975, *27*, 240–242.

Monaghan, H.P., Krafchick, B.R., MacGregor, D.L., & Fitz, C.R. Tuberous sclerosis complex in children. *American Journal of Diseases in Childhood*, 1981, *135*, 912–917.

Moolten, S.E. Hamartial nature of the tuberous sclerosis complex and its bearing on the tumor problem: Report of a case with tumor anomaly of the kidney and adenoma sebaceum. *Archives of Internal Medicine*, 1942, *69*, 589–623.

Muir, W.A., Knoke, J., Martin, A. Vignos P. & McErlean, A. Improved detection of Duchenne muscular dystrophy using discriminant analysis of creatine kinase levels. *American Journal of Medical Genetics*, 1983, *14*, 125–134.

Muts-Homsma, S.J.M., Muller, H.P., & Geraedst, J.P.M. Klinefelter's syndrome and acute nonlymphocytic leukemia. *Blut*, 1981, *44*, 15–20.

Nicolis, G.L., Hsu, L.Y., Sabetghadom, R., Kardon, N.B. & Chernay, P.R. Klinefelter's syndrome in identical twins with the 46, XX chromosome constitution. *American Journal of Medicine*, 1972, *52*, 482–491.

Nielson, J., Sillesen, I., & Hanson, K.B. Fertility in women with Turner's syndrome: Case report and review of the literature. *British Journal of Obstetrics & Gynaecology*, 1979, *86*, 833.

Nielsen, J., Sorensen, A.M., & Sorensen, K. Mental development of unselected children with sex chromosome abnormalities. *Human Genetics*, 1981, *59*, 324–332.

Nyhan, W.L. Cytogenetic diseases. *CIBA Clinical Symposia*, 1982, *35*, (1), 1–32.

O'Callaghan, T.J., Edwards, J.A., Tobin, M., Basab, K. & Mookerjee, M.D. Tuberous sclerosis with striking renal involvement in a family. *Archives of Internal Medicine*, 1975, *135*, 1082–1087.

Park, E., Bailey, J.D., & Cowell, C.A. Growth and maturation of patients with Turner's syndrome. *Pediatric Research*, 1983, *17*, 1–7.

Parker, C.E., Mavalwala, J., Melnyk, J., & Fish, C.H. The 48, XXYY syndrome. *American Journal of Medicine*, 1970, *48*, 777–781.

Penchansky, L., & Krause, J.R. Acute leukemia following a malignant teratoma in a child with Klinefelter's syndrome. *Cancer*, 1982, *50*, 684–689.

Phornphutkul, C., Rosenthal, A., & Nadas, A.S. Cardiac manifestations of Marfan syndrome in infancy and childhood. *Circulation*, 1973, *47*, 587–596.

Peress, M.R., Sosnowski, J.R., Mathur, R.S., & Williamson, H.O. Pelvic endometriosis and Turner's syndrome. *American Journal of Obstetrics & Gynecology*, 1982, *144*, 474–476.

Prader, A., Labhart, A., & Willi, H. Ein Syndrom von Adipositas, Kleinwuchs, Kryptorchismus, und Oligophrenie nach Myatonieartigem, Zustand im Neugeborenalter. *Schweizerische Medizinische Wochenschrift*, 1956, *86*, 1260–1261.

Pyeritz, R.E., Gott, V.L., McDonald, G.R., Achuff, S.C., Brinker, J.A., Haller, J.A. & Hutchins, G.M. Surgical repair of the Marfan aorta: Technique, indications, and complications. *Johns Hopkins Medical Journal*, 1982, *151*, 71–82.

Pyeritz, R.E., & McKusick, V.A. The Marfan syndrome: Diagnosis and management. *New England Journal of Medicine*, 1979, *300*, 772–777.

Pyeritz, R.E., Murphy, E.A., & McKusick, V.A. Clinical variability in the Marfan syndrome(s). *Birth Defects*, 1979, *15*, (5B), 155–178.

Raboch, J., Mellan, J., & Starka, L. Klinefelter's syndrome: Sexual development and activity. *Archives of Sexual Behavior*, 1979, *8*, 333–339.

Ratcliffe, S.G., Bancroft, J., Axworthy, D., & McLaren, W. Klinefelter's syndrome in adolescence. *Archives of Diseases in Childhood*, 1982, *57*, 6–12.

Reece, E.A., Gimovsky, M.L., & Petrie, R.H. Tuberous sclerosis in pregnancy, *American Journal of Obstetrics & Gynecology*, 1981, *141*, 467–468.

Reed, S. *Counseling in Medical Genetics* (3rd ed.). New York: Alan R. Liss, 1980.

Riccardi, V.M. Neurofibromatosis: An overview and new directions in clinical investigation. *Advances in Neurology*, 1981a, *29*, 57–63.

Riccardi, V.M. Pathophysiology of neurofibromatosis. *Journal of the American Academy of Dermatology*, 1980, *3*, 157–166.

Riccardi, V.M., Von Recklinghausen neurofibromatosis. *New England Journal of Medicine*, 1981b, *305*, 1617–1626.

Riccardi, V.M., Kleiner, B., & Lubs, M.L. Neurofibromatosis: Variable expression is not intrinsic to the mutant gene. *Birth Defects*, 1979, *15* (5), 283–289.

Roberts, W.C., & Honig, H.S. The spectrum of cardiovascular disease in the Marfan syndrome: A clinico-morphologic study of 18 necropsy patients and comparison to 151 previously reported necropsy patients. *American Heart Journal*, 1982, *104*, 115–135.

Robins, P.R., Moe, J.H., & Winter, R.B. Scoliosis in Marfan's syndrome: Its characteristics and results of treatment in thirty-five patients. *Journal of Bone & Joint Surgery*, 1975, *57*, 358–568.

Roth, J.C., & Epstein, C.J. Infantile spasms and hypopigmented macules: Early manifestations of tuberous sclerosis. *Archives in Neurology*, 1971, *25*, 547–551.

Salbenblatt, J.A., Bender, B.G., Puck, M.H., Robinson, A. & Webber, M.L. Development of eight pubertal males with 47, XXY karyotype. *Clinical Genetics*, 1981, 20, 141–146.

Schlegel, R.J., Aspillaga, M.J., Neu, R., & Gardner, L.I. Studies on a boy with XXYY chromosome constitution. *Pediatrics*, 1965, *36*, 113–119.

Scott, O.M., Hyde, S.A., Goddard, C.M., & Dubowitz, V. Prevention of deformity in Duchenne muscular dystrophy. A prospective study of passive stretching and splintage. *Physiotherapy*, 1981, *67*, 177–180.

Shapiro, L.R., Wilmont, P.L., Breholl, P., Lebb, A., Martino, M., Harris, G., Mahoney, M. & Hobbins, J. Prenatal diagnosis of fragile-X chromosome. *Lancet*, 1982, *1*, 99.

Sillence, D. Osteogenesis imperfecta: An expanding panorama of variants. *Clinical Orthopedics*, 1981, *159*, 11–25.

Sillence, D.O., Rimoin, D.L., & Danks, D.M. Clinical variability in osteogenesis imperfecta— variable expressivity or genetic heterogeneity. *Birth Defects*, 1979a, *15*, 113–129.

Sillence, D.O., Senn, A., & Danks, D.M. Genetic heterogeneity in osteogenesis imperfecta. *Journal of Medical Genetics*, 1979b, *16*, 101–116.

Simpson, J.L. Genes, chromosome, and reproductive failure. *Fertility & Sterility*, 1980, *33*, 107–116.

Simpson, J.L., Gonadal dysgenesis and sex chromosome abnormalities. Phenotypic/karyotypic correlations. In H.Vallet, & I.H. Porter (Eds.), *Genetic mechanisms of sexual development*. New York: Academic Press, 1979a, 365–405.

Simpson, J.L. Genetic aspects of reproductive failure: Deficiencies of oocyte number (gonadal dysgenesis) and abnormalities of oogenesis (spontaneous abortion). In J.R. Givens (Ed.), *The Infertile female*. Chicago: Year Book, 1979b, 293–325.

Simpson, J.L., Blagowidow, N., & Martin, A.O. XY gonadal dysgenesis: Genetic heterogeneity based on clinical observations, H-Y antigen status and segregation analysis. *Human Genetics*, 1981, *58*, 91–97.

Simpson, J.L., Christakos, A.C., Horwith, M., & Silverman, F.S. Gonadal dysgenesis in individuals with apparently normal chromosomal complements. Tabulation of cases and compilation of genetic data. *Birth Defects*, 1971, *7* (6), 215–228.

Simpson, J.L., & Photopulos, G. The relationship of neoplasia to disorders of abnormal sexual differentiation. *Birth Defects*, 1976a, *12* (1), 15–50.

Simpson, J.L., & Photopulos, G. Hereditary aspects of ovarian and testicular neoplasia. *Birth Defects*, 1976b, *12* (1), 51–60.

Sorensen, K., Nielsen, J., Wohlert, M., Bennett, P. & Johnson, S.G. Serum testosterone of boys with karyotype 47, XXY (Klinefelter's syndrome) at birth. *Lancet,* 1981, *2,* 1112–1113.

Sutherland, G.R. Heritable fragile sites on human chromosomes. I. Factors affecting expression in lymphocyte culture. *American Journal of Human Genetics,* 1979, *31,* 125–135.

Sutherland, G.R., & Jacky, P. Prenatal diagnosis of fragile-X syndrome. *Lancet,* 1982, *1,* 100.

Thompson, T., Kodluboy, S., & Heston, L., Behavioral treatment of obesity in Prader-Willi syndrome. *Behavioral Research & Therapy,* 1980, *11,* 588–593.

Tolksdorf, M., Gutezeit, G., & Munke. M. Clinical and psychological observations in Klinefelter boys. *Clinical Genetics,* 1981, *20,* 397–398.

Turner, G., Gill, R., & Daniel, A. Marker-X chromosomes, mental retardation, and macroorchidism. *New England Journal of Medicine,* 1978, *299,* 1472.

Wachtel, S.S. The dysgenetic gonad: Aberrant testicular differentiation. *Biology of Reproduction,* 1980, *22,* 1–8.

Wilson, D.P. *Endocrine aspects of Turner's syndrome.* Tulsa, Oklahoma: Great Plains Clinical Genetics Society, 1983.

Wray, L.H., Treeman, M.V.R., & Ming, P.M.L. Pregnancy in the Turner syndrome with only 45, X chromosome constitution. *Fertility & Sterility,* 1981, *35,* 509–513.

Wu, F.C.W., Bancroft, J., Davidson, D.W., & Nicol, K. The behavioural effects of testosterone undecanoate in adult men with Klinefelter's syndrome: A controlled study. *Clinical Endocrinology,* 1982, *16,* 489–497.

Zatz, M., Karp, L.E., & Rogatko, A. Pyruvate kinase and creatine kinase in normal pregnancy and its implication in genetic counseling of Duchenne muscular dystrophy. *American Journal of Medical Genetics,* 1982, *13,* 257–262.

Lonnie Zeltzer
Samuel LeBaron
Paul Zeltzer

20

The Adolescent with Cancer

Despite concerns of some authors about the plight of the chronically ill adolescent (Adams, & Lindemann, 1974; Kaufman, 1972; Moore, Holton, & Marten, 1969; Swift, Seidman, & Stein, 1967; and Weinberg, 1970), Kellerman, Zeltzer, Ellenberg, Dash, and Rigler (1980) found that chronically ill adolescents as a group did not demonstrate psychopathology. That is, their scores on standardized measures of chronic anxiety, self-esteem, and health locus of control matched those of their healthy peers. In fact, the study found that the majority of ill adolescents were hopeful and positive about the future (Zeltzer, Kellerman, Ellenberg, Dash, & Rigler, 1980). The major finding was that chronically ill adolescents saw their problems primarily in terms of the day to day realities of their disease and its treatment.

CANCER IN ADOLESCENTS

As with any disease, there is no single set of problems that invariably affects all adolescents with cancer. Different cancers will involve different types of treatments for varying lengths of time; for example, treatment of bone tumors (e.g., osteogenic sarcoma, Ewing's sarcoma, or fibrosarcoma) might include surgery, chemotherapy, and radiotherapy—or any combination thereof. But, other than an initial diagnostic bone marrow aspiration and lumbar puncture, these patients rarely undergo ongoing medical procedures. On the other hand, adolescents with leukemia or non-

CHRONIC ILLNESS AND DISABILITIES IN CHILDHOOD AND ADOLESCENCE   ISBN 0-8089-1635-1

Hodgkin's lymphoma will typically experience multiple painful diagnostic and therapeutic procedures (e.g., bone marrow aspirations, biopsies, and administration of intrathecal medication) in addition to chemotherapy over the course of their treatment. Adolescents with stage I Hodgkin's disease might receive radiotherapy alone. Even adolescents with the same diagnosis may experience variable disease courses. A minority of patients never gain remission following diagnosis or die soon after diagnosis from overwhelming sepsis. Some patients achieve a first remission, which is maintained during the one to three years of treatment, and they continue to remain disease free off treatment. Others achieve a disease-free state following a marrow transplant. Yet others have a more chronic course, filled with numerous relapses and remissions, either during the period of active treatment or following termination of the initial treatment period.

In order to understand what youths with cancer experience, it is important to first consider the medical aspects of cancer in adolescence, at least in a general sense. Twenty years ago, the focus of a discussion on adolescent cancer would have been on the dying process rather than on assisting the teenager to live with chronic disease. The reason for this change is that 20 years ago most malignancies found in people of this age group were incurable. However, recent advances in radiotherapy and chemotherapy have greatly improved the chances for long-term survival of adolescents with cancer.

Common Cancers During Adolescence

The incidence of common childhood cancers differs in relation to the age of the child or adolescent. In infancy and early childhood, the more common cancers are those that are considered to have an embryonic origin, such as acute lymphoblastic leukemia, neuroblastoma, medulloblastoma, and Wilms' tumors. Most of these tumors have their peak incidence around or prior to five years of age. During adolescence, the most common cancer is still leukemia (Altman & Schwartz, 1978). However, with progressive age, myeloblastic leukemia becomes more common than the lymphoblastic type. Wilms' tumors and neuroblastomas do occur in adolescents; but they are rare and account for less than five percent of the malignancies in this age group. In contrast, osseous tumors, such as osteogenic sarcoma and Ewing's sarcoma, are more common during adolescence. In addition, other solid tumors, such as non-Hodgkin's lymphomas and Hodgkin's lymphomas, also become more common. In contrast to tumors of the peripheral nervous system, such as neuroblastomas, tumors of the central nervous system (CNS) account for approximately 19 percent of the tumors in adolescents (Fig. 20-1). This includes both the gliomas and the medulloblastomas. Other tumors that can occur in adolescents are germ-cell tumors, rhabdomyosarcomas, and rarer types of sarcomas.

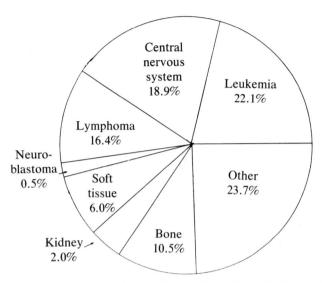

Figure 20-1. Relative Incidence of the Major Malignancies in Adolescents (From Altman, A. J., & Schwartz, A. D.: *Malignant diseases of infancy, childhood, and adolescence.* Philadelphia: WB Saunders Co., 1978, p. 3. With permission.)

Changes in Survival and Treatment

Great strides have been made in the treatment, control, and cure of cancers in children and adolescents in the past 15 to 20 years. For example, induction success for leukemia, the most common malignancy of childhood, has increased from 40 percent to over 95 percent for the lymphoblastic type. With acute myeloblastic leukemia, induction success has improved from 30 percent 15 years ago to over 80 percent today. For osseous tumors, the outlook also has improved: the initial cure rates for osteogenic sarcoma were reported as 15 and 20 percent; however, now in some centers, cure rates may approximate 90 percent. Some of these adolescents undergo limb-salvage procedures as well. Even Ewing's sarcoma has cause for optimism; whereas this tumor used to be uniformly fatal, recent advances using a combination of chemotherapy and radiation therapy have been extremely successful. In the past five years, testicular cancers have been successfully treated using multiagent chemotherapy; prior to the availability of the newer drugs, such as vinblastine, cisplatinum, and bleomycin, the tumor was almost uniformly fatal. Unfortunately, such success with other tumors, such as those in the brain, has been elusive. An increased understanding of the basic biology of the tumors is necessary before advances can be made. Perhaps one of the most significant advances in the treatment of solid tumors in adolescents has occurred in those with non-Hodgkin's lymphoma, because it can now be expected that over 80 percent will have prolonged remissions and possibly cures, compared with a previous survival rate of 40 percent. Teratocarcinomas of the ovary and the testes have also dramatically yielded to therapy, which can now claim over 75 percent complete responders.

The remainder of this discussion will focus on the adolescent with cancer as a prototype for coping with chronic disease and disability during adolescence. What is meant by coping? Several authors have viewed successful coping with chronic disease as the ability to accomplish necessary tasks while experiencing a minimal amount of uncomfortable emotions, such as anger or anxiety (Chodoff, Friedman, & Hamburg, 1964; Friedman, Chodoff, Mason, & Hamburg, 1963; Lascari & Stehbens, 1973; Townes, Wold & Holmes, 1974). However, other authors object to this definition and favor a broader one (Desmond, 1980; Moriarty & Toussieng, 1976). For example, Desmond (1980) describes coping as the "presence of effectiveness in meeting a variety of emotional and functional tasks even in the face of painful emotions." Utilizing the latter definition of coping, this chapter will focus on the unique problems and coping mechanisms of adolescents with cancer.

THE ADJUSTMENT TO CANCER AND ITS TREATMENT

Problems: A Historical Perspective

Studies concerned with the problems of adolescents with cancer generally reflect the state of the art regarding treatment of malignancies. That is, the main problems addressed in studies and reports from the 1960s and 1970s focused on the devastating effects of the disease itself. This was realistic, since at that time a majority of adolescent cancer patients died from their disease. For example, in a 1969 survey of 182 adolescents with cancer, Moore, Holton, and Marten (1969) found that the major concerns of this group of patients related to disfigurement and worries about body image and the disrupting effects of the disease on peer relationships and future planning. Plumb and Holland (1974) suggested that symptoms were the focal point around which fears of death were often displaced. However, as CNS prophylaxis and combination chemotherapy evolved in the 1970s, the outlook for survival improved dramatically. Patients were living longer, initial remissions were achieved more readily, and repeated remissions were common in those who relapsed. The side effects of the drugs then became a major focus of concern to adolescents as well as the main reason for noncompliance. It is not surprising, then, that recent studies have found problems related to treatment to be a major concern in this population. In one study of chronic illness during adolescence, those patients with cancer comprised the only group, from among five different disease categories, who reported that their treatments were worse than their disease (Zeltzer et al., 1980).

Coping: Developmental Aspects

What is known about coping with cancer during adolescence? One study of survivors of childhood cancer found that older children and adolescents experienced greater adjustment difficulties during active treatment and even subsequent to termination of treatment than did younger patients (Koocher, O'Malley, & Gogan, 1980). The impact of cancer on the adolescent has been examined from a developmental perspective as well. Many authors (Kellerman & Katz, 1977; Zeltzer, 1978; Zeltzer, 1980; Zeltzer, Zeltzer, & LeBaron, 1983) have suggested that struggles for independence can be impeded by the ill youth's greater need for reliance on parents for emotional and economic support, transportation for treatments, information related to disease and treatment, and guidance regarding activities (e.g., restricted activities if the platelet or neutrophil count is depressed). Some parents express their own anxieties by becoming overprotective of their adolescent sons or daughters with cancer, discouraging separation, and inhibiting opportunities in which the adolescent could exercise control. Needs for socialization may be frustrated by the frequency of clinic visits and chemotherapy-related disability, both of which can produce multiple school absences, decreased peer-related activity, and feelings of isolation. Body image (i.e., the need to feel attractive and socially acceptable) is a major concern during adolescence. Disfigurement secondary to surgery and radiation or, most commonly, alopecia secondary to chemotherapy may cause adolescents to feel embarrassed and unattractive, and hence may further the social isolation already experienced by the teenager (Kellerman & Katz, 1977). In fact, in interviews with adolescent amputees, it came as a surprise that loss of hair was experienced as more difficult to cope with than loss of a limb. For these adolescents, walking on crutches or using a prosthesis was seen as a physical accomplishment by peers and required less explanation than did baldness. Baldness required a decision about the purchase and use of a wig or the constant wearing of a hat or head scarf, any one of which was liable to be blown or pulled off, to fall off during sports, or to need to be taken off occasionally during activities such as swimming. Adolescents admitted to being bothered more by stares and avoidance by peers than they were by direct questioning by friends. They often did not know how to initiate a discussion about the etiology of their baldness and usually preferred to keep it a secret if possible. Because of increased reliance on the peer group for emotional support during adolescence, the need to be able to identify with peers and to feel "normal" takes on primary importance during this age period. However, the diagnosis and label of cancer may cause some adolescents to feel different than, and perhaps even inferior to, their peers.

How do Adolescents Cope?

In view of the extreme psychological and physical stress and disruption of normal development associated with cancer, several systematic studies have been undertaken to investigate how adolescents and children cope with their disease. One such study (Kellerman et al., 1980; Zeltzer et al., 1980) found that adolescents with cancer reported that they were coping well, and that they were more concerned with the day to day inconveniences than with worries about death. In general, these adolescents were found to be within normal ranges on several standardized psychological measures.

How can adolescents function in the face of seemingly overwhelming crises? One mode of adaptation postulated by several individuals working in the field (Kellerman & Katz, 1977; Moore, et al., 1969; Zeltzer et al., 1983) is the use of denial. It is proposed that adolescents with cancer generally function by paying attention to the concrete, day to day tasks (e.g., school work, medical procedures, and appointment scheduling) and by not continuously thinking about their illness. Is there any evidence for this hypothesis? Several studies suggest that adaptive denial may occur, especially during periods of enhanced stress, such as immediately following diagnosis or when the disease has newly relapsed. In a study described earlier in this chapter (Zeltzer et al., 1980), greater than 95 percent of adolescents in the sample reported that they expected things to get better for them in the future, even though more than 30 percent were in relapse at the time of the questionnaire and a significant portion of these adolescents died within two weeks to six months of testing. A questionnaire study to determine information preferences in adolescents with cancer (Levenson, Pfefferbaum, Copeland, & Silverberg, 1982) found that younger adolescents and those in active illness phases were more likely to shun additional information than were older adolescents or those in remission. The younger patients in their sample were also more likely to reject peer-group discussions with other cancer patients of a similar age and not to want their friends to know more about cancer. This information suggests that such adolescents were not ready to focus on their illness or to be given more information. Avoidance was the primary coping response for newly diagnosed, acutely relapsed, and younger adolescents. The study also found that these responses were fairly uniform across diagnostic categories and gender. Thus, age and change in health status appear to be more influencial in enhancing the use of denial by adolescents with cancer. Further support for the hypothesis of denial as a coping strategy comes from another study by Levenson, Copeland, Morrow, Pfefferbaum, and Silverberg (1983). This investigation compared parents' and adolescents' information preferences and found discrepancies between these two groups. The adolescents appeared to resist receiving cancer-related information, which their parents thought that their sons and daughters should have. Another study by Pfefferbaum, Levenson, and van Eys (1982) found that there was an even wider discrepancy between what adolescents wanted to know and what their physicians thought they should know, with the latter group wanting to provide more information than adolescents wanted to receive.

Another assumption of health care providers and parents alike is that adolescents want to take increased responsibility for their own medical care. However, it has been shown that, in general, physicians and parents want adolescents to take a more action-oriented, involved role in the management of their own disease and its treatment than most adolescents want to take (Levenson et al., 1983; Pfefferbaum et al., 1982). This desire for a more passive, dependent role on the part of the adolescent becomes especially prominent in the period immediately following diagnosis and during times of disease relapse (Levenson et al., 1982). Intermittent regression, when used selectively, has been considered to be adaptive (Adams, 1974). This consideration will be illustrated in one of the case reports later in this chapter.

If parents and physicians form the primary mechanism of environmental support for adolescents with cancer, then do the discrepancies in beliefs and expectations between the former two groups and the adolescent pose obstacles to adjustment? Spinetta and Maloney (1978) have suggested that effective mother–child illness-related communication is a critical factor in the child's ability to cope with his or her cancer. However, even they have observed discrepancies between the parents' and the child's perception of the effectiveness of that communication. In addition to the findings of the previous investigators, the authors of this chapter have also found discrepancies between parents and their adolescent offspring in the perception of the major problems facing the adolescent and the factors most helpful in coping with those problems. In a questionnaire and interview study of 16 adolescents with cancer and their families, it was found that the four major problems reported by these adolescents were (in decreasing order of distress): getting chemotherapy, hair loss, painful medical procedures, and nausea and vomiting. While mothers and fathers of the adolescents also reported that their children's pain and suffering during medical procedures and the nausea and vomiting associated with chemotherapy were major problems, they were primarily concerned with the uncertainty related to the outcome of their children's illness. Both mothers and fathers also reported that hospitalizations were very stressful; fathers were especially concerned about the amount of school their children were missing. Thus, parents tended to be more future- and goal-oriented than were their adolescent children. Consistent with the previous literature, it appears that adolescents tend to focus on more immediate, recurring sources of distress and disruption and leave worry about the future to their parents.

In this same study, adolescents reported that spending time with friends and receiving more information about their cancer were of primary help in coping with their illness. The majority of adolescents in this study were over age 14, which may explain the discrepancy between these findings and the avoidance of information primarily seen in the younger adolescents in Levenson et al.'s study (1982). The adolescents in the current sample also reported that thinking pleasant thoughts, hearing of others who did well, having someone in the clinic talk to them when they felt scared, and maintaining a sense of humor were major factors that helped them to cope with cancer. While both parents found benefits in these same coping strategies, they additionally commonly derived help from their religion. Mothers, but not fathers, reported that they received additional benefit from talking about their feelings with someone.

If there are differences in adolescents' and parents' perception of the problems relating to cancer and its treatment, and also differences in how best to cope with the illness, then how can parents best support their sons and daughters who are ill? This problem is further compounded by the belief of parents and physicians alike in the need for self-sufficiency for the adolescent patients. This expectation appears to be in direct conflict with the wishes of many adolescents, especially during acute stress situations.

The Adolescent's Behavior and the Health Care System

Nurses in an oncology clinic frequently have more contact and closer relationships with adolescent patients than do physicians. The authors asked the nurses at two large oncology centers (Los Angeles and San Antonio) to describe what they considered to be typical behavior of adolescent patients. Their first reaction was that the behavior of many adolescents was both frustrating and confusing. Teenaged patients often appear infantile at one time (e.g., whining, crying, or requiring physical restraint during a medical procedure) and manipulative the next time. The greatest area of manipulation often involved bargaining with the clinic staff over the scheduling of chemotherapy appointments; this is particularly true if conflicts arose between a patient's protocol and a planned social or school event. The nurses described a variety of adolescent responses to this situation: Some adolescents who were not verbally assertive simply did not show up for their appointments. Others bargained over the scheduling of chemotherapy. Still other patients consistently arrived late. The easiest and most rewarding adolescents to work with were the compliant ones who always received their chemotherapy on time and without complaining. The most difficult adolescent patients were those who were inconsistent—seemingly mature and taking the initiative sometimes and becoming passive, dependent, and nonverbal at others.

What these nurses and the literature are probably reflecting is the variability in the adolescent's adaptation to illness over time. Most adolescents learn from their experiences, and when they can cope well enough with one problem, then they can consider moving on to another. Acute stress periods, such as those following diagnosis, relapse, or during medical procedures and the administration of chemotherapy, can cause adolescents to temporarily regress and become dependent. During these periods, they may need to rely on parents or medical staff for support and guidance, and they may not want to take responsibility for themselves. They may need to deny their diagnosis or relapse because they are not ready to muster sufficient strength to cope as an adult might. During these times, they may not want to talk about their illness or their worries and often do not want to be educated about their illness. However, most adolescents will indicate when they are ready to take more control. Likewise, during some medical procedures, adolescents may want others in the room to initiate active direction, while at other times they shun staff- or parent-initiated intervention. Adolescents need to have the freedom to vacillate in their desire for independence and help.

BEHAVIORAL INTERVENTION FOR CANCER-RELATED PROBLEMS: MEDICAL PROCEDURES AND CHEMOTHERAPY

Because the main problems reported by adolescents generally pertain to medical procedures and chemotherapy, several investigations of interventions for pain and vomiting have been reported. While there are case reports of behavioral intervention for pain relief in pediatric cancer patients (Gardner & Olness, 1981; Olness, 1981; Zeltzer, 1980), there are only a few systematic studies (Hilgard & LeBaron, 1982; Kellerman, Zeltzer,

Ellenberg, Dash, in press; Zeltzer & LeBaron, 1982). Two of these found hypnosis effective in reducing procedure-related pain and anxiety (Hilgard & LeBaron, 1982; Kellerman et al., 1983), and one found hypnosis to be superior to nonhypnotic behavioral support (Zeltzer & LeBaron, 1982). Most investigations of behavioral intervention for nausea and vomiting have been reported in adult patients (Redd & Andrykowski, 1982). There are several case reports in younger patients (Ellenberg, Kellerman, Dash, Higgins, & Zeltzer, 1980; Hilgard & LeBaron, in press; Olness, 1981; Zeltzer, 1980) but only one systematic study of hypnosis in press (Zeltzer, Kellerman, Ellenberg, Dash, 1983). Two preliminary studies of intervention for chemotherapy have recently been completed by the authors of this chapter and will be summarized here, along with descriptions of the preceding studies.

Acute Pain and Anxiety

Katz, Kellerman, and Siegel (1980) were the first to systematically assess acute distress during medical procedures in a pediatric oncology population. They concluded that such distress was extreme and virtually ubiquitous. In their assessment, distress was measured with a procedure behavioral rating scale (PBRS), and they found that adolescents were less likely than children to exhibit stressful behaviors (i.e., adolescents had lower PBRS scores). However, as Hilgard and LeBaron (1983) noted, the assessment of distress based solely on observation of an adolescent's behavior is made difficult by the stoicism common in that age group. In the author's own experience, adolescents experience as much suffering as do children during medical procedures, but the behavioral manifestations of distress differ between the two age groups (LeBaron & Zeltzer, submitted for publication).

The first systematic studies of methods of behavioral intervention for this distress were undertaken simultaneously by Kellerman, Zeltzer, Ellenberg, and Dash (1983) at Children's Hospital in Los Angeles and by Hilgard and LeBaron (1982) at Stanford Children's Hospital. The Los Angeles group studied the effects of hypnosis in reducing pain and anxiety during bone marrow aspirations, lumbar punctures, and intramuscular injections in 27 adolescents. Patient ratings of pain and anxiety during baseline and then with hypnosis were assessed; the efficacy of hypnosis in reducing distress was confirmed in these patients. However, results for all three procedures were analyzed together. Hilgard and LeBaron (1982) limited their study to an evaluation of the effectiveness of hypnosis in reducing the pain and anxiety of bone marrow aspirations. They used both patient and observer assessments of pain and anxiety. Results of their study also suggested the efficacy of hypnosis, especially in those

patients who scored high on a standardized measure of hypnotic susceptibility.

In San Antonio, hypnosis was compared with nonhypnotic behavioral
support for reducing pain and anxiety during bone marrow aspirations and
lumbar punctures (Zeltzer & LeBaron, 1982). In this study, 33 children
and adolescents were randomized to one of two intervention groups; both
patients and independent observers rated the patient's pain and anxiety
during one to three baseline (preintervention) procedures and one to three
procedures with intervention. During baseline, bone marrow aspirations
were found to be more painful than lumbar punctures. With intervention,
hypnosis was found to be more effective than nonhypnotic behavioral
support for reducing pain and anxiety during both types of medical procedures.

Nausea and Vomiting With Chemotherapy

Nausea and vomiting with chemotherapy are major problems for many
adolescents with cancer. In one prospective study of these symptoms in
a pediatric oncology population, only eight percent of patients never experienced either nausea or vomiting (Zeltzer, LeBaron, & Zeltzer, 1983a).
Premature termination of chemotherapy because of severe nausea and
vomiting was found by Smith, Rosen, Trueworthy, and Lowman (1979)
in 33 percent of a pediatric population. Separate analysis of the adolescent
data in that study revealed an alarming 59 percent noncompliance rate.

While there are commonly held beliefs about which chemotherapeutic
agents are highly emetogenic, there are few data to document the high
versus low emesis producers. In the authors' study of 49 pediatric oncology
patients (ages 5–21 years), no commonly used chemotherapy combinations
(i.e., common to many of the Children's Cancer Study Group protocols)
could be identified that either never or always produced nausea and vomiting (Zeltzer, et al., 1983a). Furthermore, there was no association between the extent of these symptoms and the number of agents in a regimen.
Most patients' symptoms fluctuated widely even when they were receiving
repeated courses of the same agents in the same dosages (Zeltzer, et al.,
1983a; Zeltzer & LeBaron, 1983a). The implication of these data is that
there are unknown factors, besides the drugs themselves, that must influence patients' symptoms.

Since nausea and vomiting comprise a large part of the disagreeable
aspects of treatment (Seigel & Longo, 1981), oncologists often administer
antiemetics to relieve these symptoms. However, the clinical trials testing
the efficacy of these antiemetics have all been conducted in adult patients,
and benefits in children and adolescents have been consistently disappointing. Such disappointment was reflected in one survey of 56 oncology

centers. In this study only 15 percent of pediatric oncologists believed that antiemetics were effective, although 90 percent of the physicians prescribed them with chemotherapy (Penta, Poster, Bruno, & Jacobs, 1981).

Many adolescents learn to expect emesis with their chemotherapy and will often vomit prior to the administration of the agents themselves. Likewise, it is possible that adolescents who receive antiemetics with chemotherapy prior to the onset of symptoms are given a message that they should expect to vomit. It is not known whether these expectations are sufficient to actually cause increased emesis in adolescents, but some adolescents may be susceptible to such suggestions. To examine this possibility, the extent of nausea and emesis, and the extent to which these symptoms were found to be bothersome, was determined in 23 young patients during chemotherapy courses. The courses in which they received prophylactic antiemetics were then compared with matched courses (i.e., same drugs and doses) in which they were not given antiemetics (Zeltzer, LeBaron, & Zeltzer, 1983b). Significantly higher ratings for severity of nausea and vomiting and even the extent to which patients were bothered by these symptoms were found in the courses with antiemetics compared with the courses without antiemetics. The duration of symptoms was also found to be prolonged with antiemetics. Obviously, identification of the most helpful antiemetics and the patients most likely to respond to such medication awaits further study.

Behavioral intervention strategies have been explored in part because pharmacological control of emesis has been disappointing. However, the majority of behavioral studies of nausea and vomiting have taken place with adults receiving chemotherapy. The following intervention strategies have been found to be effective for anticipatory nausea and vomiting:

1. Hypnosis with guided relaxation imagery (Redd, Andresen, & Minagawa, 1982)
2. Progressive muscle relaxation with relaxation imagery (Burish & Lyles, 1980; Burish & Lyles, 1981; Lyles, Burish, Krozely, & Oldham, 1982)
3. Multiple muscle-site EMG biofeedback with relaxation imagery (Burish, Shartner, & Lyles, 1981)
4. Systematic desensitization (Morrow, Arseneau, Asbury, Bennett, & Boros, 1982)

A Los Angeles study (Zeltzer, Kellerman, Ellenberg, & Dash, 1983) of seven adolescents with cancer assessed the frequency, intensity, and duration of emesis through patient self-reports following one baseline course of chemotherapy and another matched course with hypnosis intervention. Hypnosis was found to be effective in reducing emesis following chemotherapy administration for this small sample.

The authors have recently completed two preliminary studies of chemotherapy in children and adolescents in San Antonio. In the first study, a combined behavorial approach that was aimed at focusing the patient's attention away from the chemotherapy administration and side effects resulted in a significant reduction in nausea, vomiting, and the extent to which these symptoms bothered the patients and disrupted their activities (LeBaron & Zeltzer, 1983). In this study, patients self-rated these four variables within three to five days following each chemotherapy administration. Data were collected for a mean of 2.5 courses prior to (baseline) and 2.5 matched courses with intervention for the group. A subsequent study compared the effectiveness of hypnosis with nonhypnotic supportive counseling in 19 young patients (Zeltzer & LeBaron, 1983b). Both intervention strategies were found to be effective in reducing the intensity of symptoms; hypnosis was found to be slightly more effective than supportive counseling in reducing the duration of nausea and emesis. Obviously, larger longitudinal studies of behavioral intervention for chemotherapy are necessary to determine the most effective intervention techniques and to determine the patient, family, and environmental factors that most influence receptivity to intervention.

CASE REPORTS

The following two case reports illustrate how adolescents with life-threatening diseases cope. These cases demonstrate the variable nature of coping, which in turn relates to the environmental stressors, type of support received, and developmental status and resources of the individual adolescent.

R.T., a 12-year-old boy with non-Hodgkin's lymphoma, lived with his parents and younger brother. From his diagnosis onward, R.T. was very verbal about his anxieties. He initially believed that God was punishing him with cancer because he had refused to be a member of his school's basketball team. However, his main concern was with needles, and any procedure involving them, including bone marrow aspirations, lumbar punctures, intravenous injections, and even finger sticks for blood tests. He always worried in advance and would become extremely anxious during medical procedures, usually requiring nurses to physically restrain him while he screamed and resisted.

When R.T. entered the authors' study of behavioral intervention for acute pain and anxiety (Zeltzer & LeBaron, 1982), he appeared eager for help. Prior to intervention, we met with him and learned that he loved to ride his bicycle. We also found that he scored in the high range on a standardized scale of hypnotic susceptibility, indicating that he had a good capacity for imagination. Unfortunately, his vivid imagination often turned against him prior to medical procedures;

he would imagine in great detail the "needle crunching through my bone and hurting something awful." With hypnotic intervention, he was able to make use of active, guided imagery involving an adventure on his bicycle. He experienced minimal pain and anxiety during the next several procedures, first in the presence of the therapist and then without the therapist. He had learned to talk with the nurses and his mother about interesting things during his procedures.

R.T. relapsed after nine months of chemotherapy and required frequent multiple intrathecal medications as part of his relapse protocol. During this period, as R.T. and his parents worried more about whether he was going to die, R.T. again developed extreme anxiety and resistant behavior prior to and during medical procedures. This behavior created increasing frustration in the nursing staff. The more the nurses and R.T.'s parents pleaded with or threatened him, the greater was his resistance. The authors were again asked to help him. After asking him to describe his concerns, the therapist reminded him of his strengths and "grown-up" abilities. Initially, R.T. agreed to the procedures as long as he could receive help from one of the therapists, and only if the nurse promised to perform the procedure quickly. With the support of the study team and the nurses, he was again able to cope with medical procedures. However, after three lumbar punctures involving mechanical difficulties (i.e., multiple needle insertions), R.T.'s preprocedure behavior again deteriorated. He once more refused to undergo any further procedures or chemotherapy. At this point it was assessed that further insistence would probably produce even more resistance. Thus, the staff pressure was dropped and R.T. was allowed a "cooling-off" period of no treatment for a week, giving him the chance to make some of his own decisions about the administration of his treatment. Over that time he was able to muster enough of his own resources not only to request treatment, but also to describe the manner in which he wished to receive it. He asked to receive his remaining procedures under general anesthesia. His requests were granted and he continued to keep appointments and to maintain a good relationship with the clinic staff.

During the one and one half years of his treatment, R.T. turned 14 and matured. He had found some solutions to his own acute distress and was able to develop a better relationship with the nurses. He had been referred to a child psychiatrist for psychotherapy but refused to return after two visits because he said he did not find therapy helpful. Instead, he formed his own support network, composed of the nurses, his parents, his brother, and his friends.

This case illustrates the variability of workable coping patterns over time and shows how this variation depends on changes in disease course, environmental support, and adolescent development. Despite his extreme fear, which was exacerbated by his vivid imagination, R.T. was able to master that fear and to cope with medical procedures after learning some specific helpful techniques. However, his coping abilities broke down after the magnitude of stressors exceeded his capacity to cope (i.e., his relapse, the need for frequent multiple procedures, and the technical difficulties necessitating multiple sticks for many of his procedures). An appeal to his adolescent needs for mastery helped him to cope with these added stressors for a while. However, his developmental needs for autonomy conflicted with his medical needs for treatment. In this case, the latter was especially important because without treatment R.T. would probably not have survived. It was this factor that made the nurses and R.T.'s parents push all the harder to get R.T. to comply with treatment requirements. Compliance then became the focus for autonomy struggles until the only way in which R.T. could "win" was to discontinue therapy. The relief of staff pressure through a cooling-off period allowed this adolescent to gain some control once more. He again worked out his own solutions (i.e., general anesthesia and development of a support system) and was able to cope successfully with his disease and its treatment. During all of these events, R.T. was growing and maturing. He was learning to cope by trial and error, while his own adolescent development was helping him to benefit from his experiences. His physical maturational changes, accompanied by his growth spurt, also may have influenced how the medical staff responded to him over time (i.e., he began to be treated more as an adult once he looked more like an adolescent than a child).

J.D., a 17-year-old adolescent and the oldest of five sons, was undergoing his second year of treatment for acute myelogenous leukemia when he entered the authors' study of behavioral intervention for relief of nausea and vomiting (LeBaron & Zeltzer, 1983). He described his family as close, and both his mother and father as well as some of his brothers often accompanied him to the clinic. He was a physically attractive, action-oriented adolescent who preferred sports to other activities. He was popular with his friends and enjoyed a busy social life. While finishing his last year of high school, he began working part-time in a garage. He bought a car, which he "souped-up" in the garage and enjoyed taking his friends for rides in it. On weekends he sometimes picked up a number of friends to go dancing. He told the staff that sometimes they would drive out into the countryside "to make acquaintances." He had winked with a grin and said, "I think you know what I mean."

Although J.D. enjoyed bragging about his car and his adventures with girlfriends, he appeared to be quite sensitive and concerned about his family and friends. His mother reported once in private that when she had scolded him for not completing some chores around the house, he wrote her a letter the next day to apologize and to thank her for the many things she did for him. In general, he was very conscientious about his responsibilities. In contrast to this conscientious behavior at home, J.D. preferred to portray a masculine, carefree image in the clinic, as if he could easily handle any problem. During bone marrow aspirations, for instance, he would lie on the treatment table and joke about how tough his bones had become.

One day his parents confided that J.D. had been experiencing increasing nausea and vomiting during the previous three months and that his school work and social life were now significantly disrupted by his chemotherapy. They said that J.D. had reluctantly requested help in relieving these symptoms. J.D. confirmed that he would like help; however, he then proceeded to discount and belittle the side effects and to indicate that he could handle them. The therapist asked J.D. if he felt uncomfortable to be talking about such problems, and J.D. replied, "Well, yeah, I can just hear all my friends saying, 'Oh, poor J.D., now he has to talk to a shrink.' " To J.D.'s surprise, the therapist agreed that this was indeed a strange situation. Then the therapist suggested that J.D. would be able to reduce his symptoms only with the greatest personal effort. However, the therapist also expressed the opinion that J.D. had the same physical and mental toughness and intelligence of professional athletes, and that these qualities would enable him to overcome his nausea and vomiting. The ingredients J.D. would need to help himself were techniques that other intelligent and tough patients just like him had found helpful for reducing nausea and vomiting. These remarks were intended to convey a challenge to J.D.'s love of competition, a belief that he was capable of meeting the challenge, and a perception that other patients had undergone similar experiences and that these helpful suggestions were really coming from them (his peers) rather than from the therapist.

When the therapist began to describe the possible ways in which one's state of mind might affect the severity of one's symptoms, J.D. related some examples from his own experience. He told the therapist that one evening after receiving his chemotherapy he had been lying on his living room floor feeling especially sick and miserable. Some of his friends unexpectedly came by to visit, and he decided that he was not going to let himself feel sick. Later, he noticed that he was having such fun joking with his friends that he actually had forgotten about his nausea. On another occasion, J.D. said that he went ocean fishing with his father and some friends. Each time he sat down to rest and his mind was unoccupied, he noticed that he felt seasick, whereas his feelings of nausea would disappear whenever he moved around the boat and became involved in some exciting activity.

J.D. was complimented by the therapist for having already discovered that distraction and involvement in fun activities could be effective techniques for reducing the side effects of chemotherapy. At this point, J.D. expressed discouragement and the feeling that his chemotherapy would go on forever and that perhaps the nausea and vomiting would worsen. The therapist complimented J.D. again for being sensitive enough to notice his own feelings of discouragement; these feelings would make the goal of reducing his side effects even more of an exciting challenge. J.D. was encouraged not to give up, but rather to get "psyched up" like an athlete preparing for an especially difficult contest. In this way, J.D. could be like the baseball player who is worried that he may not be able to get a hit but who concentrates so successfully that he hits a home run.

Since there was a baseball game being televised that same evening, the therapist suggested that J.D. lie on the living room floor and watch the game with his family instead of lying in bed with his emesis basin. J.D. clenched his teeth and agreed that he could be like the athlete who must concentrate on a difficult challenge. During the next clinic visit, both J.D. and his parents reported that J.D. had indeed "hit a home run." He had invited some friends over to watch the baseball game, and they spent the evening together joking and watching television. He had experienced no more vomiting and only occasional bouts of nausea since the discussion about his side effects. Several months later, his mother reported that J.D.'s nausea and vomiting virtually never reappeared and that his school work and social relationships had improved substantially.

Like the first case, this adolescent was also caught in a dilemma; independence and self-reliance were important, yet he needed help. Resolution of this conflict did not necessitate psychotherapy; rather, it required direct, practical suggestions packaged in a way that emphasized the adolescent's real strengths and not the therapist's cleverness.

Neither case should be interpreted as diminishing the appropriate role of traditional psychotherapy. The point to be emphasized is that most anxieties, conflicts, and behavioral problems in adolescents with chronic illness are responsive to a brief discussion of the problem, accompanied by a few suggestions that allow the adolescent to move in the direction of independence while simultaneously receiving help.

In summary, these cases illustrate the nature of coping during adolescence. The variability of coping mechanisms among adolescents, and even in the same adolescent at different periods, is characteristic. There are few adolescents who always cope either well or poorly. Usually the environmental situations and maturational status and needs of the adolescent dictate the form and success of the particular coping methods. The best way to help adolescents cope is to help them assess those stressors with which they are coping and to help them plan their own best strategies. An assessment of their strengths and their developmental needs will help guide the caregiver in the assistance offered.

CONCLUSION

The most important thing these authors have learned from studying adolescents with cancer is that young people are very resilient. Despite numerous psychosocial and somatic insults, most adolescents find resources within themselves for coping. The major coping mechanism appears to be a present-oriented focus and the use of what has been called "adaptive denial" (Zeltzer et al., 1980). This mechanism calls for a positive, optimistic outlook and filling one's thoughts and attention with daily tasks and concerns rather than with worries about the disease. The typical pattern when stressors overload the system is for the adolescent to temporarily regress, need nurturing, voluntarily relinquish responsibility for decision making, and often, to withdraw. However, the majority of adolescents, with support from family and medical staff, will eventually again resume control. Throughout adolescence, physical and psychological changes are taking place and the adolescent is learning something about himself or herself from each new experience. One of the primary responsibilities of health care providers is to have confidence in the adolescent's inner resources and strengths and to transmit this confidence in the support of the adolescent.

ACKNOWLEDGMENTS

This investigation was supported by PHS grant number 5 R18 CA 27376, awarded by the National Cancer Institute, DHHS. Dr. P. Zeltzer was Junior Faculty Clinical Fellow No. 542 of the American Cancer Society and was an awardee of the Robert J. and Helen C. Kleberg Foundation.

The authors wish to acknowledge the support of Dr. Howard Britton, Medical Director, and the patients and pediatric oncology staff (Clementina Geiser, M.D., Marie Garza, R.N., Sylvia Brown, R.N., Karen Richmond, R.N., and Dharma Rodriguez, M.S.W.) of the Children's Cancer Research and Treatment Center at the Santa Rosa Children's Hospital and to thank Miss Jo Ann Lieberman and Ms. Rebecca Robinson for their help in the preparation of this chapter.

REFERENCES

Adams, J.E., & Lindemann, E. Coping with long-term disability. In G.V. Coelho, D.A. Hamburg, & J.E. Adams (Eds.), *Coping and adaptation.* New York: Basic Books, 1974, 115–122.

Altman, A.J. & Schwartz, A.D. *Malignant diseases of infancy, childhood, and adolescence.* Philadelphia: WB Saunders Co., 1978, 1–15.

Boyle, I.R., di Sant'Agnesse, P.A., Sack, S., Millican, F., & Kulczycki, L.L. Emotional adjustment of adolescents and young adults with cystic fibrosis. *Journal of Pediatrics,* 1976, *88,* 318.

Burish, T.G., & Lyles, J.N. Effectiveness of relaxation training in reducing the aversiveness of chemotherapy in the treatment of cancer. *Journal of Behavior Therapy and Experimental Psychiatry,* 1980, *10,* 357–361.

Burish, T.G., & Lyles, J.N. Effectiveness of relaxation training in reducing adverse reactions to cancer chemotherapy. *Journal of Behavioral Medicine,* 1981, *4*(1), 65–78.

Burish, T.G., Shartner, C.D., & Lyles, J.N. Effectiveness of multiple muscle-site EMG biofeedback and relaxation training in reducing the aversiveness of cancer chemotherapy. *Biofeedback and Self Regulation,* 1981, *6*(4), 523–535.

Chodoff, P., Friedman, S.B., & Hamburg, D.A. Stress, defenses and coping behavior: Observations in parents of children with malignant disease. *American Journal of Psychiatry,* 1964, *120,* 743.

Desmond, H. Two families: An intensive observational study. In J. Kellerman (Ed.), *Psychological aspects of childhood cancer.* Springfield, IL: Charles C. Thomas, 1980, 100–127.

Ellenberg, L., Kellerman, J., Dash, J., Higgins, G., & Zeltzer, L. Use of hypnosis for multiple symptoms in an adolescent girl with leukemia. *Journal of Adolescent Health Care,* 1980, *1,* 132–136.

Friedman, S.B., Chodoff, P., Mason, J.W., & Hamburg, D. Behavioral observations on parents anticipating the death of a child. *Pediatrics,* 1963, *32*(604), 610.

Gardner, G.G., & Olness, K. *Hypnosis and hypnotherapy with children.* New York: Grune & Stratton, 1981.

Hilgard, J.R., & LeBaron, S. Relief of anxiety and pain in children and adolescents with cancer: Quantitative measures and clinical observations. *International Journal of Clinical and Experimental Hypnosis,* 1982, *30*(4), 417–422.

Hilgard, J.R., & LeBaron, S. *Hypnosis in the treatment of pain and anxiety in children with cancer: A clinical and quantitative investigation.* Los Altos, CA: Kaufmann, Inc., 1983 (in press).

Katz, E.R. Kellerman, J., & Siegel, S.E. Behavioral distress in children with cancer undergoing medical procedures: Developmental considerations. *Journal of Consulting and Clinical Psychology,* 1980, *48*(3), 356–365.

Kaufman, R.V. Body-image changes in physically ill teenagers. *Journal of the American Academy of Child Psychiatry,* 1972, *11,* 157.

Kellerman, J., & Katz, E.R. The adolescent with cancer: Theoretical, clinical and research issues. *Journal of Pediatric Psychology,* 1977, *2,* 127–131.

Kellerman, J., Zeltzer, L., Ellenberg, L., & Dash, J. Adolescents with cancer: Hypnosis for the reduction of the acute pain and anxiety associated with medical procedures. *Journal of Adolescent Health Care,* 1983 (in press).

Kellerman, J., Zeltzer, L., Ellenberg, L., Dash, J., & Rigler, D. Psychological effects of illness in adolescence. I. Anxiety, self-esteem, and perception of control. *Journal of Pediatrics,* 1980, *97*(1), 126–131.

Koocher, G.P., O'Malley, J.E., Gogan, J.L., & Foster, D.J. Psychological adjustment among pediatric cancer survivors. *Journal of Child Psychology and Psychiatry,* 1980, *21*(2), 163–173.

Lascari, A.D., & Stehbens, J.A. The reactions of families to childhood leukemia. *Clinical Pediatrics,* 1973, *12*(4), 210.

LeBaron, S., & Zeltzer, L. Behavioral intervention for reducing chemotherapy-related nausea and vomiting in adolescents with cancer. *Journal of Adolescent Health Care,* 1983, in press.

LeBaron, S., & Zeltzer, L. Assessment of acute pain and anxiety in children and adolescents by self-reports, observer reports, and a behavior checklist. 1983 (submitted for publication).

Levenson, P.M., Pfefferbaum, B.J., Copeland, D.R., & Silverberg, Y. Information preferences of cancer patients ages 11–20 years. *Journal of Adolescent Health Care,* 1982, *3,* 9–13.

Levenson, P.M., Copeland, D.R., Morrow, J.R., Pfefferbaum, B., & Silverberg, Y. Disparities in disease-related perceptions of adolescent cancer patients and their parents. *Journal of Pediatric Psychology,* 1983, *8*(1), 33–45.

Lyles, J.N., Burish, T.G., Krozely, M.G., & Oldham, R.K. Efficacy of relaxation training and guided imagery in reducing the aversiveness of cancer chemotherapy. *Journal of Consulting and Clinical Psychology,* 1982, *50*(4), 509–524.

Moore, D., Holton, B., & Marten, G. Psychologic problems in the management of adolescents with malignancy. *Clinical Pediatrics,* 1969, *8,* 464.

Moriarty, A.E., & Toussieng, P.W. *Adolescent coping.* New York: Grune & Stratton, 1976, 139–152.

Morrow, G.R., Arseneau, J.C., Asbury, R.F., Bennett, J.M., & Boros, L. Anticipatory nausea and vomiting with chemotherapy. *New England Journal of Medicine,* 1982, *306*(7), 431–432.

Olness, K. Imagery (self-hypnosis) as adjunct therapy in childhood cancer: Clinical experience with 25 patients. *American Journal of Pediatric Hematology/Oncology,* 1981, *3*(3), 313–321.

Penta, J.S., Poster, D.S., Bruno, S., & Jacobs, E.M. Cancer chemotherapy induced nausea and vomiting in adult and pediatric populations. *Proceedings of the American Society of Clinical Oncology,* 1981, *22,* 396.

Pfefferbaum, B., & Levenson, P.M. Adolescent cancer patient and physican responses to a questionnaire on patient concerns. *American Journal of Psychiatry,* 1982, *139,* 348–351.

Pfefferbaum, B., Levenson, P.M., & van Eys, J. Comparison of physician and patient perceptions of communication issues. *Southern Medical Journal,* 1982, *75*(9), 1080–1083.

Plumb, M.M., & Holland, J. Cancer in adolescents: The symptom is the thing. In B. Schoenberg, A.C. Carr, A.H. Kutscher, D. Peretz, I.K. Goldberg, (Eds.), *Anticipatory grief.* New York: Columbia University Press, 1974, 193–209.

Redd, W.H., Andresen, G.V., & Minagawa, R.Y. Hypnotic control of anticipatory emesis in patients receiving cancer chemotherapy. *Journal of Consulting and Clinical Psychology,* 50(1), 14–19, 1982.

Redd, W.H., Andrykowski, M.A. Behavioral intervention in cancer treatment: Controlling aversion reactions to chemotherapy. *Journal of Consulting Clinical Psychology,* 1982, 50(6), 1018–1029.

Seigel, L.J., & Longo, D.L. The control of chemotherapy-induced emesis. *Annals of Internal Medicine,* 1981, *95,* 352–359.

Smith, S.D., Rosen, D., Trueworthy, R.C., & Lowman, J.T. A reliable method for evaluating drug compliance in children with cancer. *Cancer,* 1979, *43:*169–173.

Spinetta, J.J., & Maloney, L.J. The child with cancer: Patterns of communication and denial. *Journal of Consulting Clinical Psychology,* 1978, *46,* 1540–1541.

Swift, C.R., Seidman, F., & Stein, H. Adjustment problems in juvenile diabetes. *Psychosomatic Medicine,* 1967, 29:55.

Townes, B.D., Wold, D.A., & Holmes, T.H. Parental adjustment to childhood leukemia. *Journal of Psychosomatic Research,* 1974, *18,* 9.

Weinberg, S. Suicidal intent in adolescence: A hypothesis about the role of physical illness. *Journal of Pediatrics,* 1970, *77,* 579.

Zeltzer, L. Chronic illness in the adolescent. In I.R. Shenker (Ed.), *Topics in adolescent medicine.* New York: Stratton Intercontinental Medical Book Corp., 1978, 226–253.

Zeltzer, L.K. The adolescent with cancer. In J. Kellerman (Ed.), *Psychological aspects of childhood cancer.* Springfield, IL: Charles C. Thomas, 1980, 70–99.

Zeltzer, L., Kellerman, J., Ellenberg, L., & Dash, J. Hypnosis for reduction of vomiting associated with chemotherapy and disease in adolescents with cancer. *Journal of Adolescent Health Care,* 1983 (in press).

Zeltzer, L., Kellerman, J., Ellenberg, L., Dash, J., & Rigler, D. Psychological effects of illness in adolescence. II. Impact of illness in adolescents—Crucial issues and coping styles. *Journal of Pediatrics,* 1980, *97*(1), 132–138.

Zeltzer, L., & LeBaron, S. Hypnosis and nonhypnotic techniques for reduction of pain and anxiety during painful procedures in children and adolescents with cancer. *Journal of Pediatrics,* 1982, *101*(6), 1032–1035.

Zeltzer, L., & LeBaron, S. Effects of the mechanics of administration on Doxorubicin induced side effects: A case report. *American Journal of Pediatric Hematology/Oncology,* 1984, 6(1):107–110.

Zeltzer, L., LeBaron, S., & Zeltzer, P.M.: A prospective assessment of chemotherapy–related nausea and vomiting in children with cancer. *European Journal of Cancer,* 1983, in press.

Zeltzer, L.K., LeBaron, S., & Zeltzer, P.M. A prospective assessment of chemotherapy–related nausea and vomiting in children with cancer. *American Journal of Pediatric Hematology/Oncology,* 1984, 6(1):25–37.

Zeltzer, L.K., LeBaron, S., & Zeltzer, P.M. Paradoxical effects of prophylactic antiemetics in children receiving chemotherapy. *European Journal of Cancer,* 1983, in press.

Zeltzer, L., Zeltzer, P., & LeBaron, S. Cancer in adolescence. In M.S. Smith (Ed.), *Chronic disorders in adolescence.* Littleton, MA: John Wright PSG Inc., 1983, 253–275.

Mary Jo McCracken

21

Cystic Fibrosis in Adolescence

Cystic fibrosis (CF) is the most common lethal genetic syndrome found in Caucasian children. When CF was first recognized by clinicians, the outcome was nearly always rapidly fatal. Today, with major advances in research and treatment, the majority of children diagnosed with CF will reach adulthood.

This chapter will provide a basic overview of the pathophysiology of CF, common disease complications, and psychosocial issues confronting adolescents with CF and their family. The task is to familiarize and sensitize the professional to the special problems of CF. It should be kept in mind that there is a wide variation in the extent to which individuals are afflicted with this disease. Many adolescents with CF have minimal complications; CF may then have only a minor impact on their adolescence. Others are less fortunate and are required to make major adjustments in their life-style and long-term goals. Hence, the issues discussed may not be pertinent to all adolescents with CF.

PATHOPHYSIOLOGY OF CYSTIC FIBROSIS

Cystic fibrosis, inherited through transmission of an autosomal recessive gene, is characterized by widespread dysfunction of the exocrine glands. Elevated electrolyte concentrations in sweat, a unique characteristic of CF, provide the basis for the sweat test, a reliable diagnostic tool. The production of abnormally thick, tenacious mucus from the exocrine glands leads to obstruction in numerous organs; sites of obstruction include the airways of the lung, paranasal sinuses, small intestine, pancreas, biliary system, and reproductive organs. The disease is characterized by varying degrees of organ involvement and severity, with the majority of affected individuals demonstrating pulmonary and pancreatic complications. To date, the exact biochemical defect in CF remains a mystery. Researchers are currently questioning whether single or multiple defects are responsible for the pathophysiology seen in CF.

The diagnosis of CF brings with it a commitment to life-long, daily therapy as a means of controlling disease complications and promoting optimal health. The aspects of home care are numerous, time-consuming, and demanding. The goal of management is to promote adequate pulmonary clearance of thick bronchial secretions and to offset effects of maldigestion and malabsorption due to gastro-intestinal complications. Mist tents, aerosol treatments, bronchial drainage therapy, pancreatic digestive enzyme supplements, fat-soluble vitamin supplementation, and numerous other medications and dietary requirements consume significant portions of each day and have a significant effect on the individual and on the family life-style. The cost of medical care, medications, and required dietary intake are astronomical and frequently cause considerable financial burden. Despite aggressive treatment, the nature of CF is progressive, forcing the individual to cope with major complications and premature death. Pulmonary insufficiency is the major cause of disability and mortality in CF. Malnutrition, chronic pulmonary infection, liver disease, cardiac involvement, intestinal and gallbladder obstruction, and diabetes pose additional threats with advancing age. CF is not an easy disease, for it makes itself known every day in the ongoing demands of home care, the threat of progressive complications, and the eventual premature death.

IMPLICATIONS FOR THE ADOLESCENT

Adolescence is normally a time of rapid growth physically, psychologically, and socially. Multiple tasks challenge the adolescent working his or her way from childhood toward adulthood. Developing a sense of independence and acceptance by one's peer group while consolidating a positive self-identity can create stress and turmoil for the most healthy adolescent. For the adolescent with CF, these tasks can appear insurmountable.

At a time when physical growth is rapid, obvious, and expected, the adolescent with CF often faces delays in physical maturation. The effects of pulmonary disease and pancreatic insufficiency result in small stature and lags in development of secondary sexual characteristics. The absence of pubescent changes, coupled with often being the "smallest kid in class" are painful reminders that CF makes one different. Pulmonary complications such as, chronic, productive cough, clubbed fingers and toes, barrel chest configuration, and poor exercise tolerance, create obvious physical changes, which draw attention to the adolescent with CF.

Because of pancreatic insufficiency, digestive enzyme supplements must be taken with each meal and snack. Taking pills at the lunch table or over pizza with friends can be difficult and embarrassing. This may prompt the adolescent with CF to skip medications in an effort to be like everyone else. Abdominal cramping, large amounts of flatus, and high stool output, which is greasy and contains undigested food, are part of the price the adolescent will then pay. The simple act of going to the bathroom becomes a source of embarrassment. Even with appropriate digestive enzyme supplementation, uncontrollable flatus, abdominal cramping, and foul-smelling bowel movements are frequent complaints with CF.

At a time when healthy adolescents marvel at and become increasingly interested in their body and appearance, the adolescent with CF spends much time and energy attempting to hide the physical stigmata of the disease. Shopping for clothes is painful when one is malnourished and nothing fits; undressing in the locker room with schoolmates is uncomfortably revealing, and developing heterosexual relationships is extremely threatening.

Due to the progressive nature of CF, adolescence is usually marked by an increase in complications. Inadequate clearance of pulmonary secretions results in obstructive disease and recurrent infection; chronic pulmonary infection from *Pseudomonas*, particularly mucoid strains, occurs in the majority of individuals. Additional pulmonary infections from pathogens such as *Staphylococcus aureas* or *Haemophilus influenzae* can occur at any time, creating exacerbations in othewise controlled pulmonary disease. Uncontrolled pulmonary infections frequently require hospitalization for aggressive pulmonary toilet and intravenous antibiotics. The onset of mucoid *Pseudomonas* infection in the lung is particularly difficult, since current antibiotic therapy has proved unsuccessful in eradicating this pathogen. Hence, the adolescent with CF frequently lives in a state of chronic pulmonary infection.

Hemoptysis, atelectasis, bronchiectasis, and pneumothorax are common pulmonary complications in the adolescent and young adult CF population. Chronic infection and advancing lung disease result in a frequent, productive cough, shortness of breath with exertion, exercise intolerance, and a general increase in the work of breathing. These manifestations raise the adolescent's energy requirements considerably to daily caloric intakes as high as 3000–4000 calories. Consuming such large quantities of food is difficult, particularly when infection, productive coughing, and shortness of breath suppress appetitite. Weight loss and malnutrition usually follow, further decreasing the adolescent's physical reserve and body mass.

The stress of pulmonary disease and associated exacerbations may seriously impact cardiac function. With progressive loss of pulmonary function and hypoxemia, pulmonary hypertension develops, leading to cor pulmonale. This is a particularly frightening diagnosis for the adolescent and young adult, since it not only requires additional medical intervention but is also usually associated with a poor prognosis.

Pancreatic function, already compromised by duct obstruction, may be further jeopardized. Disorganization of the islets of Langerhans, caused by fibrosis of the pancreas results in glucose intolerance in approximately five to ten percent of the CF population. The onset of diabetes in CF individuals commonly occurs in adolescence or young adulthood; treatment typically involves insulin administration by injection, coupled with appropriate dietary management. A significant diabetic–CF population has not existed for prolonged follow-up periods, and so the extent of diabetes-related complications cannot be adequately predicted. Instances of retinal vascular changes and glomerular lesions have been reported. Needless to say, the diagnosis of diabetes in CF not only complicates medical management but has the potential for serious emotional upset for the adolescent who is already struggling to cope with the chronic, life-threatening aspects of CF.

Cramping abdominal pain is a common complaint in CF and is probably due to large amounts of fecal material associated with maldigestion and malabsorption. There is an increased incidence of meconium ileus equivalent or intussusception during the adolescent and young adult years. With medical management surgery can usually be successfully avoided, but the associated pain and discomfort can prove difficult.

Sterility occurs in 98 percent of all males with CF due to anatomical changes in the body of the epididymis, vas deferens, and seminal vesicles. Sexual function is unaffected, although semen volume may be reduced. Discovery of the occurrence of aspermia in CF individuals usually takes place during the adolescent years and creates emotional turmoil and feelings of sexual inadequacy. Female reproductive organs are anatomically normal and capable of reproduction; however, ability to conceive is often hindered by abnormally thick cervical mucus, delayed menarche, and secondary amenorrhea due to nutritional deficiency and pulmonary disease. Numerous women with CF have conceived, but the stress of pregnancy is contraindicated for many CF women, except in those with minimal pulmonary dysfunction and excellent nutritional status.

For adolescents with CF, serious complications inevitably appear, forcing them to face the issues this chronic illness imposes. Hospitalization is frequently required to adequately manage disease exacerbations; and home care becomes more intensive in their attempts to maintain levels of wellness. As hard as one tries to deny the presence of CF, the reminders are frequent and impact more severe during adolescence and young adulthood.

PSYCHOSOCIAL OVERVIEW

The psychosocial impact of CF on children, their parents, and their families has been the topic of considerable research. Until recent years, most research focused on parents and younger children with CF since sizable adolescent and adult populations were relatively nonexistent. These studies, for the most part, examined the negative impact of CF on the child and its crippling effect on family functioning. The studies were fairly consistent in their conclusion that CF often results in serious psychosocial consequences for the child, parents, and family. The first major study to address the psychosocial aspects of CF was conducted by Turk (1964), who concluded that families of children with CF are exposed to a number of psychosocial stresses that prevent maintenance of usual patterns of family relationships. Poor communication among family members and between family and community were noted. A general lack of time and energy for personal, marital, and family activities was also found to be the rule.

Lawler, Nakelny, and Wright (1966) found that the majority of parents of CF children experienced considerable emotional upset, as well as marital discord. Most mothers of children with CF were clinically depressed and demonstrated repressed hostility toward the CF child for the burden he or she posed. In turn, the children with CF demonstrated marked anxiety, with significant depression and preoccupation with death. Defense mechanisms used by the children to control anxieties included denial, use of fantasy, hostility, and regression.

A study by Spock and Stedman (1966) revealed CF children to be highly anxious and in need of strength and support. They also revealed that parental anxiety and sympathy for the child commonly resulted in a more permissive, yet overprotective, home environment.

Meyerowitz and Kaplan (1967) identified marked changes in family routine, such as disruption of the mother's employment in order to care for the child with CF, and the father's taking on additional employment to offset the financial drain. Severe emotional reactions occurred in parents upon diagnosis of CF and education about the long-term cares required by the disease. Families also reported feelings of isolation from the community, as well as perceived negative reaction by the community toward their affected child.

Tropauer (1970) reported finding feelings of inadequacy, insecurity, and anxiety in children with CF. A preoccupation with death and disability was also noted, especially in adolescents. Mothers of these children experienced depression and feelings of guilt, resulting either in overprotectiveness or overt rejection. It was concluded that the adolescent with CF bears an additional vulnerability to adjustment difficulties as a result of his or her extended dependency on parents.

Four major stages of adaptation to CF are identified by McCollum and Gibson (1970). Each is characterized by severe parental emotional responses, including intense anxiety, guilt, depression, denial, and hostility. A central issue for parents throughout these stages is the potentially fatal outcome of CF. Critical issues to the CF children were a heightened sensitivity to their differences from peers and an emerging awareness of the prognosis for their condition.

Gayton, Friedman, Tarormina, and Tucker (1977) performed psychological evaluations of CF children and their parents and siblings. Personality testing of the parents revealed significant differences between mothers and fathers. A higher incidence of disturbed personality functioning was found among fathers than among mothers of children with CF. A primary effect of CF on personality functioning in mothers was an increase in depression. Assessment of family interaction indicated decreased family satisfaction and poorer family adjustment. Study results failed to support either an increased incidence of emotional disturbances among children with CF or a negative psychological impact on sibling development.

ADOLESCENT PSYCHOSOCIAL TASKS

The presence of a chronic illness in adolescence, particularly one of the magnitude of CF, cannot help but have psychosocial impact. Obvious physical changes and associated limitations due to disease pathology, extensive home cares, potential disease complications, and the threat of premature death are issues that constantly confront the adolescent with CF. The degree of impact on psychosocial functioning will understandably vary from individual to individual and according to moderating factors such as severity of illness and family adaptation. Whether youths with CF can successfully master the tasks of adolescence, despite the obstacles imposed by their disease, has been the focus of much research. Conclusions from these studies vary; some researchers identify significant emotional upset and psychosocial dysfunction, while others find little evidence of psychopathology. A discussion of the impact of CF on the developmental tasks of adolescence, as well as the results of some pertinent research follows.

Cognitive Changes

During the adolescent period, the transition from concrete to abstract hypothetical and propositional thinking occurs. Such growth in cognitive function enables the adolescent to envision the future and his or her role in life. The development of intellectual or academic interests leads to an examination of occupational choices and to educational and vocational goal setting. Such decision making can prove difficult for the adolescent with CF, who often is unsure of the future. Questions such as, How long will I live? and What limitations will CF cause for me? run through the mind of the adolescent, who is well aware of the mortality rates for the disease; despite the strongest denial mechanisms, these thoughts remain. Boyle (1976) found that attempts to discuss the future produced strong reactions of fear and avoidance in these youths. The prospect of being incapacitated or of not surviving long enough to achieve chosen goals is painful and stressful.

In the past, children with CF were not expected to reach young adulthood. Hence, decision making in regards to education and vocation were often discouraged. Now that the majority of individuals with CF survive adolescence, the need for educational and vocational counseling has become vital. Fostering academic interests can prove adaptive for the physically limited adolescent. Excelling in academics can provide a basis for self-esteem, although physical prowess may be lacking. Exacerbation of CF symptoms often results in frequent or prolonged absences from school, however, and attempts to keep pace academically with healthy peers can prove frustrating. Tutoring or homebound instruction can assist the adolescent in overcoming this obstacle if school attendance is impossible. It should be emphasized that intellectual function is uncompromised in CF.

With the development of abstract thought, issues such as the finality of death and quality of life occur (see Blum, Chapter 10). A preoccupation with death in adolescents with CF has been identified by Boyle (1976) and Tropauer (1970). Denial and avoidance are common mechanisms used to deal with this fear. Death of other CF patients frequently provokes a breakdown in coping and creates an emotional crisis. Providing the adolescent with an opportunity to discuss his or her fears of death and dying is essential. Often, in an effort to protect one another, the parents and their CF youngster avoid discussing this topic with each other. Their desire to avoid unnecessary anxiety can deprive them all of needed support. Avoidance only prevents the adolescent from working through this issue. Acknowledging the fear and providing support and the opportunity to vent thoughts and feelings regarding death will facilitate a positive adjustment.

Identify Formation

Consolidation of a positive identity is another task facing the adolescent. As self-awareness increases, adolescents spend more time focusing on physical appearance and how others perceive them. Such scrutiny can prove stressful, particularly when one's appearance differs from that of one's peers. Delays in growth and sexual maturation, along with physical changes from chronic pulmonary disease, plague the adolescent with CF. Distress, anxiety, and depression may result as the realization surfaces that CF has caused physical differences. The formation of a distorted body image—usually one that is more negative than is really the case—may occur and severely affect the CF adolescent's ability to handle physical differences. Dissatisfaction with their bodies, affected self-images, and denial of sexuality have all been documented in numerous studies of adolescents with CF (Tropauer, 1970). The realization that CF has not only delayed sexual maturation, but also affected the reproductive organs further affects body-image formation. Awareness of male sterility and pregnancy complications in females are additional insults and often lead to sexual inadequacy. The need to incorporate the physical changes from CF into a healthy self-image, with realistic assessments of strengths and weaknesses, is a challenging yet necessary task.

Overcoming denial of their illness, resolving feelings of shame and embarrassment from uncontrollable symptoms (such as cough, flatus, and shortness of breath) and delays in maturation, to see the positive aspects each has to offer, are needed for establishing self-worth and self-esteem. To see beyond physical attributes is difficult for the adolescent. Here, the support of family is invaluable. The perception that the family of the adolescent with CF has of him or her will play a vital role in the ability to overcome physical limitations and consolidate a positive self-image. If the adolescent is seen as frail, childlike, and physically abnormal by the parents, those are the conclusions the adolescent will come to as well. But, if strengths are identified and physical differences compensated for, the adolescent will be able to accept his or her body despite physical shortcomings. Therefore, parental expectations need to promote growth, development, and well-being in the adolescent, and in doing so, nurture the potential for a healthy, stable self-image.

Interpersonal Relationships

Acceptance by one's peer group and development of interpersonal relationships must also be mastered during adolescence. The need to "fit in" and be like one's peers is of primary importance to this age group. A difference in physical appearance and the presence of a chronic illness definitely make one different. The adolescent with CF faces the challenge of overcoming his or her physical differences, as well as integrating the need for frequent medications, aerosol treatments, bronchial drainage, and mist tents. It quickly becomes quite obvious that others do not cough productively throughout the day, require digestive enzyme supplements with meals and snacks, or spend time daily involved in pulmonary hygiene.

The task facing the adolescent with CF is to overcome these physical differences, while accepting the fact that there is a need for health care maintenance, and to become firmly integrated with his or her peers. A major obstacle to such integration is the adolescent's home care program. Often, such a program is extensive and can interfere with peer-group activities. The need for chest physical therapy is often a higher priority than after-school activities. Attempting to find a balance between the two can be difficult and frustrating and requires substantial flexibility and support from the adolescent's family. Often, decisions need to be made to forgo home care to allow the adolescent to attend significant events. Such flexibility is allowed within the home care program for CF. The social and physical needs of the adolescent must be weighed and a happy balance found. If home care consistently interrupts the adolescent's social life, social networking will be compromised. If unresolved, a sense of isolation can result. The adolescent will come to resent the disease, rebel against the prescribed treatment program, and experience feelings of anger and hostility.

Serious disease complications during adolescence often require frequent and prolonged hospitalizations. This causes considerable interruption of social networking with peers. It becomes increasingly difficult to maintain friendships when in the hospital. Friendships may be lost when long absences occur. Many times the adolescent's peer group may be frightened into rejection. To be a close friend of someone who is seriously ill with physical limitations and who faces a premature death, is difficult and threatening, especially for an adolescent. Friends, not knowing how to handle this situation, may use avoidance as a coping mechanism. The end result can be few peer relationships.

Inadequate peer-group involvement, whether due to the demands of a home care program, limited physical endurance, delays in maturation, or prolonged hospitalization, will have a negative effect on the adolescent. A vicious cycle can develop, resulting in social immaturity, dependency on parents, poor self-image, anger, frustration, and depression. The need to firmly establish ties with a peer group plays a vital role in mastering the tasks of adolescence and achieving autonomy.

Physical Maturation

Delays in physical and sexual maturation pose another obstacle to peer-group acceptance. The adolescent with CF often looks much younger than others of the same age and may be treated so. Not experiencing the bodily changes of adolescence concurrently with one's peers can cause pain and embarrassment. Acutely aware of these differences, the adolescent may withdraw. A sense of isolation was found to be prevalent in the adolescents with CF studied by Boyle (1976). It was felt that this isolation stemmed from peer rejection due to physical differences. The adolescents felt, however, that relating to their peer group would be easier if they themselves were less concerned with body image. McCollum (1970) also found social isolation among CF adolescents and identified retardation in growth and sexual development as the cause of this phenomenon.

In a society where male virility and female curves are stressed, the adolescent with CF, lacking these traits, may withdraw and limit peer-group involvement.

Which sex will fare better in overcoming the physical differences imposed by CF is a difficult question. The female adolescent has the option of clothes and padding to conceal deficiencies and appear more like her peers. This is not the case with males. According to Landon (1980), morphological problems in male adolescents with CF resulted in difficulty with social relationships, anxiety, self-doubt, and general emotional upset. The issue of infertility further compounds the issue. Feelings of sexual inadequacy may result and affect interpersonal relationships. Feelings of sexual inadequacy were expressed by the males in Boyle's (1976) study, while the females in that study experienced few sexual anxieties.

Autonomy versus Dependency

The struggle for independence is a well-known task of adolescence. The adolescent vacillates between dependency and independence until maturity strikes a healthy balance. The need to be independent during the adolescent years is strong, and limitations cause extreme frustration. This is equally the case for the adolescent with CF. The need and desire to be independent are just as strong, yet the disease can set the youth up for failure at this task. The fear of being unable to adequately provide for his or her own physical and financial needs is ever present. Accomplishing home cares, particularly when energy levels are low or when ill, and having the financial resources for medical expenses, in addition to the basic essentials for life (food, clothing, and shelter) are issues confronting the young adult with CF. The task of dependence is considerably more difficult if parental attitudes are negative.

Throughout childhood, a good deal of parental energy has gone into adequately providing for the special needs of the child with CF. Home care has been religiously performed in the hope of avoiding serious complications and an early death. Relinquishing control of health care is difficult for parents, especially in light of their fears of the physical consequences of failure. The overprotective parent will find it threatening to let go. A power struggle often ensues with the result that the adolescent rebels, both against parents and against the disease.

If peer-group acceptance has been compromised, the adolescent with CF faces an additional obstacle to independence. The support of one's peers is essential to achieving independence. If the adolescent lacks this support, his or her ability to overcome the obstacles of chronicity and the associated parental concerns and to gain independence will be greatly jeopardized. Failure to achieve an appropriate level of independence will result in a poor self-image and a decrease in mastery of adolescence and will hinder the development of autonomy.

Past research has documented the problem of dependency in children with CF (Tropauer, 1970). It is clear that achieving independence will be considerably more difficult for the individual with CF since the demands of the disease are often overwhelming for even the most stable of families. Yet independence with CF can be achieved. A comprehensive approach, which coordinates community services and health professional resources, will be needed to assist the adolescent.

Education in self-care by health professionals is vital for the adolescent. Self-care is the vehicle through which the adolescent will accomplish home care independently. It also involves an understanding of the disease process and a rationale for prescribed treatment upon which the adolescent will base health issue decisions. Self-care activities will also help resolve parental opposition to independence and will lighten the strain CF home care imposes upon the family unit. The struggle for independence should be nurtured gradually and should begin during preadolescence or in early adolescence. This can be accomplished through parental relinquishing of responsibility for home care at an appropriate pace. Realistic goals and priority setting should take place and should incorporate the adolescent's physical and emotional limitations. A contract should be established between the adolescent and his parents which identifies home care responsibilities of each party. By mid-adolescence, the majority of home care should be the adolescent's responsibility. Some youths will be physically well enough to assume total responsibility for their home care. Utilizing self-care skills throughout the late adolescent years will provide a period that can enhance mastery of these skills and adjustment to independence. This period will also provide the parents with evidence that their child is indeed capable of independence. An added bonus of self-care activities is the resolution of a major family hardship in CF—accomplishing home care. The parents will now be able to pursue their own goals in life and begin to find substitutions for the void that adolescent independence creates.

Once the issue of independence concerning home care is resolved, the adolescent can proceed in exploring the attainment of future goals. This will often include an independent living situation in young adulthood—a realistic goal for many young adults with CF. Community resources can be utilized to overcome the obstacles of limited finances or a deterioration in health status. Financial support is available to qualified young adults from Social Security, Services for Children with Handicaps, and local governmental agencies. Public Health Nursing or other home care agencies are established means of providing home care when individual resources are inadequate.

The message one needs to hear is that independence is a realistic expectation for the adolescent with CF. The degree of independence each individual can achieve will be influenced by disease complications and their associated limitations. However, numerous young adults with serious physical limitations as a result of CF have achieved effective levels of independence including independent living. Support from a variety of resources is available to assist the individual in accomplishing this goal.

Self-Sufficiency

Preparation for self-sufficiency is the final task of adolescence. Occupational choices are considered and basic educational and vocational goals decided upon. Adolescents must learn not only to make major decisions concerning their life but also to become accountable for their decisions and actions; they are moving into adulthood. A condition such as CF can alter the ground rules of this process. Health status, the threat of dete.ioration of health, and disease-imposed limitations can make this an extremely stressful time. Boyle (1976) found that the last years of high school produced emotional crises in adolescents with CF. Facing the decisions to be made with regard to educational and vocational goals brought a sense of futility. The uncertainty of their future makes such decision making difficult for adolescents with CF. They must acknowledge their limitations and incorporate them into any future plans. To avoid establishing goals and plans for the future is a mistake that can be the adolescent's undoing. For development to progress, life goals worth striving toward must be made. This is essential to the quality of life. The adolescent with CF who has no future plans is more vulnerable to the negative emotional impact this disease can produce.

It is difficult for the adolescent with CF to accept that the illness may pose limitations on career choices. Health will always be a top priority, and occupations suitable to the chronic pulmonary disease need to be chosen. Physical endurance and capabilities can also limit vocational choices. For these reasons, vocational counseling must be provided for all adolescents with CF. A study by Goldberg, Isralsky, and Swachman (1979) examined the issue of vocational development and adjustment in CF. The adolescents studied scored lower than normal in their vocational development. This was reflected in their vocational and educational plans and in the realism of these plans. However, they scored above normal in strength of commitment to their vocational choice, work values, and degree of awareness of occupational information. An obvious problem for these adolescents was their lack of realism in considering their physical limitations and financial constraints when making occupational choices. The study clearly shows that adolescents with CF plan to work and hold strong work values yet need support in making realistic vocational decisions.

For the adolescent and young adult with CF, work is often seen as a means of maximizing personal satisfaction. The prospect of a shortened life span makes the need for vocational satisfaction critical. Satisfaction with their work may be one of the few rewards in life for young adults with CF and thus it increases their self-esteem. It can also provide the motivation to survive times of physical crisis. Since the rewards of vocational satisfaction are great, appropriate vocational counseling is vital for the adolescent's vocational development. To select an occupation that will bring satisfaction and will be compatible with the physical limitations of CF is essential to the young adult's well-being.

With advancing age, the probability of serious disease complication increases. A deterioration in health status can interfere with the CF adolescent or young adult's performance and attendance at school or work. Often, repeated hospitalizations are required to control disease exacerbation. Such interference in educational or vocational activities is likely to prove extremely frustrating. It can become increasingly more difficult to achieve established goals in the time frame one has planned. Frequently, such exacerbation can result in physical limitations that require the individual to make changes in educational or vocational goals. Postponement of these goals until a stable health status is achieved may have to be accepted. It is not unusual for the adolescent with CF to temporarily quit school or change employment to a part-time status. An educational program may even exclude the adolescent from its enrollment list, rationalizing this action as being in the adolescent's best interests.

There have been numerous examples of job discrimination against youths and young adults with CF. Few young adults with CF are honest in acknowledging their chronic condition on job applications, due to the fear of rejection. Yet school and work are important for the adolescent and young adult with CF. Schools and places of employment must sensitize themselves to the special needs of this population. They will usually be rewarded by excellent performance and high standards of quality, since the individual with CF has overcome multiple challenges to participate and places high value on educational and vocational activities.

CONCLUSIONS

The adolescent with CF faces many obstacles in the mastery of adolescence. Maladjustment can result in anxiety, social dependency, self-doubt, and general emotional upset. Although this outcome is a possibility for the adolescent with CF, it is not inevitable. Research has documented the presence of both positive adaptation (Bywater, 1981; Straker & Kuttner, 1980; Drotar, Doershuk, Stun, Boat, Boyer, & Matteus, 1981) and psychopathology in many adolescents with CF. Numerous adolescents with CF are able to overcome the multiple hardships imposed by their disease with resilience and workable coping mechanisms. Several factors will have influence on the CF youth's mastery of adolescence and entrance into adulthood psychosocially well adjusted.

The importance of effective family communication has been identified as vital to facilitating a positive adjustment to CF (Turk, 1964; Tropauer, 1970; Bywater, 1981). Health professionals must be responsible for stressing the importance of effective communication within families. The health professional must help to create an environment that is conducive to the discussion of the psychosocial problems by the family and the individual. Communication with peers and community must be explored if self-sufficiency is to result. How much of one's diagnosis to share, with whom, and at what point in the relationship are constant questions.

Education holds a valuable place in the CF care plan for both parents and teenagers. Parents need adequate education on the pathophysiology of the disease, growth and development rationale for treatment, and potential complications. Additionally, nutrition education is critical for both parent and teen so as to maximize physical development (see Story, Chapter 8).

The teenager needs to understand the principles of the disease and how to adequately provide for his or her own health care needs. Self-care activities facilitate the adolescent's movement to self-sufficiency. Encouragement, realistic goal setting, and vocational counseling are necessary for overcoming the obstacles imposed by CF.

The promotion of independence and autonomy cannot be overemphasized. Medical science will have accomplished little by prolonging life for those with CF if that life is deficient in quality. The development of autonomy and independence is needed in order to accomplish a positive life adjustment. Without these two factors, the adolescent will be at a loss both psychologically and socially and, thus, unable to fully experience the rewards of life.

In summary, the diagnosis of CF brings major changes to the life of its victims and their families. This condition makes unique demands, which can result in psychosocial deficits or psychopathology. This, however, is not inevitable. Numerous adolescents with CF and their families make a positive adjustment. Past research has documented significant psychosocial problems in the CF individual and family. More recent research suggests that individuals with CF can make a positive adjustment and that emotional disturbances and maladjustment are not the inevitable result of

CF. The fact that CF poses a considerable challenge to its victims and their families is obvious, but many rise to the challenge and develop resilience and effective coping mechanisms in overcoming the obstacles of the disorder. Healthy development is a realistic goal.

The future for the individual with CF is optimistic; research is continuously providing the medical professional with more effective tools for controlling disease complications and health professionals are becoming increasingly sensitive to the hardships this disease imposes and are providing increasingly appropriate interventions to facilitate healthy adaptation.

REFERENCES

Boyle, R.R., Tisant'Agnese, P.A., Sack, S., Millican, F., & Kulczycki, L.L. Emotional adjustment of adolescents and young adults with CF. *Journal of Pediatrics*, 1976, *88*, (2), 318–326.

Bywater, E.M. Adolescents with CF: Psychosocial adjustment. *Archives of Diseases in Childhood*, 1981, 56, 538–543.

Drotar, D., Doershuk, C.F., Stun, R.C., Boat, T.F., Boyer, W., & Matteus, L. Psychosocial functioning of children with CF. *Pediatrics*, 1981, *67*,(3), 338–343.

Gayton, W.G., Friedman, S.B., Tarormina, J.F., & Tucker, F. Children with CF: Psychological test findings of patients, siblings and parents. *Pediatrics*, 1977, *59*, 888–894.

Gayton, W.F., & Friedman, S.B. Psychosocial aspects of CF: A review of the literature. *American Journal of Diseases of Childhood*, 1977, *126*, 856.

Goldberg, R.T., Isralsky, M., & Swachman, H. Vocational development and adjustment of adolescents with CF. *Arch Phys Med Rehabil*, 1979, *60*, (Aug.), 369–374.

Landon, C., Rosenfeld, R., Northcraft, G., & Lewiston, N. Self image of adolescents with CF. *Journal of Youth and Adolescence*, 1980, *9*, (6), 521–528.

Lawter, R.H., Nakelny, W., & Wright, N.A. Psychological implications of CF. *Canadian Medical Association Journal*, 1966, *94*, 1043–1046.

McCollum, A.T., & Gibson, L.E. Family adaptation to the child with CF. *Journal of Pediatrics*, 1970, *77*, 571–578.

Meyerowitz, J.H. & Kaplan, H.B. Familial responses to stress: The case of CF. *Soc Sci Med J*, 1967, 249–266.

Spock, A. & Stedman, D.J. Psychological characteristics of children with CF. *RC Medical Journal*, 1966, *27*, 426–428.

Straker, G., & Kuttner, M. Psychological compensation in the individual with a life-threatening illness: A study of adolescents with CF. *South African Medical Journal*, 1980, *57*, 61–62.

Tropauer, A., Franz, M.N., & Dilgard, V.W. Psychological aspects of the care of children with CF. *American Journal of Diseases of Childhood*, 1970, *199*, 424–432.

Turk, J. Impact of CF on family functioning. *Pediatrics*, 1964, *34*, 67–171.

Sue V. Petzel, Irene Bugge
Warren J. Warwick, Jeffrey R. Budd

22

Long Term Adaptation of Children and Adolescents with Cystic Fibrosis: Identification of Common Problems and Risk Factors

As advances in diagnosis and medical management lead to increases in expected longevity for children with cystic fibrosis (CF), preventive mental health efforts have become increasingly important. Recent behavioral health research has concentrated on identifying the psychosocial risks of this chronic, fatal disease and determining how to reduce the adaptive problems in affected children. Identifying the tasks and problems and the effective response strategies common to those with physical illnesses, including CF, has been recommended as a means of helping affected individuals and their families to improve their coping abilities (Hamburg, 1974; Lipowski, 1970; McCollum & Gibson, 1970; Moos & Tsu, 1977).

Moos and Tsu (1977) developed a model of the multiple social, psychological, and physical factors that contribute to the outcome of severe physical illness. This model integrates task and problem identification with other factors related to coping with physical illness as a life crisis. The term "outcome" is used to represent how the individual recovering from or adapting to physical illness attains a new psychological and physiological equilibrium. Moos and Tsu describe the outcome of physical illness as dependent on the following six variables:

1. The individual's perception of his or her illness.
2. The adaptive tasks presented by the illness.
3. The coping skills used in responding to the disease.
4. Background and personal factors.
5. Illness-related factors.
6. Physical and social environmental factors.

A number of personal, illness-related, and environmental factors affect adaptation by families in which there is a child with CF. Some studies suggest that more adaptive problems occur for children who are male, whose diagnosis is delayed until later in the disease course, whose health is deteriorating, whose family is of lower socioeconomic status, or whose parents are less educated (Drotar, 1978; Meyerowitz & Kaplan, 1967; Sultz, Schlesinger, Mosher, & Feldman, 1972; Tavormina, Boll, Dunn, Luscomb, & Taylor, 1981; Tavormina, Kastner, Slater & Watt, 1976; Tropauer, Franz, & Dilgard, 1977). In studies of children with CF, reports of school problems, problems coping with death, parental overprotectiveness, and family financial difficulties are common (Drotar, 1978; Meyerowitz & Kaplan, 1967; McCollum & Gibson, 1970; Spock & Stedman, 1966; Sultz et al., 1972; Tavormina et al., 1976; Tropauer et al., 1977). These studies also point out more frequent stress reactions and medical management problems with younger children and decreasing compliance and increasing social isolation with adolescents.

Studies concur that social and psychological factors affect the outcome in CF. However, several methodological limitations make it difficult to identify the extent to which adaptive problems are to be expected in coping with CF. First, the selection of children for study often is not random, so the incidence figures for the psychological and social problems for children with CF may not be accurate. Second, psychosocial factors that may affect outcome are not defined clearly or consistently from study to study. Third, the changing influence of social and illness-related factors as the child grows older or as the disease progresses ususally is not considered. An exception to this last criticism is McCollum and Gibson's (1970) study of the family's adaptive process over time which showed that families adapt to CF in four stages: prediagnostic, confrontational, long term, and terminal.

The goals of this study of CF children were as follows:

1. To identify the incidence of adaptive problems in the long-term adaptation phase of the illness.
2. To use these problem situations to study the effect of child and parent-characteristics (personal, illness-related, and social factors) on the frequency and difficulty of problems.

3. To determine the relative importance of the factors that influence the evolution of adaptive problems.
4. To develop a systematic method for identifying children at risk for these problems.

METHODS

Subjects

One child with CF and one parent from each of 40 families were studied. Subjects were chosen from among the 300 CF patients followed at three-month intervals at the University of Minnesota CF Clinic. Parents were contacted in the CF clinic the day their child was seen for a routine medical examination. The assumption was that clinic attendance would ensure a random sample of regular clinic patients; however, this method may oversample patients with disease severity requiring more frequent follow-up and undersample those patients less reliable for follow-up. Forty of forty-two parents contacted agreed to participate. To meet selection criteria for this study the child had to be of school age and diagnosed at least three years prior to selection. The study group was selected so that 50 percent of children were of each sex and 50 percent of each sex were above and below 12 years of age. All were Caucasian.

The mean age of the children was 12.2 years, with a range of 5.9 years (SD = 4.0). Mean age of children at diagnosis was 1.6 years (SD = 1.5). Mean age of mothers (n = 39) was 40.0 years (SD = 9.9) and of fathers (n = 33), 43.6 years (SD = 10.4). Based on Hollingshead's (1965) two-factor index of social position (high = 1, low = 5), mean socioeconomic status (SES) was 3.8 (SD = 0.9), representing the upper-middle income range. Mean number of children per family was 3.1 (SD = 1.9). Eighty percent (n = 32) of parents were married and 20 percent were unmarried (single/divorced/widowed/separated).

Procedure

Parent Measures

One parent for each child with CF completed a background information form and a 73-item parent questionnaire. The questionnaire was developed using the behavioral–analytical method of test construction (Bugge, 1981; Goldried & D'Zurrila, 1969). Based on a review of the literature, interviews with parents of CF children, and interviews with professionals working with CF patients, 91 problem situations commonly confronting parents were identified and written in role-play format (Bugge, 1981). For the present study, the 91 role-play situations were reduced, eliminating 18 items that either a parent or professional reviewing the items found confusing or redundant. The resulting 73 role-play situations were presented to parents who indicated whether each problem was (yes) or was not (no) a problem for them during the past year. The final 73 items represented the following seven problem areas:

1. Treatment—tasks or situations associated with medical procedures (e.g., medications, nutrition, mist tent).
2. Physical realities—tasks or situations associated with genetic, physical, or health consequences or future planning.
3. Hospitalization—tasks or events dealing with pre-, intra-, and posthospitalization.
4. Death—situations dealing with the CF child's own death or the death of others with CF known to the child.
5. School—tasks or events associated with relationships and behavior in school.
6. Family—situations associated with sibling, parental, marital, and extended family relationships.
7. Friends—tasks or situations associatd with peer relationships (e.g., acceptance, isolation).

Based on Moos and Tsu's (1977) model of adapting to chronic illness as a life crisis, three of these problem areas (treatment, physical realities, and hospitalization) are associated with illness-related tasks and therefore represent a set of illness-related problems. The tasks in the other four areas (school, family, friends, and death) are more general and more relevant to all types of life crises and therefore represent a second set of general problems. These seven specific problem areas, and one additional area—*financial* (a sufficient number of financial problems had not been identified to be organized into an independent cluster)—were rank ordered by the parent from most (1) to least (8) difficult. A difficulty score for each of the eight problem areas was obtained by summing and averaging the rank order for each area for all patients. A frequency score for each problem area and an overall problem frequency score for each patient were obtained by summing the number of *yes* responses within each and across all of the seven problem clusters, respectively. In addition, since the number of items in each of the seven problem areas varied, the mean frequency of the three most highly endorsed items/area was used as an index of relative frequency for each of the seven problem areas. A relative frequency score for each area was then obtained by totaling the number of *yes* responses for all patients.

Health Measures

Estimates of health status were obtained from the medical chart and included percent predicted weight,* and percent predicted pulmonary function.† Mean percent predicted weight for all children was 90.4 (SD = 13.8). Mean percent predicted pulmonary function was 79.1 (SD = 17.8). These two measures were used because they monitor the two major disease complications—pulmonary and digestive tract problems. The clinic director, who had followed the patients since diagnosis, rated all 40 patients on a scale of 5 (high) to 1 (low) for family coping and for compliance. Mean compliance for all children was 3.2 (SD = 1.1) and mean coping was 3.2 (SD = 1.2). While physician rating is a notoriously weak measure of compliance, in an exploratory study of this type it was felt that it represented a better measure than self-report or appointment-keeping behaviors. Outcome measures of weight and pulmonary function can serve as another, although indirect, measure of compliance.

RESULTS

Identification of Common Problems

The mean number of problems endorsed per patient was 18.4 (SD = 11.6) or 23 percent of the 73 presented problems. The treatment cluster of problems was the area within which the highest percentage of items was endorsed per patient, with a mean of 35.5 percent. A mean of 23.3 subjects endorsed each of the top three items in the treatment area. These three leading treatment items, therefore, were endorsed 58 percent of the time. For the remaining problem areas, the number of subjects endorsing each of the leading three items ranged from a mean of 19.3 (48.3 percent) to 7.1 (18.3 percent) in the following order: hospitalization, physical realities, school, family, and death. Of the eight problem clusters ranked for difficulty, death was seen as the most difficult (mean rank = 6.1), followed in decreasing order by treatment, hospitalization, physical realities, financial, friends, family, and school. These findings, interpreted using Moos

---

* Percent predicted weight is based on sex and height norms from a sample of 300–400 normal children.
† Percent predicted pulmonary function represents the average of four measurements of lung function, obtained from a standard spirometry test as a percentage of their expected values and also based on sex and height norms (Warwick, 1977, 1980). These four measurements are forced vital capacity, peak flow, the average of the forced expiratory volume at 1.0 and .75 seconds, and the average of three measures of mid-expiratory flow.

and Tsu's model (1977), indicate illness-related problems are of relatively high frequency, while general problems are of low frequency.

General Determinants of Outcome

Relationships within Personal, Social, and Illness-Related Factors

One of the assumptions underlying the use of several personal, social, and illness-related measures is that they assess different factors contributing to outcome. Inspection of an intercorrelation matrix revealed no significant relationship between the three personal variables (age, sex, and compliance) or between the three social variables (SES, marital status, and family coping). The two health variables, percent predicted weight and percent predicted pulmonary function, showed significant positive correlations. Of the relationships between variables across the three groupings, the most significant was the positive correlation found between family coping, defined as a social factor, and compliance, defined as a personal factor. These two variables represented clinical observations, and their intercorrelation may represent either real association or perception of basically the same factor. The only other significant relationship across the variable groupings was between sex and percent predicted weight. This parameter was lower for females than for males (p = .047) reflecting the well-known increased morbidity and earlier mortality of females with CF.

Relationships Between Factors and Problem Frequency or Difficulty

The relationships between personal, social, and illness-related factors and the number of problems are presented in Tables 23-1, 23-2, and 23-3. T tests were performed for sex and marital status while regressions and correlation coefficients were calculated for the other factors.

Personal Factors: Sex, Compliance, and Age.

As shown in Table 22-1, no statistically significant differences were found between total number of problems, number of problems by area, and difficulty of problems for males compared with those for females except that females rated treatment significantly more difficult (p = 0.025; all other t tests, p> .05). For both males and females treatment was the problem area of highest frequency, family and physical realities were intermediate in frequency, and school, hospitalization, death and friends were low in frequency. Problems associated with death were more frequent for females, and problems with friends were more frequent for males.

Table 22-1

Comparison of Frequency and Difficulty (Rank Order) of
Problem Areas for Males (n = 20) and Females (n = 20)

| | Frequency | | | | Difficulty | | | |
| | Males | | Females | | Males | | Females | |
Problem area	Mean (SD)	Relative order	Mean (SD)	Relative order	Mean (SD)	Relative order	Mean (SD)	Relative order
Illness-related problems								
Treatment	7.4 (4.3)	1	6.8 (3.7)	1	4.6 (1.7)	3	5.9* (5.9)	1
Physical realities	3.8 (2.9)	2	3.8 (2.5)	3	3.8 (2.0)	5	5.1 (2.3)	3
Hospitalization	1.2 (2.0)	5	1.0 (1.6)	5	4.8 (2.1)	2	4.5 (2.1)	5
General problems								
Death	0.6 (1.1)	7	1.2† (1.0)	6	6.5 (2.2)	1	5.8 (2.6)	2
Family	3.0 (2.5)	3	4.0 (3.2)	2	3.5 (2.2)	6	3.2 (2.6)	7
Friends	1.2 (1.2)	6	.6 (.9)	7	3.0 (1.8)	7	3.7 (2.7)	
School	1.9 (2.1)	4	2.2 (2.2)†	4	2.5 (2.5)	8	2.7 (1.4)	8
Financial	na	na	na	na	4.1 (2.1)	4	4.5 (2.4)	4
Total problems	18.4 (11.4)	na	18.2 (11.0)	na	na	na	na	na

na = not applicable
* $t(34) = 2.34$, p = .025
† $t(37) = 1.90$, p = .065

Death and treatment were ranked as difficult by both males and females.
School, friends, and family were rated least difficult. Other problem areas
were rated as intermediate in difficulty by both males and females.

Although the total frequency (Table 22-2) and difficulty of problems
by area (Table 22-3) were not significantly associated with age, frequency
of problems with death and physical realities was found to increase with
advancing age. Hospitalization, treatment, and total problem frequency
significantly increased with decreasing compliance (Table 22-2).

The personal factors studied demonstrated strongest association with
specific problem frequency, some association with overall problem frequency, and no association with problem difficulty. Compliance dem-

Table 22-2

The Relationship of Illness-Related, Social, and
Personal Factors to Frequency of Problems (n = 40)

Multiple R	Illness-Related problems			General problems				Total problems
	Treat- ment R	Physical realities R	Hospital- ization R	Death R	School R	Family R	Friends R	R
Illness-related factors								
%wt	−.05	.12	−.29	.06	.17	.23	.02	.02
%pft	.33*	.19	−.02	−.02	.28	.32*	.21	.32*
Social factors								
Family coping	−.29	−.05	−.16	.14	.04	.01	−.03	−.20
SES	−.09	−.31	.04	−.16	−.31	−.18	−.22	−.26
Marital status	t	t	t	t	t	t	t	t
Personal factors								
Age	.16	.34*	.30	.48†	.15	.25	.21	.30
Compliance	.49†	−.18	−.34	−.39*	−.20	−.08	−.26	−.39*
Sex	t	t	t	t	t	t	t	t

* p ≤ .05; † p ≤ .01
%wt = percent predicted weight
%pft = percent predicted pulmonary function
t = t test

onstrated a strong negative relationship with both specific and overall problem occurrence and was most highly correlated with illness-related rather than general problems. Less compliant children with CF have more problems in general and particularly more problems with hospitalization and treatment. Overall problem frequency appears to be independent of sex and age. Death represents a special problem; it is difficult but infrequent and is more of a problem with advancing age, with decreased compliance, and it is possibly more of a problem for females than for males.

Social Factors: Marital Status, SES and Family Coping.

There were no statistically significant differences between total number and frequency of problems by area (Table 22-2) or difficulty of problems (Table 22-3) for children living with married parents compared with those living with a single parent (divorced, separated, single, or widowed) (all *t* tests, p > .05). Total number of problems and number and difficulty of

Table 22-3
The Relationship of Illness-related, Social and
Personal Factors to Difficulty of Problems (n = 40)

	Illness-related problems			General problems				
	Treatment	Physical realities	Hospitalization	Death	School	Family	Friends	Financial
Multiple R	R	R	R	R	R	R	R	R
Illness-related factors								
%wt	−.13	.40*	.06	.23	.06	−.03	.07	−.07
%pft	.05	.16	−.08	.16	.13	.16	.27	−.27
Social factors								
Family coping	−.09	−.04	−.28	−.17	.04	−.08	.00	.08
SES	−.29	−.05	−.22	.21	−.11	.09	.13	.19
Marital status	t	t	t	t	t	t	t	t
Personal factors								
Age	.26	−.20	.06	−.28	.00	−.08	.04	−.04
Compliance	−.25	.28	−.26	−.06	−.09	−.06	.04	−.04
Sex	t	t	t	t	t	t	t	t

* p ≤ .05
%wt = percent predicted weight
%pft = percent predicted pulmonary function
t = *t* test

problems by area also were not significantly associated with SES or with family coping (Tables 22-2 and 22-3) (p > .05). Problem frequency within all areas did not change with increasing physical realities (r = −.31, p = .06) and school experiences (r = −.31, p = .06) for their children. These results suggest that problem frequency and difficulty for young people with CF are independent of the sociodemographic factors of parental marital status, SES, and estimates of family coping.

Illness-Related Factors: Percent Predicted Weight and Percent
Predicted Pulmonary Function.

The results in Table 22-2 indicate that the total number of problems and the number of problems by area were not significantly associated with percent predicted weight. However, total number of problems and problem frequency in the treatment and family areas were found to correlate with percent pulmonary function. A greater number of total, treatment, and family problems were reported for healthier children. Difficulty was not significantly associated with percent predicted pulmonary function, neither was it significantly associated with percent predicted weight in the area of physical realities. Problems in this category were more difficult for healthier children. These results suggest that percent predicted pulmonary function is positively associated with frequency of total, treatment, and family problems but is not associated with problem difficulty. Percent predicted weight is not associated with problem frequency or difficulty of most problems except for a very selective association with difficulty of physical reality problems.

Interactions Between Factors and Problem Frequency or Difficulty.

All social, personal, illness-related factors were poor predictors of perceived problem difficulty. Percent predicted weight, family coping, and family interactions were poor predictors of specific and total problem frequency. Significant interactions were found for total number of problems and for only two specific problem areas: treatment and death. The interaction between age, percent predicted pulmonary function, and compliance was the strongest predictor of total problem frequency. The interaction of these three variables accounted for 41 percent of the variance in the total number of problems. The interaction between age, percent predicted pulmonary function, and compliance best predicted the number of problems in the treatment area, while age and compliance were sufficient for achieving a similarly good prediction of death problems. Healthier, older, and less-compliant patients reported a greater number of overall problems; these problems primarily were treatment or death related. Socioeconomic status also interacted with percent predicted pulmonary function and compliance and with age and compliance to predict a total number of problems and number of treatment problems. Less-compliant, higher-SES, and healthier patients reported a greater number of total problems; these problems are primarily treatment related.

DISCUSSION

The children with CF in this study had been diagnosed at an early age, their health was relatively stable, and they represented a cross-section of ambulatory school-age CF patients.

In the long-term adaptation phase of this disease, a number of common problems occur for affected children and their families. Some children are at higher risk for these problems than others.

Based on this study, illness-related problems tend to be more frequent and difficult than general problems. Treatment problems are significant and represent the most frequent and the second most difficult problem area. Death, as suggested by others (McCollum & Gibson, 1970; Spock & Stedman, 1970; Tropauer et al., 1970), was shown to be an especially difficult problem. The importance of school-related problems for children with CF (Drotar, 1978; Lawler, Nakielny, & Wright, 1966) was partially substantiated by this study, as this problem area was demonstrated to have intermediate frequency but low difficulty.

The greater incidence of overall problems—mainly in the treatment and death areas—for the older, less-compliant youth may represent increasing resistance to treatment. Increased resistance or rebellion against therapeutic efforts by the adolescent CF patient has been suggested by others (Drotar, 1978; Lawler et al., 1966; Tropauer et al., 1977). The current results show resistance to treatment in the adolescent to be associated with more satisfactory health and higher SES. In other words, chronic illness has a cumulative effect upon overall problem frequency for the noncompliant child, especially for the relatively healthy noncompliant child of higher SES.

Previous studies have reported an increased incidence of compliance and social and physical management problems in older children with CF (Lawler et al., 1966; McCollum & Gibson, 1970; Meyerowitz & Kaplan, 1967; Tavormina et al., 1976). However, in the current study, the child's age did not independently affect the overall incidence of problems, neither was increasing age independently associated with increased incidence of most specific problems. Only problems with death and physical realities increased with age, while difficulty of all problems was independent of age. The positive association between age and problems with death and physical realities probably reflects the older child's increased cognitive development, especially the increased capacity for formal operational thought and time perspective (Piaget & Inhelders, 1958). These capacities are likely to increase a child's ability to question or reflect upon the meaning of health as well as the meaning of life and death. Such questioning characterizes the content of the items about death and physical realities. For the healthier CF child, the increased difficulty of physical-reality problems, the increased frequency of treatment and family problems, and the increased frequency of overall problems with increasing age appears similar to reports that less noticeably ill children experience more difficulties (Tavormina et al., 1981). The paradox presented by apparent satisfactory health in the presence of chronic disease appears to be a special problem for chronically ill children and their parents, especially as the child grows older.

Previous studies have reported that boys with CF have more problems than girls (Sultz et al., 1972; Tavormina et al., 1981; Tavormina et al.,

1976). In this study, the child's sex was independent of problem frequency. However, treatment problems were judged more difficult by girls than boys. This special difficulty may reflect the nature of the mother–child relationship. Treatment procedures for children with CF actively involve parents, particularly the mother (McCollum & Gibson, 1970), and mothers were the primary respondents in this study. Studies suggest that the reciprocal intensity of the mother–child relationship can lead to the mother's identification with the child. Thus, more than the father, the mother may be threatened by the child's death (Natterson & Knudson, 1960). In the current study, the intensity or difficulty of treatment issues appears to have increased when the ill child was a girl. Increased sharing of responsibility for treatment with other family members might reduce difficulty of treatment situations, at least as experienced by the mother of girls with CF. Additional understanding of the role of the parent–child relationship in coping with CF, including the effect of same and cross-sex variables, is also relevant.

Previous studies suggesting that chronically ill children of lower SES have more school-related problems than their higher SES peers have been interpreted to mean "better educated parents [are] . . . able to compensate the handicapped child more successfully by more effective motivation and educational assistance" (Sultz et al., 1972, p. 99). In this study, problem incidence was independent of SES. However, children whose parents had the least education and were of lower SES tended to report fewer rather than more school-related problems. It may be that increased parental education increases the importance of the child's school experiences for the parents; the child's uncertain future necessarily limits and frustrates the parents' expectations and hopes, and a greater number of school-related problems are perceived by the parents. This interpretation is tentative, and the association between problem incidence and SES needs clarification.

Marital status was not associated with the number or difficulty of problems. Regardless of marital status, mothers may be responsible for parenting the chronically ill child. That the mother is the primary parent is also suggested in other studies of children with CF (McCollum & Gibson, 1970; Tavormina et al., 1981). Therefore, from the viewpoint of the mother, the major respondents in this study, little change in problem incidence or difficulty may be perceived when the father is actually absent from the family by separation, divorce, or death.

Frequency of problems was associated with various social, personal, and illness-related factors, but difficulty was associated with few. The correlates of problem difficulty probably are represented by other determinants affecting outcome as suggested by Moos and Tsu (1977), but they are not included in this study. For example, the individual's perception of their illness and the coping skills that they select, as well as additional social, illness-related and personal factors represent other determinants that are not identified and measured in this study, but which also may be critical to the development of problems with physical realities, hospitalization, school, family, and friends.

Of the two health status scores used, percent predicted weight was a poor predictor of the number of problems compared with percent predicted pulmonary function. The former correlate probably was not associated with problem frequency because the patient group was relatively homogeneous for this parameter. Those CF patients who have significantly lower scores of percent predicted weight generally have been chronically ill for an extended period and, because of frequent hospitalizations, such patients were less likely to be selected for this study. Moreover, the range of variation compatible with stable health is relatively small compared with the percent predicted pulmonary function score, which can show wide variations in relatively healthy CF patients.

OBSERVATIONS AND CONCLUSIONS

The relationships between specific problems, age, and health status can be used by health professionals to anticipate with parents the problems that may develop as their child with CF grows older and as the disease progresses.

The strong negative association between compliance and problem frequency, and especially frequency of problems with treatment, suggests that intervention–education efforts targeted specifically at decreasing problem frequency are likely to be associated with increased compliance.

A list of effective solutions is available for each of the problem situations used in the current study (Bugge, 1981). This group of problems with solutions provides the content base with which to teach families effective solutions to problems that arise with their children who have CF. As Hamburg (1974) described, "People can benefit from specific information regarding tasks and strategies relevant to their current circumstances." Developing a new pattern of action that is likely to be effective tends to change emotional responses. The more effective the action, the greater is the relief from distress.

Different instructional methods will be useful in helping parents anticipate and cope with different problems. Behavioral rehearsal and modeling are likely to be useful for instructing parents in coping with those problems that occur frequently, are viewed as difficult, or for which a variety of role-play situations and effective solutions have been generated (e.g., treatment issues). Parents will be less motivated to rehearse or model problem solutions for problems that are not viewed as frequent (e.g., death) or difficult (e.g., school). For these issues and parents, feedback regarding the incidence of adaptive problems and factors that affect their incidence may provide instructional benefits other than skill building, such as increased acceptance of and reality testing regarding common issues. However, improved coping can be achieved in many ways in addition to improving a parent's problem–solving skills. For example, some parents who under–report the frequency of problems may find information about the incidence of common problems helpful in accepting the reality of problems when they do occur. They may also find it a source of reassurance that they are experiencing relatively few problems.

Moos' and Tsu's (1977) model of coping with chronic disease as a life crisis describes several adaptive tasks closely related to the clusters of problems used in the current study. Integrating these tasks with the results of this study identifies additional coping techniques for children with CF. For example, based on Moos' and Tsu's model, problems with death are associated with preparing for an uncertain future. Teaching the older child with CF this adaptive task is relevant even when explicit issues of death are not reported as part of day to day living.

The education and health promotion possibilities of this CF questionnaire may be extended by its adaptation to microcomputer technology. Use of the microcomputer has been demonstrated to be a useful method of health education (Ellis, Raines, & Hakanson, 1982). Adaptation of the CF questionnaire to the microcomputer, including problem situations and solutions, would assist children with CF and their parents to actively seek information and feedback, to prepare for probable difficulties, and to develop new problem-solving efforts by practice and rehearsal.

The developed instrument is relevant to one specific disease: cystic fibrosis. These results, however, demonstrate the feasibility of using Moos' and Tsu's (1977) model of outcome and a list of problems developed by the behavioral–analytical method to study the diverse factors contributing to the outcome of other diseases. The current results represent one step in the more rigorous study of the psychosocial factors that affect outcome of chronic physical illness and in the development of health education tools for families and their chronically ill children.

REFERENCES

Bugge, I. *Development of a behavioral role-play test to measure parental coping with chronic illness (cystic fibrosis)*. Unpublished doctoral dissertation, University of Montana, 1981.

Drotar, D. Adaptational problems of children and adolescents with cystic fibrosis. *Journal of Pediatric Psychology*, 1978, *1*, 45–50.

Ellis, L.B., Raines, J.R., & Hakanson, N. Health education using micro-computers: One year in the clinic. *Preventive Medicine*, 1982, *11*, 212–224.

Goldried, M.R., & D'Zurrila, T.A. A behavioral-analytic model for assessing competence. In C.D. Spielberger (Ed.), *Current topics in clinical and community psychology* (Vol. 1). New York: Academic Press, 1969.

Hamburg, D.A. Coping behavior in life-threatening circumstances. *Psychotherapy and Psychosomatics*, 1974, *23*, 13–25.

Hollingshead, A.B. *Two factor index of social position*. New Haven, Connecticut: Yale Station, 1965.

Lawler, R.H., Nakielny, W., & Wright, N.A. Psychological implications of cystic fibrosis. * *Canadian Medical Association Journal*, 1966, *94*, 1043–1046.

Lipowski, Z.J. Physical illness, the individual and the coping processes. *Psychiatry in Medicine*, 1970, *1*, 91–102.

McCollum, A.T., & Gibson, L.E. Family adaptation to the child with cystic fibrosis. *Journal of Pediatrics*, 1970, *4*, 571–578.

Meyerowitz, J.H., & Kaplan, H.B. Familial responses to stress: The case of cystic fibrosis. *Social Science and Medicine*, 1967, *1*, 249–266.

Moos, R.H., & Tsu, V.D. The crisis of physical illness: An overview. In R.H. Moos (Ed.), *Coping with physical illness*. New York: Plenum Publishing Corporation, 1977.

Natterson, J.M., & Knudson, A.J. Observations concerning the fear of death in fatally ill children and their mothers. *Psychosomatic Medicine*, 1960, *22*, 456–465.

Piaget, J., & Inhelder, B. *The growth of logical thinking from childhood to adolescence*. New York: Basic Books, 1958.

Spock, A., & Stedman, D.J. Psychological characteristics of children with cystic fibrosis. *North Carolina Medical Journal*, 1966, *27*, 426–428.

Sultz, H.A., Schlesinger, E.R., Mosher, W.E., & Feldman, J.G. *Long-term childhood illness*. Pittsburgh: University of Pittsburgh Press, 1972.

Tavormina, J.B., Boll, T.J., Dunn, N.J., Luscomb, R.L., & Taylor, J.R. Psychosocial effects on parents of raising a physically handicapped child. *Journal of Abnormal Child Psychology*, 1981, *9*, 121–131.

Tavormina, J.B., Kastner, L.S., Slater, P.M., & Watt, S.L. Chronically ill children: A psychologically and emotionally deviant population? *Journal of Abnormal Child Psychology*, 1976, *4*, 99–110.

Tropauer, A., Franz, M.N., & Dilgard, V.W. Psychological aspects of the care of children with cystic fibrosis. In R.H. Moos (Ed.), *Coping with physical illness*. New York: Plenum Publishing Corporation, 1977.

Warwick, W.J. Pulmonary function in healthy Minnesota children. Spirometry studies. *Minnesota Medicine*, 1977, *60*, 435–550.

Warwick, W.J. Pulmonary function in healthy Minnesota children. Flow-volume studies. *Minnesota Medicine*, 1980, *63*, 191–195.

Susan D. Klein
Roberta G. Simmons
Carol R. Anderson

23

Chronic Kidney Disease and Transplantation in Childhood and Adolescence

This chapter represents the results of a multifaceted longitudinal research project conducted at the University of Minnesota to investigate the impact of chronic kidney disease and transplantation. Data from several interrelated studies make it possible to construct a meaningful description of the influence of the disease and transplantation on the development of the adolescent and young adult.

POPULATIONS AND METHODS

Original Study

Chronically Ill Children

In order to assess the effects of the disease, the authors interviewed a population of 72 chronically ill patients (ages 8–20 years, mean age 13.6 years) who were attending the pediatric renal clinic from 1972 to 1973. Criteria were established to exclude acute, short-term illnesses. First, a duration criterion of at least one year from time of diagnosis was applied in selecting cases. Second, the physician rated the severity and chronicity of the disease in each individual included in the study; generally, all patients with one of the following diagnoses were interviewed: chronic pyelonephritis, chronic glomerulonephritis, polycystic kidney disease, congenital interstitial nephritis, diabetic glomerulosclerosis, chronic end-stage renal disease (undetermined etiology), hypoplasia, or lupus erythematosus.

The research questionnaires, which included both closed- and openended items, consisted of a large group of multiple-choice questions designed to measure aspects of the individual's self-image (to be discussed later), as well as a group of items dealing more specifically with the individual's illness and its influence on his or her life. Since this project also focused on understanding the effects of chronic disease on family members and on assessing familial patterns of coping, 65 mothers and 44 normal siblings were also interviewed. Complete findings of this research may be found in Klein (1975).

Child Transplant Recipients

At the same time, a group of 52 children and adolescents (ages 8–19.2 years) who had maintained a transplanted kidney for at least one year were interviewed (mean period since transplantation, two and one half years). Fourteen of them (age 16 or older) were given an adult questionnaire, and 38 of them (ages 8–15) were administered the same questionnaire as the chronically ill children. Thus, the adjustment of the transplanted children can be directly compared with that of the chronically ill children.

In tandem with these quantitative surveys, a psychiatrist conducted in-depth assessments of all subjects from both groups at several points both pre-transplantation and post-transplantation (Bernstein, 1977). The psychiatrist was able to follow 100 patients fully; some were too young to respond to the structured questionnaires, and others had been ineligible for these questionnaires because they had not yet survived a year. A detailed description of both the psychiatric assessment techniques used and the results of this psychiatric study may be found in Bernstein (1977).

Comparison Groups

The adjustment of the chronically ill and the transplant patients may be compared with that of two control populations. First, 44 normal siblings, closest in age to the group of chronically ill patients, were interviewed via a similar questionnaire; they comprise one comparison group. Second, Rosenberg and Simmons (1972) used many of the same quantitative measures of psychological adjustment in their large study of normal Baltimore school children (n = 1918). For this analysis, the authors attempted to make the Baltimore sample more comparable to the Minnesota population by including in the control group only white children ages 10 to 18 (n = 621).

A major study of adult transplant patients at the University of Minnesota was conducted concurrently. All patients age 16 and older who received tranplants between 1970 and 1973 were interviewed before transplantation, about three weeks after, and again one year post-transplant using the adult questionnaires. The extensive structured questionnaires asked about many aspects of the patient's quality of life, including daily activities, symptoms, family and other relationships, and work. A complete description of the methodology and results of this study may be found in Simmons, Klein, and Simmons (1977).

Follow-up Study

From 1978 to 1980, a long-term follow-up study was done of all patients who had received transplants between 1970 and 1973, who still retained a functioning kidney, and who agreed to again participate in the study. The responses of these patients (now five–nine years post-transplant) provide a picture of what life is like over the long term for the kidney transplant patient. Thirty of the 52 pediatric transplant patients originally interviewed fit the criteria for the follow-up study; that is, they had received a transplant between 1970 and 1973 and still retained a functioning kidney. Three of the 30 were still under 16 and thus received the child's questionnaire; 8 additional children who were too young to respond to the earlier surveys were also interviewed using the child's questionnaire. Two patients refused to participate, and the remaining 25 of the 30 were interviewed via the adult questionnaire, since they were 16 years of age or over. Thus the total response rate for the group who received transplants as children was 28 of 30, or 93%. In the long-term follow-up study, those who received transplants as children and are now age 16 years or more can be compared with 85 nondiabetic individuals who had received transplants as adults.

Measures of Self-Image and Adjustment

A central focus in studying these populations was the assessment of psychosocial adjustment in terms of self-esteem and other dimensions of self-image. The social–psychological scales for adults were replicated from Rosenberg (1965), Rosenberg and Simmons (1972), Kohn (1969), and Coleman (1966). The children's studies focused on many of the same dimensions of the self-picture as were used in the adult studies. However, the questions and scales were modified for use in children ages 8 years and above, and reliability and validity were tested in previous research (Rosenberg & Simmons, 1972).

Reliability was again satisfactorily established for the chronically ill children by Klein (1975). Dimensions of emotional well-being measured for children and adults are listed in Table 23-1. For more complete information on these measures and their reliability, see Simmons, Klein, and Simmons (1977).

Table 23-1
Dimensions of Emotional Well-Being Measured
in Children (Age 8 and Above) and Adults
(Age 16 and Above)

Children	Adults
Happiness or depressive affect	Happiness or depressive affect
Anxiety	Anxiety
Self-image	Self-image
Self-esteem	Self-esteem
Self-consciousness	Preoccupation with self
Stability of the self-picture	Identity stability
Sense of distinctiveness	
Show true feelings	
Satisfaction with appearance	Satisfaction with appearance
Perceived popularity	Satisfaction with social roles
	Control over destiny
	Independence-dependence

Methods: Summary and Aims

In examining the quality of life of children and adolescents suffering
from kidney disease, three studies from the University of Minnesota will
be considered, in summary:

1. A study of 72 chronically ill children and their families which was
   conducted in 1972–1973.
2. A study conducted in 1970–1974 of all individuals who were given
   kidney transplants as children, 52 of whom had reached one year
   post-transplant, currently had functioning kidneys and were of
   the proper age (8–19 years) to receive quantitative questionnaires.
3. A follow-up study conducted in 1978–1980 of all individuals given
   kidney transplants between 1970 and 1973, who still had functioning kidneys from five to nine years later.

The latter study includes 11 children who were below age 16 at the
time of the follow-up and received virtually the same questionnaires as
the chronically ill children, and 25 late adolescents and young adults who
received adult questionnaires. These 25 individuals who received transplants in childhood or adolescence can be compared with 85 individuals
who were originally transplanted as adults and were now also from five
to nine years post-transplant.

In each study, the authors will attempt to document the extent to
which the illness and treatment interfered with physical, emotional, and
social well-being and to identify factors that affect adjustment to chronic

illness and to a kidney transplant. In particular, how do age (childhood versus adolescence versus adulthood) and sex affect this adjustment? To what extent do age differences seem to reflect the normal developmental process of adolescence rather than special processes related to illness? We turn first to the study of 72 chronically ill children and adolescents.

FINDINGS

Influence of Chronic Illness on Children and Adolescents

Extent of Impact

Physical and social well-being. Chronic kidney disease clearly takes a toll on the physical well-being of children and adolescents, as evidenced in their answers to multiple-choice questions (Klein & Simmons, 1977). Compared with their normal siblings, the 72 chronically ill children were more likely to perceive that they were ill (p < .001), less likely to consider themselves as very healthy (p < .001), and more likely to mention their health when asked about their worries. Unlike their normal siblings (n = 44), the 72 patients interviewed also reported that they tired more easily than others (p < .001). The mothers of the chronically ill children (n = 65) indicated that these children were less active and less able to compete physically. Only about 68 percent of the ill children reported that they participated in gym class, and of these, only about two thirds engaged in all of the regular athletic activities.

The school is the center of much of a child's life, and other researchers have shown that ill children often have academic problems (Pless & Roghmann, 1971; Sultz, Schlessinger, Mosher, & Feldman, 1972). Absenteeism serves as a universal indicator of interference with school life. Over a third of the mothers of the chronically ill children reported that absenteeism was a problem, with 25 percent of the ill subjects missing more than five days a month, whereas none of the normal siblings missed so many days. It appears that their illness also jeopardized the quality of their academic performance: about one quarter of the children stayed back at least one year, and half of them needed a tutor. Although rates for normal children are not available for comparison, these rates for absenteeism and below-grade performance seem high.

In spite of the liabilities associated with a lack of energy and limited physical activities, a series of questions about number of friends and frequency and type of social activities showed virtually no difference between the sick children and their normal siblings.

Emotional well-being.   It was expected that the chronically ill children would show more negative emotional adjustment, particularly in self-image. In a study of Baltimore school children Simmons, Rosenberg, and Rosenberg (1973) found that several aspects of self-image were negatively affected at the onset of adolescence. A drop in self-esteem and an increase in depression and self-consciousness occured around ages 12 to 14, and for some measures, there was improvement in late adolescence. Simmons et al. (1973) also reported this stage to be more difficult for girls than for boys. Thus the authors predicted that preadolescent and adolescent individuals who were chronically ill would show even greater disruption in their adjustment than the healthier control group.

The relatively few quantitative studies of the adjustment of chronically ill children are contradictory in their findings; some show little difference between ill children and normal controls (Collier, 1969; Crain, Sussman, & Weil, 1966); others indicate that about one third of all chronically ill children develop secondary social and psychological problems (Haggerty, Roghmann, & Pless, 1975; Pless & Roghmann, 1971). One of the more recent studies comparing healthy adolescents with adolescents with chronic or serious diseases shows no difference between the two groups on quantitative measures of self-esteem and anxiety, although youngsters with certain diseases demonstrate less control over their health (Kellerman, Zeltzer, Ellenberg, Dash, & Rigler, 1980; Zeltzer, Kellerman, Ellenberg, Dash, & Rigler, 1980).

Comparing chronically ill children, their normal siblings, and the normal control groups on nine social–psychological scales;* the major differences found in this study of the children with chronic kidney disease pertain to their body image, or satisfaction with their looks. Only in this one aspect did the chronically ill children appear to suffer in comparison with healthy children. Thirty-nine percent of these children considered themselves not satisfied with their looks, compared with only 28 percent of the normal siblings and 22 percent of the Baltimore controls (p < .05 for the comparison of these three groups). In fact, 39 percent of the ill children perceive themselves as too short in comparison with 23 percent of their siblings, a figure reflecting the retardation of growth caused by some kidney diseases.

Other dimensions of emotional adjustment and self-image appear to be surprisingly undamaged for the total sample of chronically ill children. Self-esteem, self-consciousness, stability of self-image, a sense of distinctiveness, felt ability to reveal true feelings, self-estimates of popularity,

---

*Happiness; self-image/self-esteem; self-consciousness; stability of self-picture; sense of distinctiveness; body image; relationship to others/show true feelings; estimate of popularity; anxiety.

and reported anxiety were all within the normal range. See Simmons, Klein, and Simmons (1977) for further data.

For most of the chronically ill children, the level of happiness also appeared to be no lower than that of the controls. Yet there were a few patients who showed severe evidence of depression according to their mother or physicians. All of these were adolescents rather than younger children, and all had more serious diseases. There were four chronically ill adolescents who made suicide threats or attempts. Two of these suicidal youngsters were heading for kidney transplantation, and both had watched a relative die after an unsuccessful transplant. The other two suicidal patients were among the ten patients who had lupus erythematosus, a particularly severe disease that affects other body systems as well as the kidney.

Factors Affecting the Adjustment of the Chronically Ill Children

Although it appears that chronic renal illness is not a serious psychological stressor for children generally, there are certain subgroups that are more severely affected by the disease experience. The major factors that increase the vulnerability of a patient include adolescent age, severity of illness, female sex, and dissatisfaction with appearance. The family's reaction and pattern of coping also appear to be important to the child.

Seriousness of illness. It was hypothesized that among the chronically ill youngsters, those who are more seriously ill would show greater disturbance of the self-picture and lower levels of happiness. In one of the related studies it was shown that transplanted adults with greater health problems showed less favorable social–psychological adjustment (Simmons et al., 1977). For the authors' study of children, there were two relatively objective and one subjective measure of severity to be correlated with various measures of the child's adjustment. The two relatively objective judgments of severity were made by the physician and the child's mother, and the third reflects the child's own perception of his disease. Although objective severity of the disease does appear to affect the child, several dimensions of self-image remain unaffected (Klein & Simmons, 1977). The child's own definition of the severity of the disease, however, correlates more highly and significantly with almost all of the measures of psychological adjustment, such that the more severe the disease, the more unfavorable the adjustment (significant Pearson correlations range from 0.18 to 0.43). The child's own subjective definition accounts for more of the variance in the child's adjustment than either the physician's definition or that of the mother. Based on a canonical correlation of each adjustment definition to all of the nine social-psychological scales discussed earlier, the percent variance explained by the child's own definition is 35 percent (p ≤ .01), compared with 14 percent by that of the physician and 19 percent by that of the mother.

These findings are similar to those reported by Zeltzer et al. (1980) and Kellerman et al. (1980). See also Zeltzer et al., Ch. 16). They found that physician measures of severity did not relate to measures of psychological adjustment, whereas the perceived impact of the illness did correlate with self-esteem and anxiety. Thus the child's own interpretation of the severity of the condition seems to be more important for his or her psychological health than are external judgments. Because information about the predisease status of the children is not available, however, there can be no certainty regarding causal direction. It seems reasonable to conclude that those who perceive the disease to be a great problem react with lower happiness and less favorable aspects of self-image. However, Zeltzer et al. (1980) and Kellerman et al. (1980) found perceived high impact of illness correlated with high anxiety and low self-esteem in healthy adolescents who had nonserious, acute diseases as well as in adolescents with serious and chronic diseases. Thus, it may be that children who initially have lower self-esteem and are less happy are more likely to perceive kidney disease as a major problem than are those with better self-images.

Age and sex.   The age and sex of the individual have been found to affect the self-image of the normal child, as mentioned earlier. A drop in adjustment occurs in early adolescence, sometimes followed by recovery in later adolescence, and females appear to be at a greater disadvantage than males on several self-image dimensions, although not on happiness (Simmons et al., 1973). The age-related changes in self-image and depression for chronically ill children appear to be similar to those for normal youths (Klein & Simmons, 1977). Also, in comparison with males, ill females show less stability of the self-concept (p = .02) and less satisfaction with looks (p = .06) but greater happiness (p = .03). In sum, effects of age and sex on self-image seem to reflect normal developmental differences rather than the effects of chronic illness.

Given normal developmental trends, it is not surprising that female adolescent patients react more negatively than their male counterparts to the effects of kidney disease on their looks. Studies of normal children show that in adolescence, though not necessarily earlier, valuation of looks is higher among girls than among boys (Simmons & Blyth, in process; Simmons & Rosenberg, 1975). Thus, it is understandable that ill female adolescents are more likely to be dissatisfied with their looks.

Satisfaction with appearance.   Furthermore, one would expect the child's own subjective experience or satisfaction with appearance to affect his or her total adjustment. It has already been shown that the most significant difference between chronically ill and normal children relates to satisfaction with body image. It would not be surprising if, in a society that so highly values good looks, children who are dissatisfied with their appearance show more negative general adjusment.

In fact, although the relationships are small, chronically ill children who are less satisfied with their looks do show slightly more negative adjustment in other ways (less stability of self-picture, $r = .18$, $p = .07$; less ability to reveal true feelings, $r = .15$, $p = .10$; and lower self-esteem, $r = .11$, NS). Dissatisfaction with the body image is an even greater problem for children who have received transplants, an issue to be discussed later. Again, of course, the causal direction can only be hypothesized— it is possible that a global negative attitude affects both self-esteem and evaluation of looks, rather than the child's evaluation of his or her appearance influencing other dimensions of adjustment.

The family and adjustment to illness. Family background factors seem to have general consequences for the self-image of children rather than specific effects on ill children. In general, chronically ill middle-class children and their siblings appear to have a better self-image than members of lower-class rural families. In addition, large family size appears to be associated with detrimental self-image effects, although this finding is not totally consistent (Klein & Simmons, 1977).

The way in which the family copes with the child's illness is significant for the child's adjustment. Children who take responsibility for their own care, in contrast with those who do not assume a major burden of self-care, demonstrate significantly more positive adjustment along a number of dimensions.[†] The way in which the mother of the ill child manages her role is also important. If the mother indicates confusion and difficulty in managing the treatment of the sick child, the child is likely to score negatively on several dimensions of adjustment.

Finally, children who reported that their mothers held them in high esteem scored more favorably on scales of self-esteem, self-consciousness, self-stability, satisfaction with looks, happiness, and ability to reveal feelings.[‡] In fact, it is the authors' hypothesis that the special protection of the ill child by the mother is one of the reasons for the surprising finding

---

[†]Controlling for severity of disease and age, it has been found that the following partial correlations between children's assumption of their own care and dimensions of adjustment: high stability ($r = .15$); low anxiety ($r = -.19$, $p = .08$); more ability to reveal feelings ($r = .41$, $p = .001$); more satisfaction with appearance ($r = .35$, $p = .004$); less perception of self as different ($r = -.15$). Correlations for the other four scales in Table 23-1 indicate no relationship. In general, unmentioned scales show nonsignificant findings.

[‡]There were no differences on other scales except for sense of distinctiveness (children whose mothers think more highly of them tend to view themselves as more distinctive).

that such children score as high as normal youngsters on most scales. The ill children are somewhat more likely than normal controls to believe their mother holds them in highest esteem, to see themselves as their mother's favorite, and to report their mother as the family member to whom they are closest (Klein & Simmons, 1977).

Influence of Kidney Transplantation on Children and Adolescents: Original Study—1970–1974

Extent of Impact

Physical and social impact. There are two sources of information, as noted earlier, for the 1970–1974 study of post-transplant children:

1. Quantitative questionnaires administered to 52 youngsters (ages 8–19) who were at least one year postsurgery.
2. Psychiatric evaluations over time of all children ever transplanted at the University of Minnesota up to that time (n = 100) (Bernstein, 1977).

These transplant recipients had more serious illness and experienced more significant medical procedures than most of the chronically ill children described earlier. As a result of the severity of their illness, their physical appearance is more likely to have been significantly compromised.

There are, primarily, two problems related to transplantation that affect the child's appearance: physical size and side effects of medication. Severe kidney disease often retards growth, and although transplantation may reverse this pattern, Bernstein, the psychiatrist who evaluated the children in the Minnesota study, noted that "growth is variable and frequently disappointing" (Bernstein, 1977, p. 128). This problem is particularly apparent during adolescence.

In 1974, 20 percent of the adolescent males age 15 or over were under five feet tall; 21 percent of the females were under four and one half feet tall. In the follow-up study in 1980, 21 percent of the males ages 16–27 were under five feet, but none of the females was under four and one half feet tall.

The second major cause of problems with appearance is related to the continual need for medications to prevent kidney rejection--including steroids and immunosuppressive drugs. The cushingoid appearance that is sometimes a side effect of these drugs is characterized by an abnormally round, or moon-shaped, face and a protruding abdomen. Bernstein (1977) observed at one point that about 20 percent of the 81 surviving transplant recipients she was evaluating had a notable cushingoid appearance. Other appearance problems for the children who had received a transplant occurred much less frequently and included deformities caused by bone disease and delayed sexual maturation. It appears that distortions in physical appearance can be a major problem in severe kidney disease and kidney transplantation in adolescence.

It would, however, be an error to focus merely on the negative physical effects of kidney transplantation. Kidney transplantation is a therapeutic intervention designed both to save the individual's life and to enable him or her to experience a higher quality of life than with alternative therapies for end-stage kidney disease. In fact, Bernstein (1977) reports that an increase in physical energy is one of the most remarkable changes following transplantation.

According to Bernstein (1977), this renewed vigor has differing effects on children of various ages. It results in the most dramatic flowering of physical abilities, personality traits, and cognitive skills in the youngest patients (those below age 5) who have been ill most, if not all, of their lives. Preadolescent and older adolescent children show positive but less striking gains. Thus it appears that the change from pretransplant to posttransplant may not be as dramatically positive for the adolescent patient as it is for younger patients.

In terms of school attendance, almost all youngsters with functioning kidneys were in school without major problems, with the exception of three grade school children who had medical difficulties and two teenagers in good health who had dropped out. While grade school children reported a few problems with peers, adolescents were more often subject to teasing, especially because of differences in appearance (Bernstein, 1977, pp. 140–141). Adolescence has been characterized as a time of intensification of the desire for peer conformity and the intolerance of differences (See Sebald, 1977, pp. 250–251), and there is some evidence of such a process occurring in at least a few transplant patients.

Emotional well being. Post-transplanted children of appropriate age (8–15) were measured with the same social–psychological scales as the chronically ill children. Surprisingly, children who have received transplants appear to do as well as normal controls on most scales. Once again, satisfaction with looks is the only dimension on which these children fare poorly (Simmons et al., 1977).

Measures of adjustment on social–psychological scales are available, as are clinical evaluations (Bernstein, 1977) of the incidence of major psychiatric problems among all children who received transplants by 1973. Table 23-2 demonstrates this incidence and will be discussed in the next section of the chapter.

Table 23-2
Total Number of Individuals Who Received Transplants
as Children Demonstrating Major Psychological Problems
(Psychiatric Study 1970—1974)

	Current age				
	0–5 years (n = 9)	6–11 years (n = 23)	12–18 years (n = 35)	19–24 years (n = 33)	Total number* (n = 100)
At time when kidney function is adequate	0	0	2	1	3 (3%)
At time when there is threatened kidney failure	1	4	15	2	22 (22%)
After kidney failure†	0	1	2	1	4 (4%)
Total number	1	5	17	4	29 (29%)
Percentage of children demonstrating problems	11%	22%	49%	12%	29%

* See Bernstein (1977), page 132.
† Twenty-two patients rejected their kidneys and returned to the kidney machine.

Factors Affecting the Adjustment of Transplant Recipients

The same factors that jeopardized chronically ill children appear to
have similar effects on post-transplant youngsters. First of all, the severity
of health problems after transplantation has emotional ramifications. As
Table 23-2 demonstrates, these youngsters are particularly likely to develop
psychological problems when the function of their new kidney is threatened. Insofar as the psychiatrist could determine, only three children developed severe emotional problems when kidney function was adequate.

Second, the adolescent patient seems emotionally vulnerable in comparison with patients of other ages. As Table 23-2 shows, Bernstein (1977)
found the incidence of major emotional problems to be low among the
youngest patients (11 percent), somewhat greater among those 6–11 years
old (22 percent), and highest among adolescents (49 percent). One of the
most severe reactions—suicidal thinking—as far as we know, occurred
only among adolescents: seven adolescents revealed suicidal thinking at
intervals, and one of these (a boy) completed a suicidal act after his transplanted kidney was immunologically rejected and he had to return to the
artificial kidney machine (dialysis) to maintain life.

Third, dissatisfaction with one's body image appears to interfere with
the child's general psychosocial well-being. When the disease is thought
invisible, adjustment is high; once the youngster believes the disease is
visible, general adjustment seems lower. Post-transplant children who feel

satisfied with their appearance are better adjusted in many other ways than are those who are dissatisfied. In comparison with other children, those who are less satisfied with their appearance show lower self-esteem ($r = .43$, $p = .005$); more self-consciousness ($r = -.34$, $p = .03$); a greater sense of distinctiveness ($r = -.22$, $p = .10$); higher anxiety ($r = -.34$, $p = .05$); less happiness ($r = .28$, $p = .05$); less self-reported peer popularity ($r = .27$, $p = .07$); and less stability of the self-picture ($r = .30$, $p = .05$). (Similar findings are shown by Simmons et al., 1977 for adult transplant recipients.) In addition, children who are dissatisfied with their looks are less likely to have friends of the same or opposite sex or to socialize with peers after school (Bernstein, 1977).

Furthermore, among those youngsters who showed serious psychiatric adjustment problems, there were several adolescent girls who reacted severely to medication-related distortions of appearance (Bernstein, 1977). One such 16-year-old girl was so distressed that she discontinued the medications that prevented her from immunologically rejecting her new kidney; she subsequently died. Again, then, appearance issues appear to be particularly salient for female patients.

Finally, lack of family support may place a child at risk in terms of adjustment. Earlier it was suggested that special maternal attention might be responsible for the high level of adjustment among chronically ill children. Among transplanted youngsters, three of the ones with suicidal tendencies, including the boy who actually committed suicide, were from disrupted families that failed to give the teenager emotional support as he or she faced a crucial medical complication.

Follow-Up Study: The Long-Term Impact of Kidney Transplantation

In addition to the above studies conducted in the early 1970's, in 1978–1980 the authors conducted a long-term follow-up of all patients transplanted between 1970 and 1973 who still had functioning kidneys. At the time of the long-term follow-up, the study participants were five to nine years post-transplant. Patients age 15 and below ($n = 11$) received virtually the same children's questionnaire as the chronically ill children, whereas older patients received the adult version.

Children Age 15 or Less at the Follow-Up

At the time of the long-term follow-up the average age of these children was 11.4 years (range = 8–15), most of them having received their transplant at about age 5. While the number is too small for complex analyses, their high level of school adjustment is similar to that reported in the transplant patients studied in the early 1970s. All of these patients are attending school, and only three report that the transplant prevents their participating fully at school. All report they go to gym, and 10 of the 11 participate in the regular gym activities, although they do not appear to engage in extracurricular team sports.

While it is too early to determine the eventual growth of these children, their small size is perceived as a problem. Several of the 11 report being teased about their appearance (six specifically mention shortness). Once again, the greatest emotional cost of the transplant appears to be related to body image, a cost that may be even greater in older adolescents.

Late Adolescents and Young Adults at Time of Follow-Up

Physical well-being.   Twenty-five patients who received transplants between the ages of 8 and 19 were between 16 and 27 years old at the time of the long-term follow-up and still had functioning kidneys: 10 were still adolescents (ages 16–19) and 15 were young adults (20–27). The issue of concern here is the level of adjustment of these young people who have spent some part, if not all, of the key adolescent years as transplant patients. On some measures their long-term adjustment can be compared to that of patients who originally received transplants when adults. First of all, what is their level of physical well-being?

For most people, late adolescence and young adulthood are times of maximal health, marked by few health worries. How well do these 25 patients feel? Seventy-six percent of them say they feel as healthy as most people. Yet 40 percent of them report having some kind of medical difficulty in the year preceding the interview year, and 29 percent were hospitalized during that period. Five of the 25 patients were noted to be chronically rejecting, a condition in which the kidney graft gradually deteriorates and dialysis or another transplant is needed. In comparison with the long-term patients who received transplants when adults and are now somewhat older, these 25 young people seem to feel better and experience fewer symptoms of uremia (nausea, weakness, headaches, tiredness, pain, swelling, eyesight problems, and mental confusion). Twelve percent of these late adolescents–young adults indicate they are pretty worried, and 64 percent say they are a little worried about their health now, while only 24 percent report they are not worried. In comparison with healthy peers who do not have to cope with a lifetime of medication and the possibility of kidney rejection, these young people seem at some physical disadvantage, yet their outlook is generally positive.

Vocational rehabilitation.   Late adolescent–young adult transplant patients are far more likely to be vocationally rehabilitated than the patients who were adult transplant recipients (see Table 23-3). Compared with the

Table 23-3
Work–School Status of Transplant Patients According to Age

Current age	Males				Females				Total			
	Patients who received transplants as children or adolescents		Patients who received transplants as adults		Patients who received transplants as children or adolescents		Patients who received transplants as adults		Patients who received transplants as children or adolescents		Patients who received transplants as adults	
	16–19	20–27	26–44	45–62	16–19	20–27	26–44	45–62	16–19	20–27	26–44	45–62
Working or going to school full-time (%)	86	100	77	57	100	50	33	25	90	73	60	38
Part-time (%)	14	0	0	14	0	12	27	20	10	7	10	18
Not working or going to school (%)	0	0	23	29	0	38	40	55	0	20	30	44
	100	100	100	100	100	100	100	100	100	100	100	100
	(7)	(7)	(22)	(14)	(3)	(8)	(15)	(20)	(10)	(15)	(37)	(34)
	(NS)				(NS)				(p < .10)			

443

oldest group of adults, their vocational rehabilitation appears particularly high. Table 23-3 shows that of young adults who were adolescents when they became recipients (now age 20–27), seventy-three percent are working or in school full-time, compared with 60 percent of those who were adults when they became recipients (now age 26–44) and compared with only 38 percent of those adult recipients who are now age 45–62. Although the numbers are quite small, the findings are the same in looking at males and females separately.

Emotional well-being. Late adolescent-young adult patients seem to fare quite well emotionally, as have all of the other patient groups examined. They report themselves to be reasonably happy with their life in comparison with control groups. Table 23-4 shows that 34 percent of individuals in a nationwide normal control group report that they are very

Table 23-4
Happiness of Transplant Patients and Control Group

"Taken all together, how would you say things are these days—would you say you are very happy, pretty happy, or not too happy?"			
	Very happy (%)	Pretty happy (%)	Not too happy (%)	Total (%)
Nationwide sample*				
1. 1980	34 (496)	53 (771)	13 (195)	100 (1462)
Transplant recipients (age 16 and above)				
2. Pretransplant	18 (30)	58 (99)	25 (42)	100 (171)
3. 1 Year Post-transplant	57 (85)	36 (54)	7 (11)	100 (150)
5–9 Years Post-transplant				
4. Those who received transplants as children or adolescents	28 (7)	72 (18)	0	100 (25)
5. Those who received transplants as adults	37 (31)	49 (41)	14 (12)	100 (84)

* Report of General Social Surveys, The National Opinion Research Center; personal communication, Tom Smith (3/17/83). (Also see Bradburn, N. M. *The structure of well-being.* Chicago: Aldine, 1969, p. 40.)
Chi-square: between all groups: $p < .001$
            between recipients pretransplant, 1 year-post-transplant, and 5–9 years posttransplant: $p < .001$
            between recipients 1 year post-transplant and 5–9 years post-transplant: $p < .001$

happy in response to a widely used multiple-choice question; approximately the same percentage of these 25 patients (28 percent) also indicate they are very happy (Row 4). While these late adolescent–young adult patients are a little less likely to report being very happy than are the long-term older patients who were adult transplant recipients (Row 4 and 5—28 percent versus 37 percent), they are also less likely, at the other extreme, to indicate they are not too happy (0 percent versus 14 percent). More important, neither of the 5–9 year post-transplant groups shows the elation demonstrated by patients at one year post-transplant who had recently been rescued from a terminal illness (Row 3—57 percent). Neither 5–9 year post-transplant group shows the unhappiness of the pretransplant patients (Row 2—Only 18 percent). However, in-depth psychiatric evaluations are not available for these patients at 5–9 years post-transplant. Therefore an assessment of suicidal tendencies is lacking unless they are uncovered by the structured questionnaires.

The 25 patients in the late adolescent–young adult group can be further compared with the older transplant patients using adult versions of the psychological scales presented earlier[s]. Unfortunately, a normal control population is unavailable for comparison with these measures. On most scales there are no significant differences between the younger and older post-transplant patients. The younger group who received transplants as adolescents or children does, however, show significantly lower stability of the self-concept than does the group of older patients ($p < .05$).

Factors Associated with Adjustment of the Late Adolescent–Young Adult Transplant Recipient

The factors that affected the adjustment of these 25 patients are very similar to those that affected the adjustment of the children with chronic kidney disease and the post-transplant children. The following factors are related to several dimensions of negative adjustment: current health status, physical appearance, and gender.

First, patients who were free from medical difficulties within the past year are more likely to show a high degree of independence (71 percent versus 56 percent), control over destiny (57 percent versus 40 percent), and self-esteem (64 percent versus 50 percent); furthermore, they are more likely to indicate low levels of depressive-affect (93 percent versus 60 percent) and low self-preoccupation (71 percent versus 50 percent)[||].

---

[s]Control over destiny; stability; independence; self-esteem; anxiety; depression; preoccupation with self. Adult scales are coded so that a high score is favorable.

[||]There is no relationship to the other two psychological scales, anxiety and stability. Partial correlations controlling for gender are not smaller in size than the zero-order correlations between medical difficulties and scores on the social–psychological scales. Thus, the findings do not disappear when gender is controlled.

Second, the authors checked satisfaction with physical appearance via the following questions: How do you feel about the way you look now? Are you very happy, pretty happy, not very happy, or not at all happy with your physical appearance?

Response to this question indicates that dissatisfaction with appearance is associated with negative adjustment on six of the seven scales, although some of the correlations are small. Those who are more unhappy with their looks show greater depression (r = −.56, p ≤ .01); lower self-esteem (r = −.33, p ≤ .10), as well as lower control over destiny (r = −.16, n.s.); higher anxiety (r = −.15 n.s.); higher self-preoccupation (r = −.12, n.s.); and lower independence (r = −.13 n.s.). Furthermore, those who are more satisfied with their looks are more likely to be vocationally well-rehabilitated, employed, or going to school full-time (r = .35, p ≤ .05).[#] As with the chronically ill children, the late adolescent–young adults' subjective dissatisfaction with appearance seems critical to their general adjustment. Once the disease has become visible, it appears to have greater significance for overall adjustment.

Third, gender of the late adolescent–young adult is related to differences in adjustment along six of the seven measures of psychological adjustment. The young males show slightly more anxiety than do the females. However, females show less control over destiny (p = .04), lower stability of identity, less independence, greater preoccupation, less happiness, and lower self-esteem (Table 23-5). Findings hold when level of medical problems is controlled.

These gender disadvantages for the female are not apparent in older patients who were adult recipients. In fact, older women seem to fare better psychologically than do older men over the short term after transplantation. At a year post-transplant, the women showed significantly lower anxiety, depression, greater stability of self-image, and greater control over destiny (Simmons et al., 1977). Most of these differences between older men and women persisted at 5–9 years post-transplant, although most are no longer statistically significant (Table 23-5).

In addition to indicating more negative psychological adjustment, when level of medical problems was controlled, young women show

[#]The direction of all of these relationships remains the same when partial correlations are run controlling for the extent of medical problems in the past year and controlling for gender. Usually the sizes of the correlations also remain similar. However, the correlations between satisfaction with looks and independence and between satisfaction with looks and self-preoccupation virtually disappear when medical problems are controlled. It should also be noted that most subjects indicate they are fairly happy with the way they look, while the number choosing very happy or not happy is small. Thus these findings have to be regarded as somewhat tentative due to the small numbers of cases.

Table 23-5

Social-Psychological Scales According to Age and Sex
(5–9 years Post-Transplant)

	Median scores			
	Late adolescent–young adult patients		Patients who received transplants as adults	
	Male (n = 14)	Female (n = 11)	Male (n = 41)	Female (n = 44)
Control over destiny	3.500	1.900*	2.900	3.333†
Stability	2.800	1.000	3.250	3.389
Independence	2.850	2.500	2.828	2.783
Self-esteem	5.500	5.000	4.917	5.800‡
Anxiety**	1.500	2.500	2.250	2.333
Depression**	4.833	4.500	4.000	4.773
Preoccupation with self**	2.800	2.500	2.731	2.848

* Median test (Siegel, 1956) between younger males and females: p < .05
† Among all four groups: p < .10
‡ Between older males and females: p < .10
** All seven scales have been coded so that a high score indicates favorable adjustment. A high score in this case indicates low anxiety, low depression, low preoccupation with self.

greater damage to body image, feel less healthy, and are more negative about the transplant than are other transplant patients. Young women who received transplants as children or adolescents are most likely to report that the transplant has affected their looks (91 percent); in fact, the interviewer's independent ratings show that these patients are the most likely to be very cushingoid (43 percent). The young women are the least likely (73 percent) of any group to feel more healthy than they did before their transplant. They are also the least likely to be happy that they had a transplant (64 percent) and are by far the least likely (36 percent) to report that the years since the transplant have been better then they had expected. On all of these variables on which the young women are at a disadvantage in comparison with the young men, the older women rate as positively or more positively than do the older men. Thus young women seem to suffer because of their age and period in the life cycle.

As we noted earlier, chronically ill children and female child transplant recipients also show some disadvantages compared with their male counterparts, particularly in relation to body image. This also holds true in normal female adolescents (Bush, Simmons, Hutchinson, & Blyth, 1977-1978; Rosenberg & Simmons, 1975; Simmons & Rosenberg, 1975). In addition, there is some evidence that normal adult women cope less well psychologically than do men (Bush et al., 1977-1978). Yet, once illness strikes, older women show relatively higher levels of adjustment compared with men of their age with the same health problem, according to this and other studies (Simmons et al., 1977).

It is hypothesized that the social roles of older women and the relative lack of protective social and familial supports for late adolescent–young adult women may help to explain some of these differences.

Social roles and support. There appears to be no difference between the late adolescent–young adult group and older adults in the satisfaction they report with various social relationships. A very high proportion of both groups indicate satisfaction with recreation, social life, and relationships with friends. High levels of satisfaction were also reported for relationships with spouse and children. However, relatively few of the late adolescent–young adult group have these important relationships. Whereas 86 percent of the older adults have spouses and 80 percent have children (n = 85), only 20 percent (two males and 3 females) of these young adults are married, and only 8 percent have children (n = 25). Not only do the younger people lack the security and support of the marital relationship, there is also a certain amount of anxiety about whether they can marry and have children. Of the 20 unmarried late adolescents and young adults, 11 report having dated in the past few months, and 3 say they have a particular girlfriend or boyfriend. While it is difficult to determine normal rates, it appears this may be a low level of social activity for this age group. Individuals who have a kidney transplanted during a significant stage in their adolescence may have particular difficulty in establishing relationships with the opposite sex, while individuals who receive a transplant later have already established such relationships prior to becoming seriously ill.

In particular, the young women seem to be faring the worst, although the small number of cases limits definitive conclusions. Eight of the 11 respondents who say they are dating are male. Thus nearly half of the young women (5 out of 11, or 45 percent) are neither married nor dating (compared to 4 out of 14 males, or 29 percent).

As discussed earlier, the family was found to provide positive support for the chronically ill child. During the transition to independence in late adolescence and early adulthood, however, this protection becomes less available. The individual is at a normal hiatus between his or her family of origin and a new family to be created. Thirty-two percent of the late adolescents and young adults do not live with their family, in contrast to only 5 percent of the older adults. The late adolescents and young adults are also less likely to report that their family is very close (56 percent versus 81 percent). This normal transitional period may be particularly stressful for the young adult who has a transplant. Realistically, he or she has health problems that cannot be completely ignored in an effort to become independent and productive.

Young women are perhaps more vulnerable to the lack of family roles than are young men. The males are more likely to be employed or going to school on a full-time basis (64 percent of females versus 93 percent of males). Thus fewer young women have a job to provide security and satisfaction. Sex-role expectations in this society generally point to the importance of family roles as a source of satisfaction for women. Older women have the roles of wife, homemaker, and mother, which continue to be important after transplantation, and their adjustment is more positive.

In sum, individuals who become transplant recipients in adolescence generally fare well over the long term; however, less high adjustment occurs in individuals whose health is less good, in females, and in patients who are dissatisfied with their appearance. Family support may also play a role. One factor that does not make a difference is age within the late adolescent–young adult group, although the small sample size precludes definite conclusions. If adolescents (ages 16–19) are compared with young adults (20–27), no significant differences can be found on the psychological scales, and those differences that do exist are inconsistent in direction.

Compliance and Associated Factors in the Late Adolescent– Young Adult

There is one more issue for this age cohort that should be discussed. It has been found that adolescents have particular problems with compliance (see Blum, Chapter 10). Patients who have a transplant are faced with a never-ending need to take medications in order to prevent the new kidney from being rejected immunologically. In addition, these medications may have visible side effects that appear more negative to patients of this age. Thus, it might be expected that late adolescent–young adult patients will have particular problems taking their medications as directed. Korsch, Fine, & Negrete (1978) have shown that noncompliance can be a significant cause of kidney rejection in children.

Among all the Minnesota patients (age 16 and above) who are now 5–9 years post-transplant, compliance is higher among those patients who originally received transplants at an older age. Only about half of the late adolescents and young adults report that they never miss their medications, and almost one quarter miss them once a week or even more often. The danger in this kind of behavior is that it can lead to kidney rejection and even death. The older patients, who were transplanted at a later age, seem more aware of this danger, or perhaps they deny the danger less. In any case, they seem less willing to take chances.

The compliance behavior of those in the late adolescent–young adult group appears to follow a pattern very different from that of the older adults. On the basis of the health-belief model (Becker & Maiman, 1975), it could be hypothesized that asymptomatic patients may not be as motivated to take their medications as those with symptoms, since they may be less likely to believe that their condition is serious and that failure to follow the prescribed action could affect their well-being. Older adults act as expected: those who have uremic symptoms are more likely to comply than those with no symptoms. Those in the late adolescent–young adult group behave exactly opposite: the ones who are symptomatic, both male and female, miss their medications more often.

This difference between the young and older adults is shown in response to several related questions. Having medical difficulties within the past year, chronically rejecting a kidney, and being hospitalized are related to greater compliance in the older-adult group, but not in the late adolescent–young adult group. For example, among older patients, 100 percent of those who were hospitalized during the past year report they never miss their medications, compared with only 73 percent of those who were not hospitalized (p < .10). Among the late adolescent–young adult patients, less than half comply to this extent and whatever difference occurs between hospitalized and nonhospitalized patients is the reverse of that in the older adult group. By several indicators, then, those of the late adolescent–young adult patients who are feeling better and see themselves as relatively healthier are more likely to comply. Although we cannot untangle the direction of causal relationships here, it appears that the noncompliant patients within this age cohort may actually be making themselves sicker. Since there are relatively few young patients with medical problems, however, their compliance problems may well go unrecognized by the physicians. Their behavior may reflect denial, acting out, or self-destructive motivations. But because of its potentially serious consequences, it is important to understand as much as possible about it.

Although case numbers become quite small, satisfaction with body image appears to have important effects on compliance in late adolescents and young adults; whereas among older patients it does not seem as important. Only 5–6 percent of older patients, who were transplanted as adults, miss their medication often, regardless of whether they feel that the transplant has changed their looks. In contrast, in late adolescent–young adult patients, medications are missed often by 29 percent (5/17) of those who say the transplant has altered their looks but by none (0/4) of those who say their looks are unchanged. Similarly, of older patients who were transplanted as adults, 77 percent report that they never miss medications regardless of whether they are happy or unhappy with their appearance. Among the late adolescent–young adult patients, 59 percent (10/17) of those who are happy with their appearance report that they comply perfectly and never miss their medications, but none (0/4) of those who are unhappy with their appearance report that they comply to this extent. All four of these patients report that they miss their medications occasionally, if not often.

Since young females are the patients who seem most likely to exhibit negative side effects of the medication, it is not surprising that they report the poorest compliance. Only 30 percent of the young women report that they never miss their medications. Among older adults there is no reported difference between the sexes (Table 23-6).

Table 23-6
Comparison of Compliance in Late Adolescent–Young
Adults and Older Adults According to Sex

	Late adolescent–young adult patients (Age 16–27)			Patients who received transplants as adults (Age 26–72)		
	Male (%)	Female (%)	Total (%)	Male (%)	Female (%)	Total (%)
Miss medications						
Never miss	64	30	48	76	78	77
Occasionally* miss	27	30	29	18	16	17
Often miss†	9	40	24	6	6	6
	100	100	100	100	100	100
	(n = 11)	(n = 10)	(n = 21)	(n = 34)	(n = 37)	(n = 71)

Chi-Square among all four groups: $p < .05$
* Occasionally means that the patient may be late with medications or may miss no more often than once a month.
† Often means that the patient misses at least once a week and sometimes as often as every day.
Chi-square: $p = .07$

Noncompliance may be one link in a vicious circle. Those patients who are more ill are also more likely to need high dosages of drugs, and the higher the dosage of drugs, the greater the distortions of appearance. Those who show these distortions of appearance are more likely to feel dissatisfied and are therefore less inclined to take the medications. As a result of this noncompliance, the patient may become even more ill and require still more drugs. Thus the negative cost of compliance (in terms of appearance) is higher to the sicker patient, who needs more of the medications to maintain the transplanted kidney.

In this light it is understandable why late adolescent–young adult patients who are not vocationally rehabilitated are more likely to miss their medications. They may be sicker originally, on higher dosages, and tempted more to noncomply, which further compromises their level of health and rehabilitation. Again, older adults act differently; those who are partially or not at all vocationally rehabilitated are more compliant. Also in the late adolescent–young adult patients, noncompliance appears to be associated with psychological maladjustment on all seven scales: e.g., those who miss their medications show less control over destiny (29 percent versus 70 percent), lower self-esteem (46 percent versus 80 percent), and lower self-preoccupation (40 percent versus 80 percent). The older adult noncompliers do not consistently show such maladjustment.

Thus, the late adolescent–young adult patients who are not taking their medications appear at risk both psychologically and physically. They are not feeling well, they are generally unhappy and specifically unhappy with their appearance, they seem to think less highly of themselves, and they tend to be female. This problem of noncompliance may be particularly difficult to solve because of interdependence of these factors; i.e., the medications tend to create appearance problems and unhappiness, but without them the patient will not be able to maintain health.

SUMMARY AND DISCUSSION

Overall, children and adolescents who are coping with chronic kidney disease appear psychologically resilient. In spite of physical limitations, their adjustment appears to be comparable to that of normal youngsters and to be subject to normal developmental changes related to age and sex. Other studies of crisis and stress point to a bifurcation of psychological reaction: some individuals emerge from the experience strengthened and matured, while others are significantly weakened and suffer impaired mental health (Simmons et al., 1977). Among the patients and families in the studies reported in this chapter, many spontaneously report a positive growth in maturity and a greater appreciation of life after the illness. Such a reaction may help to explain the high level of adjustment in these children, adolescents, and young adults.

Nevertheless, some areas of adjustment are problematic for these patients, and certain types of patients experience marked distress. The most significant difference between the chronically ill and other children involves the body image; they are less likely to be satisfied with their appearance. Aside from dissatisfaction with appearance, other factors related to poor adjustment include severity of disease (particularly as perceived by the child), adolescence, and female sex.

The short-term adjustment (about two and one half years post-surgery) of pediatric transplant patients appears to be very similar to that of the chronically ill children. No differences are found in comparison with normal children except in terms of greater dissatisfaction with body image, which is more extreme than among the chronically ill. The sources of this dissatisfaction are retarded growth and cushingoid side effects of the immunosuppressive medications. Children who are dissatisfied with their appearance have significantly lower self-esteem and show negative adjustment along other psychosocial dimensions. Also, psychiatric evaluations indicate that patients who are in the adolescent age period are more at risk psychologically than are older or younger patients. Generally, however, the patients show a remarkable increase in energy and high levels of rehabilitation in terms of resumption of school and other activities.

Previously, there have been little data available to measure the long-term quality of life for children and adolescents who have received a kidney transplant. The data presented here on 25 late adolescent–young adult patients who become transplant recipients during childhood or adolescence provide objective indicators of the physical success of treatment at that age. The vast majority are still alive five and ten years later (81 percent and 74 percent) and about half maintain the original transplanted kidney. The young adult patients show higher rates of vocational rehabilitation 5–9 years post-transplant (73 percent) than individuals who received transplants as adults. This level of rehabilitation is considerably more positive than the level of 50 percent for job or school performance reported by Poznanski et al. (1978) in their study of the quality of life of 18 children and adolescents who survived at least two years post-transplantation. In addition, the late adolescent–young adult patients seem to feel very well in comparison with older adults. As a group, they show a positive level of physical well-being and productivity and a positive outlook on life.

In terms of emotional adjustment as well, the late adolescent–young adult group compares favorably with the group of older adults. Only in terms of stability of self-concept do the younger patients, who received transplants as children or adolescents, appear to be at a disadvantage.

In comparing this late adolescent–young adult cohort with older individuals who received transplants as adults, the authors cannot separate the effects of current age from the effects of age at transplantation. The aim has been to determine how individuals who became transplant recipients when young—and thereby experienced a significant disruption of adolescence—adjust over the long term. How do they cope with the challenges of later developmental periods—late adolescence, young adulthood? To the extent that they react differently than do older post-transplant patients, it is uncertain whether to attribute the difference to their younger age now or to the fact that they experienced the transplant when they were an adolescent. Insofar as they are coping comparatively well, the issue becomes less urgent.

Yet certain late adolescent-young adult patients seem at greater psychological risk than others. Three of the same factors that negatively affect younger children are also related to more negative adjustment in these late adolescent-young adult patients: poor health status, dissatisfaction with appearance, and female sex. Patients who are experiencing more health problems show lower self-esteem and lower control over destiny. In the original studies it was found that during the first year after transplant, patients and their families were very aware of the favorable contrast between their post- and pretransplant health status. As the memory of the pretransplant period recedes 5–9 years later, however, it is likely that the young adults in the follow-up study compare themselves more with other healthy people rather than comparing their current health status with their own pretransplant condition. In comparison with normal peers, they are clearly at some disadvantage.

Dissatisfaction with appearance remains a major problem over the long term. Although it has been suggested that the cushingoid effects of medication dissipate over time, they appear to persist in some cases, and they are most noticeable in young women. Dissatisfaction with body image is associated with poor psychological adjustment and may, in fact, interfere with successful social maturation.

The young women are more at risk on this count than any of the other groups. Again, it is unclear whether this vulnerability is related to their current life period or due to the disruption of adolescence by the transplant, or both. In any case, they show more negative psychological adjustment than do young men, whereas older women are not at a disadvantage in comparison with older men. The young women are more dissatisfied with their appearance than are the young men; they feel less healthy; they are less positive about their transplants and are more likely to miss taking their medications. In their study of noncompliance, Korsch et al. (1978) also reported that adolescent females are more likely to stop their medications.

The family also appears to be an important factor in explaining the adjustment of transplant patients of all ages. There are two aspects of the family that seem especially relevant: the patient's role in the family and the family support he or she receives. These may be particularly important variables in explaining why very young chronically ill and transplanted children fare so well psychologically. The authors have hypothesized that the child's functional role is less vulnerable to illness than is that of the adult. Children and adolescents are not expected to maintain a job or take care of a house and family, nor are they expected to be independent. At the same time, the family is supportive of the ill child; mothers in particular seem to provide special attention while reassuring the child of his or her normalcy (Klein & Simmons, 1977). When the family is unable to be supportive of the chronically ill child or the child who has received a transplant, psychological and behavioral problems often result; in fact, most of the suicidal adolescents previously mentioned had families who were nonsupportive. Korsch et al. (1978) also report that noncompliant patients tend to have families who do not play a positive role in helping the patients adapt to the transplant.

The child's protected status in the family appears to be reduced as the child grows up. The situation shifts as the older adolescent is faced with the transition to young adulthood and the need to assert independence and assume responsibility for himself or herself. The relative lack of social supports and family security among the late adolescent–early adult patients is clear: about 32 percent of them are not living with their family; only five of the 25 young adults are married. Females seem to have less contact than males with the opposite sex, yet such contact may be more important to their sense of self than it is to the males. Being married and having children are often important goals of young women. A young woman who is dissatisfied with her appearance and not dating may become intensely unhappy. In addition to this social disadvantage, the young women are less likely than the men to be employed full-time. Thus they often lack a job, which can provide some satisfaction, security, and alternative compensation for absent social and family interactions.

The periods of the life cycle from childhood through adolescence to adulthood are marked by psychological changes, new developmental tasks, and shifts in priorities. It is important that medical care providers be aware of these developmental changes. In particular, the problems of the adolescent and the young adult patient are different from those of older adults. Because the physicians see more older adult patients, it is likely that they tend to react to the patients entering young adulthood as adults, without recognizing the special developmental problems that these patients—especially the young women—may face. After patients have survived the first year's adjustment to a transplant, the tendency is to watch mainly for physical problems. Yet the identification of the patient who is at psychological risk may, in fact, be essential to his or her survival. There appears to be a continuing need for a team approach that involves mental health professionals in the long-term management of child transplant recipients (Drotar, Ganofsky, & Makker, 1979; van Leeuwen & Matthews, 1975).

In spite of documentation of the frequency of noncompliance with medical treatment, Korsch et al. (1978) noted that noncompliance had not been generally recognized as a cause of kidney rejection among transplant patients. These data suggest that noncompliance is a greater problem among adolescent and young adult patients than it is among older adults. The patients in the Korsch study who were identified as noncompliers were patients who had actually discontinued their medications. Data from this study suggest there may be an even larger group of patients who often miss taking their medications. Furthermore, the motivations for compliant behavior seem very different in the young than in the older adult.

Patients who became transplant recipients when they were children or adolescents have a physical advantage over older patients. As a group they seem to be coping well with the transition to adulthood and have achieved a high level of productivity. Yet there are some patients (particularly young women) who are clearly at risk emotionally and socially, and their problems may, in fact, result in lowered compliance and, ultimately, transplant failure. It is in this population that development of appropriate assessments and interventions might be particularly advantageous.

ACKNOWLEDGMENT

This work is supported in part by a National Institute of Mental Health Research Development Award 5 K05 MH41688 to the second author and National Institute of Arthritis, Metabolism, and Digestive Diseases grants 9 R01 AM28618 and 2 P01 AM13083.

REFERENCES

Becker, M., & Maiman, L. Sociobehavioral determinants of compliance with health and medical care. *Medical care*, 1975, *13*, 10–24.

Bernstein, D.M. Psychiatric assessment of the adjustment of transplanted children. In R.G. Simmons, S.D. Klein, & R.L. Simmons (Eds.), *Gift of life: The social and psychological impact of organ transplantation*. New York: Wiley Interscience, 1977, 119–147.

Bradburn, N.M. *The structure of psychological well-being*. Chicago: Aldine, 1969.

Bush, D.E., Simmons, R.G., Hutchinson, B., & Blyth, D.A. Adolescent perception of sex roles in 1968 and 1975. *Public Opinion Quarterly*, 1977–1978, *41* (4), 459–474.

Coleman, J.S. *Equality of educational opportunity*. Washington, DC: U.S. Government Printing Office, SUDOCS: FS5.238:38000 1966.

Collier, B.N., Jr. Comparisons between adolescents with and without diabetes. *Personnel and Guidance Journal*, 1969, *47* (7), 679–684.

Crain, A.J., Sussman, M.B., & Weil, W.B., Jr. Family interaction, diabetes and sibling relationships. *International Journal of Social Psychiatry*, 1966, *12* (1), 35–43.

Drotar, D., Ganofsky, M., & Makker, S. Comprehensive pediatric management of severe reactions of children to dialysis and transplantation. *Dialysis & Transplantation*, 1979, *8* (10), 983–986.

Haggerty, R.J., Roghmann, K.J., & Pless, I.B. *Child health and the community*. New York: Wiley, 1975.

Kellerman, J., Zeltzer, L., Ellenberg, L., Dash, J., & Rigler, D. Psychological effects of illness in adolescents. I. Anxiety, self-esteem and perception of control. *Journal of Pediatrics*, 1980, *97* (1), 126–131.

Klein, S.D. *Chronic Kidney Disease: Impact on the child and family and strategies for coping*. Unpublished doctoral dissertation, University of Minnesota, August, 1975.

Klein, S.D., & Simmons, R.G. The psychosocial impact of chronic kidney disease on children. In R.G. Simmons, S.D. Klein, & R.L. Simmons (Eds.), *Gift of life: The social and psychological impact of organ transplantation.* New York: Wiley Interscience, 1977.

Kohn, M. *Class and conformity: A study in values.* Homewood, IL: Dorsey, 1969.

Korsch, B., Fine, R., & Negrete, V.F. Noncompliance in children with renal transplants. *Pediatrics,* 1978, *61* (6), 872–876.

Pless, I., & Roghmann, K. Chronic illness and its consequences: Observations based on three epidemiologic surveys. *Journal of Pediatrics,* 1971, *79* (3), 351–359.

Poznanski, E., Miller E., Salquero, C., & Kilsh, R. Quality of life for long-term survivors of end stage renal disease. *Journal of the American Medical Association,* 1978, *239(22),* 2343–2347.

Rosenberg, F.R., & Simmons, R.G. Sex differences in the self-concept in adolescence. *Sex Roles: A Journal of Research,* 1975, *1* (2), 147–159.

Rosenberg, M. *Society and the adolescent self-image.* Princeton, NJ: Princeton University Press, 1965.

Rosenberg, M., & Simmons, R.G. *Black and white self-esteem: The urban school child.* Washington, DC: American Sociological Association, 1972.

Sebald, H. *Adolescence: A social psychological analysis* (2nd ed.). Englewood Cliffs, NJ: Prentice-Hall, 1977.

Siegel, S. *Non-Parametric Statistics for the Behavioral Sciences.* New York: McGraw Hill, 1956, 174–184.

Simmons, R.G., & Blyth, D.A. *Moving into adolescence: The impact of pubertal change and school context.* Monograph in process.

Simmons, R.G., Klein, S.D., & Simmons, R.L. *Gift of life: The social and psychological impact of organ transplantation.* New York: Wiley Interscience, 1977.

Simmons, R.G., & Rosenberg, F. Sex, sex-roles, and self-image. *Journal of Youth and Adolescence,* 1975, *4* (3), 229–258.

Simmons, R.G., Rosenberg, F., & Rosenberg, M. Disturbance in the self-image at adolescence. *American Sociological Review,* 1973, *38* (5), 553–568.

Sultz, H.A., Schlessinger, E.R., Mosher, W.E., & Feldman, J.C. *Long term childhood illness.* Pittsburgh: University of Pittsburgh Press, 1972.

Van Leeuwen, J., & Matthews, D. Comprehensive mental health care in a pediatric dialysis-transplantation program. *Canadian Medical Association Journal,* 1975, *113*, 959–962.

Zeltzer, L., Kellerman, J., Ellenberg, L., Dash, J., & Rigler, D. Psychological effects of illness in children. II. Impact of illness in adolescents—Crucial issues and coping styles. *Journal of Pediatrics,* 1980, *97* (1), 132–138.

Index